SIXTH EDITION

Handbook of
Patient Care in
Vascular Diseases

SIXTH EDITION

Handbook of Patient Care in Vascular Diseases

Editors

Todd E. Rasmussen, MD, FACS
Professor of Surgery and Associate Dean for Research
F. Edward Hébert School of Medicine - "America's Medical School"
Uniformed Services University
Attending Vascular Surgeon
Walter Reed National Military Medical Center
Bethesda, Maryland

W. Darrin Clouse, MD, FACS
Associate Professor of Surgery
Harvard Medical School
Division of Vascular and Endovascular Surgery
Massachusetts General Hospital
Boston, Massachusetts

Britt H. Tonnessen, MD, FACS
Attending Vascular Surgeon
The Vascular Group, PLLC
Poughkeepsie, New York

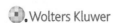. Wolters Kluwer

Philadelphia • Baltimore • New York • London
Buenos Aires • Hong Kong • Sydney • Tokyo

Acquisitions Editor: Keith Donnellan
Editorial Coordinator: Tim Rinehart
Marketing Manager: Julie Sikora
Senior Production Project Manager: Alicia Jackson
Design Coordinator: Terry Mallon
Art Director: Jennifer Clements
Senior Manufacturing Coordinator: Beth Welsh
Prepress Vendor: SPi Global

Sixth edition

9 8 7 6 5

Printed in the United States of America

Library of Congress Cataloging-in-Publication Data
Names: Rasmussen, Todd E., editor. | Clouse, W. Darrin, editor. | Tonnessen, Britt H., editor.
Title: Handbook of patient care in vascular diseases / editors, Todd E. Rasmussen, W. Darrin Clouse, Britt H. Tonnessen.
Description: Sixth edition. | Philadelphia : Wolters Kluwer, [2019] | Includes bibliographical references and index.
Identifiers: LCCN 2018043097 | ISBN 9781451175233
Subjects: | MESH: Vascular Diseases—diagnosis | Patient Care | Vascular Diseases—physiopathology | Vascular Diseases—therapy | Handbooks
Classification: LCC RD598.5 | NLM WG 39 | DDC 617.4/13—dc23 LC record available at https://lccn.loc.gov/2018043097

We dedicate this edition to those who have
helped us along the way, to the different kinds
of learners and providers of vascular care, and to
our wonderful, if not challenging, patients.

Todd E. Rasmussen

W. Darrin Clouse

Britt H. Tonnessen

FOREWORD FOR THE SIXTH EDITION

Excellence in vascular care comes from several angles. The first is attentive, safe selection of patients for procedures that are likely to help them. The second is adherence to principles of care that deliver good, long-term outcomes. The third is recognizing complications early so intervention prevents morbidity and mortality.

When this *Handbook* was conceived and written originally in 1980–1981, three surgeons exemplified the principles that sustain the current edition: Drs. R. Clement Darling II, David C. Brewster, and Clifford J. Buckley. They were my role models and inspiration to record their thoughts on achieving excellence in vascular care. Subsequent editions have tweaked these principles and added new knowledge.

Remarkably this edition will appear almost four decades after the first. The current authors are accomplished vascular surgeons. They share the common background of Mayo Medical School and the Mayo Clinic where the needs of the patient come first. They have excelled in various academic, military, and community practices. This diversity and depth of experience is the foundation of this new edition.

If I were a young vascular specialist, I would read every word of this concise guide. As a senior vascular specialist, I will read every word to update my knowledge! In my experience, this *Handbook* is essential. Wherever I travel in the world, colleagues ask, "When is the next edition coming?"

Now, we can say that the sixth edition of *Patient Care of Vascular Diseases* is here, and you do not want to miss its traditions and innovations. You will be a better specialist by reading it!

John (Jeb) Hallett, MD
David C. Brewster, MD

For three and a half decades, the *Handbook of Patient Care in Vascular Diseases* has served as a guide for health care providers of many disciplines and for those at different levels of education and training. As with the original, this edition is rooted in the fundamentals of pathophysiology and a well-preformed history and physical exam. More than most patients, those with vascular disease have an interesting story to tell and physical signs to go with it. Our job is to listen to the story and look for evidence of disease. Then, and on a selective basis, we can use advanced technologies to diagnose or exclude the condition and pursue treatment.

An informed and orderly approach is especially important given that few conditions involve as many costly and potentially risky diagnostics or can result more consequential (life and limb-threatening) problems as vascular disease. We speak from experience that failure to approach these patients in a thoughtful and disciplined manner can result in unneeded and expensive procedures, suboptimal or adverse outcomes, or both.

There have been many changes in the care of patients with vascular disease in the 10 years since the last edition of the *Handbook*. For one thing, vascular disease is more common today than in 2008. In 2011, the baby boomer demographic began turning 65 years old, and in 10 more years, 20% of the U.S. population will be older than 65. Because the prevalence and incidence of vascular disease are both sharply increased with age, there are just more patients alive today with this condition.

To provide better care for this larger number of patients, new training models have been developed with dozens of "0-5" vascular surgery residencies now in place in the U.S. aimed at providing students a training opportunity directly out of medical school. There are also new training opportunities for physicians and nonphysicians (e.g., nurses, nurse practitioners, and physician assistants) in vascular medicine and different accreditation processes for noninvasive vascular labs and the physicians who interpret the studies. Most practices and centers have made changes to better integrate these various parts of care into a multidisciplinary team—be it in the clinic, in the lab, on the ward, or in the operating room or radiology suite. Caring for the vascular patient is now more of a team effort!

In the setting of these changes, this sixth edition is written to provide a basic understanding of vascular disease and cardiovascular risk, noninvasive vascular testing, and the risks of using radiation for imaging. The *Handbook* has updated chapters and guidelines, provides a simple review of endovascular devices, and concludes with a set of *logical care outlines* for conditions common to our patients; conditions such as arterial occlusive and aneurysm disease, dialysis access, and venous thrombosis and thromboembolism.

The *Handbook* is still brief so that it can be a handy resource carried in the pocket of a white coat or scrubs, thrown on a table in the medical student or resident lounge or nurses' station, or on the duplex machine in the vascular lab. A far cry from the spiral-bound first edition, this modern version includes a complimentary e-book that can be read on one's favorite device (e.g., computer, tablet, or smartphone) or listened to with its Read Aloud feature.

In 1979-1980, Dr. John "Jeb" Hallett, a vascular surgery fellow at the Massachusetts General Hospital (MGH), conceived the idea of a *Handbook of Vascular Surgery* similar to the cardiac surgery handbook from the MGH. With encouragement and support from his mentors, Drs. R. Clem Darling and David C. Brewster, Dr Hallett wrote the first edition of this *Handbook* during his military service as Chief of Vascular Surgery at Wilford Hall Air Force Medical Center. As students of Dr. Hallett at Mayo Medical School, we have been recruited over the years to sustain this practical resource. With innovation in mind, we present the current edition to you and hope that it guides you to excellent outcomes for your vascular patients.

T. E. R.
W. D. C.
B. H. T.

CONTENTS

BASIC CONCEPTS

Like other disease processes, a number of basic principles guide the management of most vascular problems. These include *obtaining a history, performing a physical examination,* and *gathering information from other diagnostic testing.* Following these principles, one can provide logical and appropriate patient care; neglect one of these steps and a clinical scenario may become confusing and the patient's care misguided. In the first two chapters of this handbook, we outline and emphasize these basic concepts. Because the handbook covers both arterial and venous diseases, we have organized the basic concepts around these two disease groups. Each chapter is subdivided under the headings "Magnitude of the Problem," "Basic Anatomy," "Etiology," "Pathophysiology," and "Natural History."

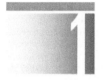

Arterial Disease

I. **MAGNITUDE OF THE PROBLEM.** Peripheral arterial disease (PAD) is one of the most common causes of death and disability worldwide. As a disease process related to age, PAD will become more prevalent in decades to come. Specifically, the first of the 82 million Americans in the "baby boom" demographic turned 60 years old in 2006, and the number of people over the age of 65 is anticipated to increase 100% by 2032. Physical disability resulting from the consequences of PAD is just as important to consider as mortality resulting from the condition. For example, approximately 800,000 people in the United States have a stroke each year, and many are left with a permanent neurologic deficit, which is devastating to both the patient and the family. Patients with arterial disease may also be limited by chest pain (angina pectoris), exertional leg pain (claudication), extremity ulceration (tissue loss), respiratory insufficiency (COPD and lung cancer), and even amputation (Chapter 13).

Advances in the diagnosis and successful treatment of PAD have occurred, and now include broader use of duplex ultrasonography (US) and less invasive endovascular techniques (Chapters 5, 9 and 10). Progress has also been made in the identification of clinical risk factors and development of new types of medications that allow prevention or reduction of arterial disease in many patients (Chapters 6, 7 and 8). Despite these advances, many patients are unwilling to modify their lifestyles or comply with medication use, and as such, arterial disease will remain a leading health problem during the career of most providers practicing today.

II. **BASIC ANATOMY.** The peripheral arterial system refers to non-cardiac arteries, including the thoracic and abdominal aorta and branches thereof as well as arteries of the neck and the extremities. The arterial network is a complex organ system that must withstand the dynamics of pulsatile flow for the life of an individual. The wall of the artery consists of three layers, or tunics, referred to as the *tunica intima, tunica media,* and *tunica adventitia* (Fig. 1.1A). Each of these three layers plays a unique part in arterial function to allow delivery of oxygenated blood throughout the body. Although the makeup of each layer varies slightly, depending on the location of the artery in the body, all must function and remain intact in the setting of health.

A. **The Intima.** The inner lining of the artery is a single layer of cells referred to as the **intima**. These endothelial cells perform unique functions via receptors on their surface. Secretion of proteins, such as endothelin, and other substances, such as nitric oxide, regulates vessel tone and affects platelet aggregation and formation of thrombus. Like other cells in the body, endothelial cells require oxygen for survival and function, and receive this from the flowing blood (i.e., luminal blood supply). Underlying the intima is a thin matrix of elastic fibers called the **internal elastic lamina**.

B. **The Media.** The middle layer of the artery is formed by smooth muscle cells and variable amounts of elastin and collagen. The amount of elastic tissue within the media decreases proportionally to the smooth muscle content as arteries become more peripheral (e.g., further from the heart). Central arteries such as the thoracic aorta with greater elastic content are termed *elastic arteries* while *muscular arteries,* such as the femoral or carotid arteries, have greater smooth muscle content in the media. The media primarily responds to signals from endothelial cells of the nearby intima. Under normal conditions, the media provides structure to the vessel and is responsible for variations in vessel tone. In the setting of injury or disease, the media is the main location for cellular response including proliferation of smooth muscle cells and migration of other cell types into the media (e.g., macrophages and fibroblasts). The media has a dual source of nourishment receiving oxygen via diffusion from the circulating blood (luminal oxygen supply) and by small vessels that penetrate the outer wall, which are termed **vasa vasorum** (abluminal oxygen supply). A second **external elastic membrane** forms the outer border of the media separating it from the adventitia.

C. **The Adventitia.** The outermost layer of an artery is the adventitia, which is composed mainly of the long fibrous structural protein called collagen as well as autonomic nerves that supply the smooth muscle cells of the media. Additionally, the vasa vasorum courses along and through the adventitia. Although the adventitia may appear thin and without substance, it is a key element in the total strength of the arterial wall. In muscular arteries, the adventitia may be as thick as the media itself. In such arteries, surgical closure of the arterial wall or anastomosis of a synthetic graft to the vessel should incorporate the adventitial layer; failure to do so may result in anastomotic breakdown.

III. **ETIOLOGY.** The etiology of nearly all acquired arterial disease is **atherosclerosis.** The term atherosclerosis comes from the Greek terms *athero,* meaning gruel or paste, and *sclerosis,* meaning hardening. Arteriosclerosis refers to any hardening of the artery or loss of its elasticity, and is often used interchangeably with atherosclerosis, although technically atherosclerosis is a form of arteriosclerosis.

The etiology of atherosclerosis is a complicated immune-mediated process that begins at the interface of endothelial cells and the circulating blood. The etiology has not been linked to one causative factor, but rather to a combination of *mechanical* (e.g., shear stress and hypertension), *circulating* (e.g., lipids, glucose, or insulin), and *environmental* (e.g., tobacco use) factors. Together, these elements reach a threshold in certain genetically predisposed persons and initiate the disease process of atherosclerosis. The development of atherosclerosis may be thought of as occurring in several stages (Figure 1.1).

A. **Response to Injury.** Under normal circumstances, the endothelial lining provides a nonsticky surface through which circulating blood may flow. However, this layer of cells may be damaged by mechanical forces such as hypertension or circulating factors such as metabolites from cigarette smoke or oxidized lipids. Damage to the endothelial cells causes the lining of the vessel to become sticky, and white blood cells (monocytes and T cells) and platelets (thrombocytes) begin to adhere in an attempt to repair the injury (Fig. 1.1A and B).

Experimental and clinical observations also indicate that early endothelial injury is more prone in areas of blood-flow separation and low **shear stress** (Fig. 1.2). The layer of blood adjacent to the intima is referred to as the **boundary layer** and, although flow in the center of the artery is **laminar**, this outer area of boundary layer separation has slower, more

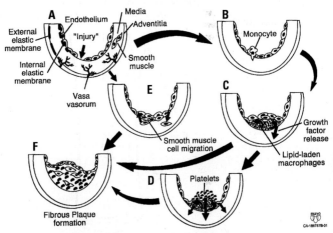

FIGURE 1.1 Pathogenesis of atherosclerosis. Endothelial "injury" or dysfunction can be initiated by a variety of forces: hyperlipidemia; free radicals caused by cigarette smoking, hypertension, and diabetes mellitus; genetic alterations; and elevated plasma homocysteine. Monocytes **(A)** attach to injured endothelium **(B)**, secrete growth factors **(C)**, and finally migrate into the subendothelial layer. Lipid-laden macrophages become part of the fatty streak. Endothelial disruption attracts platelets **(D)** that secrete platelet-derived growth factor (PDGF). Smooth muscle cells in the proliferative atheromatous lesion may also secrete growth factors such as PDGF. Increased endothelial turnover results in enhanced growth factor production. Smooth muscle cells are stimulated to migrate into the intimal layer **(E)**. Smooth muscle and "injured" endothelial cells turn up their growth factor production. Fibrous plaques **(F)** evolve from fatty streaks. Atheromas develop from fatty streaks to fibrous plaques that can degenerate eventually into complicated plaques with surface ulceration, hemorrhage, and embolization. This fibrous plaque rupture and ulceration appear to be related to macrophages releasing proteolytic enzymes. (Adapted from Ross R. Atherosclerosis—an inflammatory disease. *N Engl J Med.* 1999;340:115-126.)

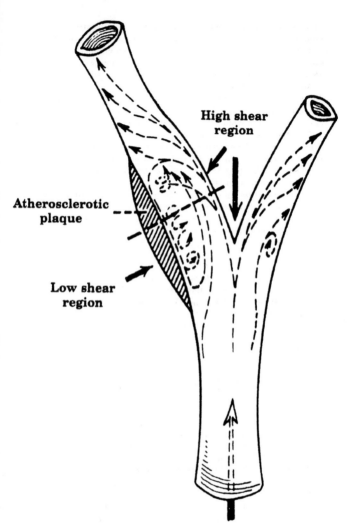

FIGURE 1.2 Patterns of low and high shear stress. Atherosclerotic plaques, which usually localize to the outer wall at arterial bifurcations, tend to develop at areas of boundary layer separation and low shear stress. (Adapted from Malek AD, Alper SL, Izumo S. Hemodynamic shear stress and its role in atherosclerosis. *JAMA*. 1999;282:2035-2042.)

disturbed currents. These areas of low shear force (<4 dyne/cm^2) have also been shown to induce endothelial dysfunction and generally occur at the outer walls of arterial branch points. Depending upon the magnitude and length of time over which any one of these insults occur, the process may be self-limiting and result in healing of the vessel lining.

Alternatively, and in more severe or chronic cases, the injury process continues and alters the permeability and activity of the endothelial layer. From this point, adherent cells as well as the endothelial cells secrete substances that initiate an *immune-directed* process within the media of the vessel wall—immune directed in the sense that inflammatory cells of various types (monocytes, T cells, and macrophages) and the factors they secrete (cytokines) play a central role in directing the process. In response to cytokines, cells not typically in the media, such as macrophages, T cells, and fibroblasts, migrate into the media in the area of injury (Fig. 1.1C–E). Smooth muscle cells in the media proliferate and alter their function with regard to production of the extracellular matrix and calcium metabolism, while macrophages engulf oxidized lipids and become lipid-laden macrophages, or **foam cells.** While the intent of this reaction is to "heal" the vessel damage, the result is often formation of the earliest atherosclerotic lesion referred to as an atherosclerotic plaque or "fatty streak." These lesions can occur early in life and are composed primarily of inflammatory cells, cholesterol, low-density lipoproteins, and calcium. Whether or not these early plaques progress to more advanced pathologic lesions depends upon several clinical, environmental and genetic factors. Research has shown that cigarette smoking accelerates formation and progression of these early lesions and that exercise, risk-factor modification, and medications such as statins cause such lesions to remain stable or regress.

B. **Advanced Atherosclerosis.** In scenarios in which the injury response progresses, it is thought that the immune response remains activated or "turned on." This may be due to local factors, such as foam cell death and increased oxidative stress; circulating factors, such as elevated lipids, glucose levels, or metabolites of cigarette smoke; or genetic factors related to the immune-response genes. Additionally, the observation that advanced atherosclerotic plaques occur mostly at *arterial branch points* suggests that differences in local shear stress related to turbulent flow may also act as an accelerating factor. Whatever the cause, the end result is propagation of the immune response within the wall of the artery, leading to deposition of calcium between the vessel layers and formation of an intermediate lesion termed the **fibrous cap** (Fig. 1.1F). Capped fatty deposits, also termed **atheromas,** can extend into the lumen of the artery, causing the artery to narrow or become unstable and open or rupture, releasing debris into the bloodstream (embolization). Atheromas are also active as they secrete cytokines, which lead to a condition termed **vascular remodeling.** Remodeling is a process in which smooth muscle cell proliferation continues and activates a set of enzymes (**matrix metalloproteinases**) able to destroy the structural proteins of the vessel wall. One or two specific metalloproteinases cause breakdown of the structural proteins in the media and adventitia resulting in weakening of the artery and dilation of the arterial segment. While such dilation initially compensates for the luminal narrowing (stenosis) caused by atheroma or plaque, the process eventually leads to aneurysm formation if unchecked. In chronic and advanced atherosclerotic lesions, the elasticity of the arterial wall is lost and the process ultimately narrows the vessel lumen causing flow limitations, or continues to break down the structural components of the arterial wall to form an aneurysm.

Although intimal thickening and calcification of the arteries are to some degree a "normal aging process," the variability or spectrum of disease among individuals is a topic with many unanswered questions. Why is it that in the same patient one may find early and complicated lesions as well as arterial segments completely unaffected? Why is it that atherosclerosis appears to lead to occlusive lesions in some individuals but arterial aneurysms in others? Why are some arterial segments prone to aneurysm formation while others appear protected against aneurysm formation?

IV. **PATHOPHYSIOLOGY.** To make the pathophysiology of atherosclerosis more understandable, one may think of three main categories of clinical consequences:

1. Formation of a flow-limiting blockage within the artery (*stenosis*)
2. Dilation of the artery (*aneurysm*)
3. Release of atheroma down the arterial stream (*embolization*)

A. **Occlusive Disease.** Atherosclerosis becomes symptomatic by gradual occlusion of blood flow to the involved extremity or end organ. Symptoms occur when a **critical arterial stenosis** is reached. Blood flow and pressure are not significantly diminished until at least 75% of the cross-sectional area of the vessel is obliterated (Fig. 1.3). This figure for cross-sectional area can be equated with a 50% reduction in lumen diameter. The formula for the area of a circle (area = 3.14 × radius²) explains the relationship between vessel diameter and cross-sectional area.

Factors other than radius also influence the significance of an arterial stenosis, but to a lesser extent (**Poiseuille's law**). These include the length of stenosis (i.e., longer segments become critical earlier), blood viscosity, and peripheral resistance. In situations where resistance is decreased beyond a fixed stenosis (vasodilation), velocity and turbulence across that stenosis increase, resulting in a decrease in pressure across the lesion (**Bernoulli's principle**) (Table 1.1). Evidence also suggests that a series of subcritical stenoses can have an additive effect, similar to a single critical stenosis although not linear. Thus, three subcritical stenoses (30%, 40%, and 10%) may not have the same effect as a single 80% narrowing of a vessel.

The hemodynamic concepts pertaining to blood velocity across a stenosis are important in understanding patient symptoms and physical

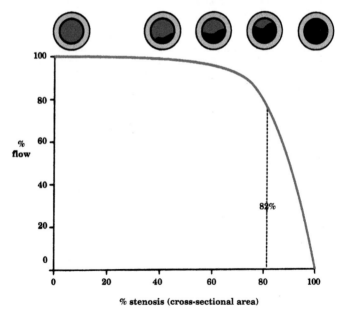

FIGURE 1.3 Critical arterial stenosis. Blood flow remains relatively normal across an arterial stenosis until at least 75% of the cross-sectional area is obliterated (50% diameter reduction).

Principle	Definition	Equation	Terms of Equation
Bernoulli's	Relationship between pressure, gravitational (potential) energy, and kinetic energy in an idealized fluid system. In moving blood through arteries, the portion of total fluid energy lost is dissipated in the form of heat.	$P_1 + \rho g h_1 + \frac{1}{2}\rho v_1^2 = P_2 + \rho g h_2 + \frac{1}{2}\rho v_2^2 +$ heat	P = pressure $\rho g h$ = gravitational potential energy $\frac{1}{2}\rho v_2^2$ = kinetic energy
Law of Laplace	Arterial wall stress and therefore risk of aneurysm rupture is directly proportional to vessel diameter and arterial pressure.	Wall stress = $P \times d/t$	P = systolic blood pressure, d = vessel diameter, t = vessel wall thickness
Poiseuille's	Relationship between flow and the pressure difference across the length of a tube, its radius, and the fluid viscosity. The most important determinant of flow is radius.	$Q = \pi r^4 (P_1 - P_2)/8L\eta$	Q = flow r = radius of vessel $P_1 - P_2$ = potential energy between 2 points L = distance between 2 points η = viscosity coefficient
Reynolds number	A dimensionless quantity that defines the point at which flow changes from laminar (streamlined) to turbulent (disorganized). If Re >2,000, disturbances in laminar flow will result in fully developed turbulence. In normal arterial circulation, Re is usually <2,000.	$Re = \rho v d/\eta$	Re = Reynolds number d = tube diameter v = velocity ρ = specific gravity η = viscosity
Resistance (rearranged Poiseuille's law)	Analogous to Ohm's equation of electrical circuits (resistance = pressure/flow)	$R = P_1 - P_2/Q = 8\eta L/\pi r^4$	R = resistance $P_1 - P_2$ = pressure drop Q = flow η = viscosity L = length of tube r = radius of tube

TABLE 1.1 Basic Principles of Fluid Dynamics

examination findings. For example, these concepts help in the diagnosis of patients who complain of extremity pain with exertion (i.e., claudication), yet have a normal examination, including ankle-brachial index (ABI), while at rest in the office. Having a grasp of hemodynamic principles allows the provider, in such cases, to recognize the importance of a provocative test, such as measuring the ABI after a period of walking, in confirming or excluding the diagnosis of vascular claudication.

Under normal conditions (i.e., no arterial stenoses), a person's ABI will increase with and immediately following walking. However, if the patient in the above scenario has significant arterial occlusive disease (stenoses), the ABI will *decrease* in the symptomatic extremity with exercise. In this situation, Bernoulli's principle shows that with exertion comes vasodilation in the extremity, which increases velocity and turbulence across any fixed stenosis and results in a pressure decrease across the stenosis. This decrease in pressure during exertion manifests as a decreased exercise ABI and symptoms of claudication. Hence, a stenosis may be noncritical at rest, but manifest as critical with a provocative test such as exercise.

B. Aneurysm Disease. Arterial aneurysms arise as a consequence of the loss of structural integrity of the vessel wall, namely degradation of the network of structural proteins such as elastin and collagen in the mid and outer layers of the arterial wall. Over time, this weakening results in dilation and aneurysm formation (*aneurysm = 1.5 times the normal diameter of the vessel*). Once an aneurysm forms, laminar flow is disturbed in this irregularly shaped vessel, turbulent blood flow increases, and there is accumulation of **mural thrombus** (i.e., clot) within the aneurysm. Although the amount of mural thrombus can at times be considerable, it does not offer strength to the aneurysm or prevent expansion or rupture, and it is a risk for embolization or even aneurysm thrombosis (occlusion).

The etiology of arterial aneurysms is not fully understood but shares pathways with the etiology of atherosclerosis already discussed in this chapter (Fig. 1.4). Unique to aneurysm formation, however, is the important role of the proteolytic enzymes referred to as **matrix metalloproteinases** (MMPs) and **temporary inhibitors of matrix metalloproteinases** (TIMPs). The balance between the activity and inhibition of these enzymes appears to be negatively altered in predisposed individuals. This phenomenon, in

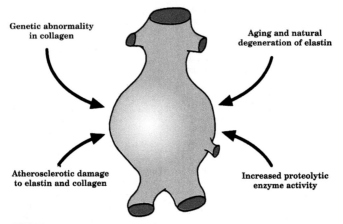

Genetic abnormality in collagen

Aging and natural degeneration of elastin

Atherosclerotic damage to elastin and collagen

Increased proteolytic enzyme activity

FIGURE 1.4 Factors contributing to the multifactorial pathogenesis of arterial aneurysms.

association with the inflammatory response associated with atherosclerosis, results in loss of arterial wall structural integrity and leads to aneurysm formation.

The tendency for arterial aneurysms to form in certain locations, such as the abdominal aorta, can be partially explained by differences in arterial content and hemodynamic factors. It is accepted that the elastin content of arteries is greatest during childhood and that the more distal abdominal aorta has proportionally less elastin content than the paravisceral or thoracic aorta. Consequently, in individuals affected by atherosclerosis, the abdominal aorta is proportionally more susceptible to elastin degradation and, therefore, aneurysm formation when compared to other arteries higher in either elastin or smooth muscle content.

Additionally, it is known that a pulse wave arrives at any vessel bifurcation and that a portion of this pressure is reflected back against the arterial wall proximal to the bifurcation. Minimal reflections occur when the sum of the cross-sectional areas of the daughter arteries (e.g., iliacs) to the parent artery (i.e., aorta) is 1.15 or greater. With advancing age, this sum decreases even in aortas without atheromatous change, and so more pressure is reflected back to the wall of the infrarenal abdominal aorta. The result is a partial standing wave in the abdominal aorta, the chronicity of which may contribute to the commonality of aneurysms in this and other locations.

Lastly, it is proposed that there is a relative paucity of vasa vasorum in the abdominal aorta, which also may contribute to its relative susceptibility to aneurysm formation. It is hypothesized that the blood supply to the media and adventitia of the aorta is adversely affected by atherosclerosis, specifically through obliteration of these vasa vasorum. Areas in which the concentration of these nutrient vessels is less, such as the abdominal aorta, are considered more susceptible to weakening of the artery and aneurysm formation. Congenital defects in the integrity of the vessel collagen and elastic content are found in certain connective tissue disorders, such as Marfan syndrome and Ehlers-Danlos syndrome type IV; these unique conditions will be described in later chapters.

The risk of aneurysm rupture is described by the **law of Laplace**, which places arterial wall stress in relation to vessel diameter and arterial pressure: Wall stress = P × d/t. Aneurysm rupture occurs when the intraluminal pressure exceeds the tensile strength of the wall of the artery. The risk of rupture, therefore, is proportional to aneurysm diameter (d) and intraluminal or systolic blood pressure (P) and inversely related to wall thickness (t).

V. **NATURAL HISTORY.** Peripheral arterial disease is considered a diffuse, slowly progressive "polyvascular" disease; polyvascular in the context that, if present, atherosclerosis affects all arteries of the body to some degree. During early adult life, arterial disease usually remains asymptomatic and undiagnosed. However, if the diagnosis is made, the disease process should be considered to be present in multiple circulations, most notably the coronary. It is accepted that coronary death is the most common cause of mortality in patients with symptomatic and asymptomatic atherosclerotic disease, and should therefore be considered in all patients with arterial disease, even if only apparent in the legs.

Additionally, if atherosclerosis is diagnosed in one area of the vasculature, a careful history and physical examination will often reveal evidence of significant disease at other peripheral sites. For example, a patient may present with calf claudication but also have an unknown abdominal aortic aneurysm on routine physical examination. The diffuse nature of atherosclerosis requires that the initial patient evaluation includes a baseline examination of the entire vascular system.

The natural history of atherosclerosis is variable. Some patients are minimally bothered by its presence, while others are incapacitated. Although atherosclerosis may follow a progressive course, the natural history can be altered favorably in most cases by appropriate risk factor modification, use of medication, and invasive treatment in certain cases. Although not curative, properly selected interventions can offer excellent palliation of and symptomatic relief from the atherosclerotic process. Subsequent chapters will emphasize aspects of the natural history of atherosclerosis, so that providers can select patients who are most likely to benefit from medical, endovascular, and open surgical intervention.

Selected Readings

Ailawadi G, Eliason JL, Upchurch GR Jr. Current concepts in the pathogenesis of abdominal aortic aneurysms. *J Vasc Surg.* 2003;38:584-588.

Aziz M, Yadav KS. Pathogenesis of atherosclerosis: a review. *Med Clin Rev.* 2016;2:1-6.

Bhatt D, Steg P, Ohman E, et al. International prevalence, recognition and treatment of cardiovascular risk factors in outpatients with atherothrombosis. *JAMA.* 2006;295:180-189.

Goessens BMB, van der Graaf Y, Olijhoek JK, Visseren LJ; SMART Study Group. The course of vascular risk factors and the occurrence of vascular events in patients with symptomatic peripheral arterial disease. *J Vasc Surg.* 2007;45:47-54.

Hackman DG. Cardiovascular risk prevention in peripheral arterial disease. *J Vasc Surg.* 2005;41:1070-1073.

Hiatt WR, Armstrong EJ, Larson CJ, Brass EP. Pathogenesis of the limb manifestations and exercise limitations in peripheral artery disease. *Circ Res.* 2015;116:1527-1539.

Hobeika MJ, Thompson RW, Muhs BE, Brookes PC, Gagne PJ. Matrix metalloproteinases in peripheral vascular disease. *J Vasc Surg.* 2007;45:849-857.

Kuivaniemi H, Ryer EJ, Elmore JR, Tromp G. Understanding the pathogenesis of abdominal aortic aneurysms. *Expert Rev Cardiovasc Ther.* 2015;13:975-987.

Libby P, Bornfeldt KE, Tall AR. Atherosclerosis: successes, surprises and future challenges. *Circ Res.* 2016;118:531-534.

Norgren L, Hiatt WR, Dormany JA, Nehler MR, Harris KA, Fowkes FGR. Intersocietal consensus for the management of peripheral arterial disease (TASCII). *J Vasc Surg.* 2007;45(suppl S):S5A-S67.

Ross R. Atherosclerosis—an inflammatory disease. *N Engl J Med.* 1999;340:115-126.

Tabas I, Barcia-Cardena G, Owens GK. Recent insights into the cellular biology of atherosclerosis. *J Cell Biol.* 2015;209:13-22.

Venous Disease

The spectrum of venous disorders ranges from unsightly (spider veins) to uncomfortable (varicose veins) to disabling (chronic venous insufficiency). Although many venous problems are chronic, thromboembolic events are acute and can be life threatening. A solid understanding of the principles of venous disease can help the provider effectively diagnose and treat these challenging patients.

I. **MAGNITUDE OF THE PROBLEM.** The magnitude of venous disease is widespread, with at least 15% of the US population affected by simple varicose veins, and an even greater prevalence among women and the elderly. Another 5% to 10% are afflicted by **chronic venous insufficiency**, defined by skin changes in the leg related to prolonged venous hypertension in the deep and/or superficial venous system. **Venous thromboembolism** (VTE), defined as **deep vein thrombosis** (DVT), **pulmonary embolism** (PE), or both, affects 300,000 to 600,000 people in the United States annually (Chapter 19). A spectrum of **postphlebitic syndrome**, defined by symptoms of leg pain, edema, and/or ulceration, exists in all patients to some extent in the years following DVT. Pulmonary embolism is a potential life-threatening consequence of untreated DVT and is the most common cause of preventable death in hospitalized patients (Chapter 19).

Chronic venous disease is classified by the **CEAP grading system** (Table 2.1), an international reporting method, which accounts for the four key features of venous disease: clinical signs, etiology (congenital, primary, or secondary), anatomic location (superficial, deep, or perforator), and pathophysiology (reflux, obstruction, or both). This system was established in 1995 by an international Ad Hoc Committee of the American Venous Forum to encourage uniform reporting of venous disease and promote clinical study including natural history and treatment strategies.

II. **BASIC ANATOMY.** Although description of the veins has historically been limited by the lack of a standardized nomenclature, the following provides a current consensus on communicating venous anatomy.

A. **The superficial venous system** (Fig. 2.1) of the lower extremity includes the **great saphenous vein (GSV)**, small saphenous vein, and their tributaries. The GSV is occasionally duplicated in the thigh or calf. In the thigh, an anterior accessory GSV is the most constant branch. At the knee, the **saphenous nerve** becomes superficial and joins the GSV as it courses distal in the leg, an anatomic proximity that is relevant in instances where intervention on the GSV is considered. Below the knee, the posterior accessory saphenous vein drains into the GSV. Numerous medial perforating veins connect the deep calf veins (i.e., tibial veins) with the great saphenous system and are called **perforator veins**. The small saphenous vein (formerly the lesser saphenous vein) ascends along a posterior course in the calf to join the popliteal vein in the popliteal fossa in the majority of limbs (Fig. 2.2). As a normal variant, the small saphenous may continue cephalad to join the great saphenous or femoral vein.

B. **The deep veins** of the lower extremity are the paired posterior tibial, peroneal, and anterior tibial veins in the leg, which ascend with their

2.1	Basic CEAP Classification of Chronic Venous Disease

Clinical
0—no signs of venous disease
1—telangiectasias or reticular veins
2—varicose veins
3—edema only from venous etiology
4—pigmentation or eczema
5—healed venous ulcer
6—active venous ulcer

Etiology
C—congenital
P—primary
S—secondary (postthrombotic)

Anatomy
S—superficial veins
P—perforator veins
D—deep veins

Pathophysiology
R—reflux
0—obstruction
R,0—reflux and obstruction

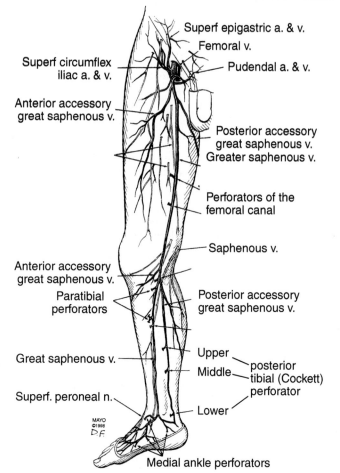

FIGURE 2.1 Anatomy of the great saphenous vein and perforators.

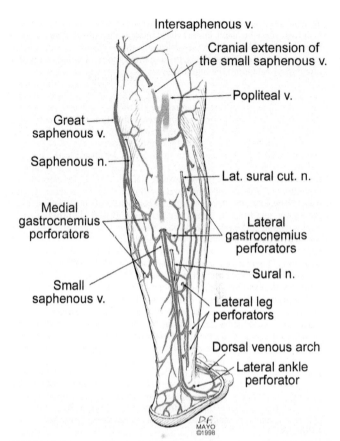

FIGURE 2.2 Anatomy of the small saphenous vein. Note the proximity of the small saphenous vein to the sural nerve. (Reprinted with permission from the Mayo Foundation.)

correspondingly named arteries. The popliteal vein becomes the **femoral vein** in the adductor canal. The **deep femoris vein** drains the lateral thigh muscles, joining with the femoral to become the common femoral vein in the groin (Fig. 2.1). The external iliac vein begins above the inguinal ligament, before its confluence with the internal iliac vein at the sacroiliac joint, which then becomes the common iliac vein.

C. **Perforating veins** connect the superficial with either the deep veins (direct perforators) or with venous sinuses in the calf (indirect perforators). Abundant perforating veins normally direct flow from the superficial toward the deep network via a system of **venous valves**. The more anatomically constant direct perforators are located in four general locations: *medial calf* (**paratibial** and **posterior tibial perforators**), *lateral calf*, *thigh*, and *foot* (Fig. 2.1). Perforators have often been assigned eponyms, but in modern nomenclature are described according to anatomic location.

D. **Venous sinuses** comprise a thin-walled, valveless, large capacitance system located in the calf musculature. When the calf muscles contract, pressure in excess of 200 mm Hg is created, propelling venous blood toward the heart. A normally functioning calf muscle pump displaces greater than 60% of venous blood within that leg into the popliteal vein with a single contraction.

E. **Venous Valves.** A unique histologic feature of many veins is the presence of valves. These bicuspid, endothelialized structures direct "one-way" flow of venous blood from the extremity toward the heart, and by their closure prevent reversal of flow or reflux. Present throughout the column of venous blood from the foot to the inguinal ligament, valves work to equalize pressure throughout the venous system. Valves are present in the both superficial and deep veins. In the lower extremity, the greatest number is located below the knee, decreasing in frequency until the inguinal ligament. A single valve in the common femoral vein or external iliac that may protect against "spillover" reflux into the GSV is absent in one-third of the population. The common iliac, vena cava, and portal venous system are devoid of valves.

F. **The vein wall** is comprised of the same layers discussed in the previous chapter (intima, media, and adventitia), although their composition and function differ slightly in the venous circulation. These differences include (a) a thin wall that is one-tenth to one-third as thick as an artery, (b) less elastic tissue, (c) an attenuated media comprised of smooth muscle and adventitia, and (d) a thickened adventitia comprised of fibroelastic connective tissue. Although veins possess vasa vasorum, they receive most of their nourishment by diffusion from the bloodstream.

G. **Upper Extremity.** As with the lower extremity, anatomic variations are far more common in the venous than in the arterial system. The **cephalic, median antebrachial, brachial,** and **basilic** veins constitute the venous system of the arm (Fig. 2.3). The cephalic and median antebrachial veins are generally considered superficial veins of the arm while the basilic and brachial veins are subfascial or deep. The superficial or deep location of upper extremity veins is particularly important as one considers formation of arteriovenous circuits (*arteriovenous fistula*) for hemodialysis access in the arm (Chapter 20). At the elbow fossa, the **median cubital vein** joins the cephalic with the basilic vein, and also receives a deep communicating branch from the forearm. The paired **venae comitantes** course with the arteries in the forearm, becoming the paired brachial veins in the upper arm. The medial brachial vein and basilic vein typically join at the axillary vein, which then becomes the subclavian vein at the border of the first rib. In contrast, the cephalic vein joins the subclavian vein at the **deltopectoral groove** of the anterior shoulder.

III. **ETIOLOGY**

A. **Venous insufficiency or reflux** results from a failure of one or more of the valves within the venous system, resulting in loss of the balance of venous pressure. In the setting of reflux, the venous system below the abnormal segment is exposed to high venous pressures from pooling of blood due to gravity. Under these circumstances, venous pressure in the lower extremity in a person who is standing can be chronically elevated and sustained as high as 150 to 200 mm Hg (when the individual is on his or her feet). This condition preferentially affects the most dependent parts of the extremity and over time leads to venous distention, seeping of blood components into the interstitial space, and the sequelae of **chronic venous insufficiency.** Venous reflux can affect any combination of the superficial, perforator, and deep veins, and can be the result of a degenerative process, as is commonly seen in varicose veins. From the histologic standpoint, varicose veins possess less elastin and less contractile force and, as a result, are more prone to dilate and become varicose in a setting of chronic venous hypertension.

Valvular dysfunction may also be acquired after a thrombotic event (i.e., blood clot) damages the valves, resulting in a fibrous contracture of the cusps and **postphlebitic syndrome. Deep venous insufficiency** usually follows thrombosis (DVT) and is sometimes a result of primary degeneration or congenital defect in the valves. Thrombosis not only adversely affects the valves of the venous system but also damages the endothelium, rendering it ineffective at preventing future clot formation. Postphlebitic

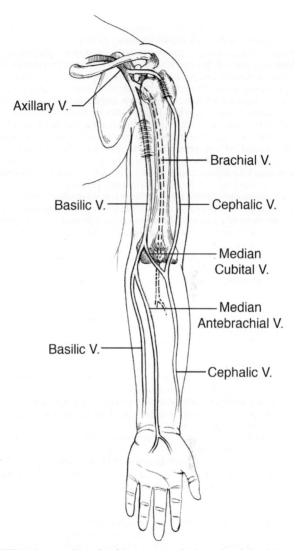

FIGURE 2.3 Anatomy of the veins of the upper extremity. Anatomic variations in the upper extremity veins, as with those of the lower extremity, are common.

syndrome develops months and years after DVT and is a result of valvular and endothelial dysfunction of the deep veins. Postphlebitic syndrome is a clinical spectrum present in all patients who have had DVT and can, in its most severe form, lead to venous hypertension, edema, subdermal scarring (**lipodermatosclerosis**), and venous ulceration. Venous ulcers occur most commonly at the medial and lateral malleoli of the leg (e.g., the most dependent), where venous pressures over time are greatest.

B. **Venous obstruction** may be due to either intrinsic or extrinsic venous disorders. Failure of the deep vein to reopen (recannulize) after thrombosis can lead to reflux as well as outflow obstruction. The most severe clinical symptoms of postthrombotic syndrome occur in limbs with a combination of reflux and obstruction. **Klippel-Trenaunay syndrome** is a congenital triad of *capillary hemangiomas* (port-wine stains), *limb hypertrophy*, and *varicose veins*. Patients with this condition may have venous obstruction as a consequence of complete (aplasia) or partial (hypoplasia) development of the deep venous system. The etiology of extrinsic venous compression can be pelvic malignancy, retroperitoneal fibrosis, and iatrogenic or congenital factors. A condition known as **May-Thurner syndrome** results from compression of the left common iliac vein underneath the right common iliac artery. This anatomic relationship is asymptomatic in most adults, but a small fraction may manifest left lower extremity edema, subtle leg asymmetry, or left-sided venous thrombosis. It is speculated that the position of the left iliac vein underneath the right iliac artery is responsible for the higher prevalence of left lower extremity venous thrombotic events compared to the right.

C. **Acute venous thrombosis** may result from a combination of three factors that comprise **Virchow's triad**: stasis, intimal injury, and hypercoagulability.

1. **Venous stasis** may result from immobilization, such as in a postoperative situation or in the setting of prolonged travel. Slow movement of blood, particularly through valve cusps, may predispose to leukocyte adhesion and local hypoxia, triggering endothelial injury and hypercoagulable factors.

2. **Minor endothelial injury** and the ensuing cascade of platelet migration and fibrin adherence are usually balanced out and overcome by the intrinsic fibrinolytic system. However, injury, as may be associated with an indwelling catheter, extremity injury, or other factors, may trigger thrombosis.

3. **Hypercoagulable states** that predispose to venous thrombosis may be genetic (hereditary) or acquired (Chapter 19). Common acquired states include the postoperative condition (transient decrease in fibrinolysis and increase in procoagulant factors), injury, malignancy, pregnancy, and oral contraceptive use. Genetic hypercoagulable states may contribute to 50% to 60% of unexplained DVTs, and should be investigated in patients with iatrogenic, familial, or recurrent thrombosis (Chapter 19).

D. **Pulmonary thromboembolism**—also referred to as PE—results when thrombus in the venous system travels to the right heart, through the tricuspid and pulmonic valves, to lodge in one or more of the pulmonary arteries. The majority of PE comes from the lower extremities, but this condition may also result from thrombus in pelvic and upper extremity veins (Chapter 19).

IV. **PATHOPHYSIOLOGY**

A. **Normal Physiology.** Venous pressure at the ankle reflects the weight of the column of blood to the level of the right atrium. Normal pressures in the standing position are 90 to 100 mm Hg, depending on height. With exercise, the calf muscle propels blood from the leg, *reducing* the venous pressure by over 70% after about 10 steps. Recovery time to refill the leg with venous blood upon cessation of exercise normally exceeds 20 seconds (mean 70 seconds) (Fig. 2.4).

B. **Superficial Venous Insufficiency.** Patients with varicose veins may only be able to reduce their ambulatory venous pressure by 30% to 40% and as such their superficial veins become dilated and uncomfortable. In some patients, as much as 20% to 25% of femoral venous outflow is refluxed into an incompetent saphenous system, resulting in this blood going back down the leg in a "circus" type motion.

C. **Deep Venous Insufficiency.** In the setting of deep venous insufficiency, ankle pressures may only decrease 20% with exercise and refill time in the leg is

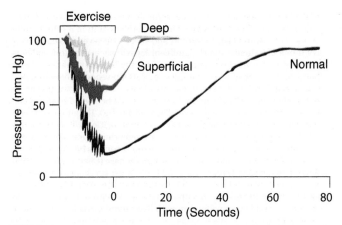

FIGURE 2.4 Ambulatory venous pressures. Normally, leg exercises cause lower extremity venous pressures to drop approximately 70% because the musculovenous pump propels blood toward the heart and competent venous valves prevent reflux. Normal return to baseline venous pressure after exercise with refilling of the calf muscle is greater than 20 seconds. Varicose veins (superficial veins) are associated with a 30% to 40% venous pressure reduction with exercise because a portion of deep venous return is refluxed down the incompetent saphenous vein. Deep venous valve incompetence results in less initial drop in venous pressure, but a more rapid restoration of venous pressure in the leg with cessation of exercise. (Adapted from Schanzer H, Peirce EC II. Pathophysiologic evaluation of chronic venous stasis with ambulatory venous pressure studies. *Angiology*. 1982;33:183-191.)

abnormally fast. Limbs with combined deep and perforator reflux, in particular, have an inefficient muscle pump and develop significant venous pooling at rest and during activity.

D. **Deep Venous Obstruction.** In patients with this condition, there may be a paradoxical increase in ambulatory venous pressures (i.e., increase instead of the expected decrease). In these cases, venous outflow obstruction may lead to **ambulatory venous hypertension** and **venous claudication**, a "bursting" sensation in the leg with ambulation. Over time, development of venous collaterals may reduce the symptoms of venous obstruction.

E. **Venous Thromboembolism (VTE) (Chapter 19).** The main physiologic consequence of this condition—also referred to as acute pulmonary embolism or PE—is hypoxemia resulting from blockage of the pulmonary arteries. Emboli to either pulmonary artery or a larger **saddle embolus** straddling the pulmonary artery bifurcation obstruct right heart outflow and lead to myocardial strain and heart failure. Large PE may lead to sudden cardiovascular collapse and death while smaller or recurrent PE may also be fatal, particularly in those with underlying conditions rendering them unable to compensate.

V. **NATURAL HISTORY.** Although acute VTE or PE can be life threatening, many venous disorders are chronic problems. It is important that both the patient and the provider understand this chronicity. In most cases, the natural history can be altered so that the patient remains productive and comfortable.

A. **Varicose Veins and Telangiectasias** (spider veins) are common and have a natural history ranging from asymptomatic and unsightly, to achiness and heaviness after prolonged standing, to swelling and itching. **Superficial thrombophlebitis** may occur, but is rarely complicated by deep venous thrombosis or PE. Large superficial varicosities can cause overlying ulceration of the skin and, in rare cases, bleeding; especially in the elderly or debilitated.

B. **Postphlebitic Syndrome** is present to some degree in all who have had a DVT. During the first 1 to 2 years following DVT, this condition most commonly consists of only mild leg discomfort and edema. However, 5 years following DVT, half of patients report significant leg edema, induration, and stasis dermatitis at or near the ankle. Five to twenty percent of patients having had a lower extremity DVT progress to develop venous ulceration. By 10 years, more than 90% have some sort of lower extremity symptoms. The natural history of postthrombotic syndrome can be altered by use of compression therapy with support hose (30 to 40 mm Hg). Thrombolytic therapy (**catheter-directed thrombolysis**) for acute, symptomatic DVT of the proximal lower extremity or iliac vein may favorably alter the natural history of postphlebitic syndrome by more quickly reducing thrombus burden, preventing venous obstruction, and reducing valvular damage (Chapters 9 and 10).

C. **Acute Deep Venous Thrombosis or DVT.** The most serious consequence of deep venous thrombosis is VTE to the lung (Chapter 19). Pulmonary embolism or PE seldom occurs when the thrombus is located below the knees, and is more common with iliofemoral thrombus. The natural course for many patients with simple DVT, even without anticoagulation, is resolution of the acute tenderness and swelling. Over a period of 3 to 6 months, the deep veins usually recanalize. Without appropriate anticoagulation, about 30% of untreated patients have recurrent thrombosis or PE with a high mortality. Most limbs with acute DVT are normal in color or have a cyanotic appearance. In more severe cases, **phlegmasia alba dolens** (turgid, white, painful leg) occurs with extreme acute venous outflow obstruction. A more severe manifestation of venous thrombosis is **phlegmasia cerulea dolens** (turgid, blue, painful leg), in which massive swelling can lead to arterial compromise and venous gangrene.

D. **Pulmonary embolism.** Because many episodes of DVT probably go undetected, the incidence of thromboembolism to the lungs is difficult to ascertain. Estimates indicate a PE rate of 5% even in adequately treated patients. Approximately one patient in 10 with a symptomatic PE dies within an hour. The remaining patients, who are adequately treated with anticoagulants, usually follow a course of resolution and return to good cardiopulmonary function within several weeks. The most important factor predicting a poor prognosis is preexisting heart disease. A minority of patients develop recurrent emboli and pulmonary hypertension with **cor pulmonale** (right heart failure).

Selected Readings

Almeida JI, Wakefield T, Kabnick LS, Onyeachom UN, Lal BK. Use of the Clinical, Etiologic, Anatomic, and Pathophysiologic classification and Venous Clinical Severity Score to establish a treatment plan for chronic venous disorders. *J Vasc Surg Venous Lymphat Disord.* 2015;3(4):456-460. doi: 10.1016/j.jvsv.2015.05.007.

Eberhardt RT, Raffetto JD. Chronic venous insufficiency. *Circulation.* 2014;130(4):333-346. doi: 10.1161/CIRCULATIONAHA.113.006898.

Garcia R, Labropoulos N, Gasparis AP, Elias S. Present and future options for treatment of infrainguinal deep vein disease. *J Vasc Surg Venous Lymphat Disord.* 2018. pii: S2213-333X(18)30120-3. doi: 10.1016/j.jvsv.2018.01.010 [Epub ahead of print].

Jacobs BN, Andraska EA, Obi AT, Wakefield TW. Pathophysiology of varicose veins. *J Vasc Surg Venous Lymphat Disord.* 2017;5(3):460-467. doi: 10.1016/j.jvsv.2016.12.014.

O'Donnell TF Jr, Passman MA, Marston WA; Society for Vascular Surgery; American Venous Forum. Management of venous leg ulcers: clinical practice guidelines of the Society for Vascular Surgery® and the American Venous Forum. *J Vasc Surg.* 2014;60(2 suppl):3S-59S. doi: 10.1016/j.jvs.2014.04.049.

Sutzko DC, Obi AT, Kimball AS, Smith ME, Wakefield TW, Osborne NH. Clinical outcomes after varicose vein procedures in octogenarians within the Vascular Quality Initiative Varicose Vein Registry. *J Vasc Surg Venous Lymphat Disord.* 2018;6(4):464-470. doi: 10.1016/j.jvsv.2018.02.008.

INITIAL PATIENT EVALUATION

The interview and physical examination provide information that directs the need for additional diagnostic testing and treatment of patients with vascular disease. Today's electronic medical record and imaging technologies tend to divert attention from the importance of talking to and examining the patient. Diagnostic tests add valuable hemodynamic and anatomic data but **do not replace the need for a careful history and physical examination as the first step in optimal patient care.** Even in this era of specialized imaging, the adage that "the patient will tell you what's wrong, if you're willing to listen" remains true.

The initial history and physical examination serve several purposes. The process enables the clinician to establish a **clinical impression** or preliminary diagnosis. Interviewing and examining the patient often provide enough information for a good clinical impression. Diagnostic tests can then be ordered in a more appropriate and efficient manner to further hone the clinical impression. The history and physical also allow the clinician to determine the **urgency for treatment.** Although some vascular problems require urgent intervention, most entail elective evaluation and treatment. This important distinction must be made on the basis of the history and physical exam and not just the appearance of vascular disease on an imaging study. Additionally, the history and physical provide an opportunity to assess the physiologic age of the patient. Comorbidities such as pulmonary, cardiac, or renal dysfunction heavily influence management strategies and outcomes in patients with vascular disease. One should not underestimate the value of the "eyeball test," review of systems, and functional status as one considers the best treatment plan. An astute clinician would also be mindful that the vascular patient may harbor an occult nonvascular disease such as gastrointestinal or pulmonary malignancy.

The initial interview establishes a **rapport or relationship** between the patient and physician. Through this process, the physician gains the trust to reassure the patient and family and to obtain insight into the patient's overall living situation. The patient's vocation, level of independent living, and whether he or she drives an automobile all weigh heavily in the management decisions related to vascular disease. Understanding a patient's socioeconomic status may guide choice of prescription medications and expectations for support following hospitalizations and procedures. For example, prescribing a low-dose aspirin, generic statin, and angiotensin-converting enzyme inhibitor lowers all-cause cardiovascular mortality in vascular patients at low economic expense.

Finally, technology has the potential to be either intrusive or beneficial in the patient-physician relationship. Face-to-face time with the patient is essential but cannot occur if the clinician conducts the patient interview while facing a computer screen. A brief recorded message on a mobile device is one example of using technology to remind a patient of medication, physical activity, or perioperative instructions. Tablets can also be used to conveniently illustrate vascular anatomy and disease processes. Communication with patients outside a typical office setting can also be enhanced by telemedicine.

The following chapters outline techniques used to examine the arterial and venous systems in the following anatomic regions: neck, upper extremity, abdomen, and lower extremity. **Inspection, auscultation, and palpation** are performed during each portion of the vascular examination.

3 History and Physical Examination of the Arterial System

I. **GENERAL EXAMINATION.** Atherosclerotic arterial disease is a diffuse process. Therefore, the physical exam—regardless of patient complaint—should include an assessment of the arterial system in the neck, the torso, and the extremities in order to identify otherwise unrecognized or asymptomatic disease. At a minimum, the physical exam should include the following:

1. Assessment of heart rate and rhythm.
2. Measurement of the blood pressure in both upper extremities.
3. Auscultation of the neck to listen for carotid and supraclavicular bruits.
4. Auscultation of the heart to listen for arrhythmias and murmurs.
5. Palpation of the abdomen to assess masses; pulsatile or otherwise.
6. Auscultation of the abdomen to listen for bruits.
7. Palpation of peripheral pulses in the extremities.
8. Use of continuous wave Doppler to listen for the presence and quality of arterial signals and, in conjunction with a manual blood pressure cuff, performance of the ankle-brachial index (ABI) (see also Chapter 5).
9. Auscultation of the femoral region to listen for bruits.
10. Inspection of all extremities to assess for the presence of edema, ulceration, gangrene, or signs of embolization to the toes (**i.e., blue toe syndrome**) or fingers.

II. **HEAD AND NECK.** Vascular disease in the head and neck relates mostly to atherosclerosis of the carotid arteries, which is a common cause of stroke (Chapter 12). Patients should be questioned about previous stroke or **transient ischemic attack** (TIA), carotid artery intervention (endarterectomy or stent), and prior duplex ultrasound of the carotid arteries. If a carotid intervention or duplex ultrasound has been performed in the past, the indications and results are important to understand. Symptoms of TIA or stroke typically relate to episodes of *unilateral* extremity weakness or paralysis. Stroke or TIA may also manifest as an inability to initiate speech (**aphasia**), inability to form words (**dysarthria**), or facial droop. The clinician should also inquire about episodes of **transient monocular blindness (amaurosis fugax)**, which would suggest occlusive disease of the carotid artery on the same side (ipsilateral) as the ocular symptoms. Amaurosis (also described as a "descending curtain or shade") results from temporary occlusion of a retinal arteriole from emboli originating from the carotid bulb passing through the **ophthalmic artery**. The differential diagnosis of amaurosis is broad and includes migraine headache, papilledema, and giant cell arteritis.

The differential diagnosis of stroke or TIA originating from the carotid arteries in the neck includes **seizure disorder**, which more commonly causes global or bilateral symptoms followed by somnolence (postictal period). Severe hypertension can lead to **small vessel cerebral infarct** or **hemorrhagic stroke**, which can be differentiated from embolic stroke from the patient's history and presentation. **Brain tumors** or **brain aneurysms** may also cause neurologic deficits but are often accompanied by other symptoms such as headache. Diffusion-weighted magnetic resonance imaging (DW-MRI) is useful in differentiating primary intracranial disease (small vessel cerebral infarct or brain tumor) from embolic TIA or stroke originating from cervical carotid disease. Syncope, lightheadedness, and dizziness are common in the elderly. **These symptoms are rarely related to carotid occlusive disease** and are more commonly due to autonomic dysfunction, arrhythmias, middle ear disease (vestibular system), or **subclavian steal syndrome**.

A. **Inspection.** Normally, the carotid pulsation is not visible. However, it may be prominent at the base of the right neck in thin patients with long-standing hypertension. Such patients are often referred for concerns of aneurysm, when in fact they have a tortuous or prominent common carotid artery. If large enough, a rare **carotid artery aneurysm** or **carotid body tumor** would be visualized in the anterior neck (i.e., cervical region).

Another observation related to carotid occlusive disease is a bright reflective defect or spot on the retina referred to as a **Hollenhorst plaque**. These plaques seen on funduscopic exam were described by a Mayo Clinic ophthalmologist in the 1960s and represent cholesterol emboli originating from atherosclerotic disease of the carotid arteries.

B. **Palpation.** The common carotid pulse is palpable low in the neck between the midline trachea and the anterior border of the sternocleidomastoid muscle. Even in the setting of internal carotid artery occlusion, there is generally a palpable carotid pulse, as the external carotid often remains patent. A diminished or absent common carotid pulsation suggests proximal occlusive disease at the origin of the carotid artery in the chest. The presence of a temporal artery pulse anterior to the ear indicates a patent common and external carotid artery.

The vertebral artery is not accessible to palpation as it lies deep at the posterior base of the neck and is surrounded by the cervical vertebrae for most of its course. Pulsatile masses at the base of the neck or in the supraclavicular fossa generally originate from the **subclavian artery**.

C. **Auscultation.** The bell side of the stethoscope is placed lightly over the middle and base of the neck while the patient suspends respirations. **Cervical bruits** are an abnormal finding and may originate from carotid stenosis or lesions of the aortic valve or arch vessels. A bruit from a carotid stenosis is usually loudest at the midneck over the carotid bifurcation. Transmitted bruits or cardiac murmurs tend to be loudest over the upper chest and base of the neck.

The presence of a cervical bruit does not necessarily mean that a carotid stenosis is present. In fact, only half of patients with carotid bruit will have stenoses of 30% or more and only a quarter will have stenoses of more than 75%. Additionally, **the severity of underlying carotid stenosis does not correlate with the loudness of the bruit**. Duplex ultrasound is standard in determining the significance of a cervical bruit and is noninvasive, inexpensive, and readily available.

III. **UPPER EXTREMITY.** Although atherosclerosis is less common in the upper than the lower extremity, arterial lesions of the subclavian and axillary arteries can develop (Chapter 17). Upper extremity occlusive or aneurysm disease may cause claudication or signs of embolization in the arm or hand. Arterial occlusive lesions of the subclavian artery are more common on the left and influenced by the length of that artery compared to the right subclavian and shear stress distribution on the aortic arch. In instances when a subclavian stenosis is *proximal* to the origin of the vertebral artery, the patient may develop **subclavian steal syndrome** (Fig. 3.1). In these cases, exertion of the arm results in a pressure decrease across the stenosis that leads to reversal of flow in the vertebral artery ("steal") causing **posterior circulation symptoms** (Table 3.1). Acute arm ischemia is most

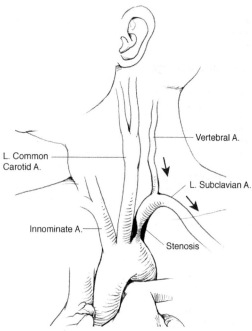

FIGURE 3.1 A proximal subclavian stenosis can result in the syndrome of subclavian steal. Flow is "stolen" retrograde from the ipsilateral vertebral artery to supply the upper extremity. Symptoms related to posterior circulation insufficiency such as ataxia, dizziness, syncope, and visual disturbances may develop and are exacerbated by arm activity.

often the result of an embolus from a proximal arterial or cardiac source. Acute thrombosis of a chronic subclavian or axillary artery aneurysm or stenosis may also result in acute arm ischemia.

A variety of nonatherosclerotic vascular diseases can affect the upper extremity (Chapter 17). **Takayasu's arteritis (pulseless disease)** is

Posterior Circulation Symptoms

Diplopia
Vertigo
Syncope
Ataxia
Dysarthria
Drop attacks
Dizziness and giddiness
Visual changes
Tinnitus and hearing changes
Nystagmus

Posterior circulation symptoms generally result from vertebrobasilar insufficiency. Subclavian steal is one such cause in patients with atherosclerotic disease. These symptoms may also occur when both vertebral arteries are diseased, or with unilateral stenosis and a contralateral hypoplastic vertebral artery.

an inflammatory condition of the arteries that occurs predominantly in young Asian women. The early stage of Takayasu's disease is characterized by an acute inflammatory response that often includes fever, malaise, and muscle aches. The later stages occur after the acute arteritis has been treated and can result in fibrotic arterial stenoses or even arterial occlusion. **Giant cell arteritis (GCA)** occurs most commonly in older Caucasian women and can affect aortic arch vessels and axillary and brachial arteries. Other symptoms associated with GCA include headaches, monocular blindness, and jaw claudication. Episodic coolness, pain, and numbness of the hand suggest **small vessel vasospasm or Raynaud's disease,** which is often triggered by an identifiable event such as exposure to the cold. The etiology may be idiopathic (primary Raynaud's) or associated with other collagen vascular diseases, frostbite, or atherosclerotic occlusive disease (secondary Raynaud's).

Thoracic outlet syndrome (TOS) may affect the upper extremities, causing vascular compromise from repetitive arm use. Pure vascular TOS is uncommon (10% of cases) and results from compromise of the subclavian artery or vein at the thoracic outlet (Fig. 4.1). At this location, the first rib, the scalene and subclavius muscles, and the clavicle form a tight space through which the subclavian vessels pass (Chapter 17). This condition is more common in young muscular individuals such as weight lifters, pitchers, and swimmers. Over 90% of TOS is related to or has a neurologic component involving the brachial plexus.

A. **Inspection.** Inspection of the upper extremity provides information about arterial perfusion. Pink fingertips with a capillary refill time of less than 2 seconds are a sign of good perfusion. In contrast, the acutely ischemic upper extremity is pallid, and may have neurologic compromise in the form of motor or sensory deficits. The main change in appearance of the extremity with chronic arterial ischemia is muscle atrophy, especially in the forearm and proximal hand. Embolization or small-vessel disease may be recognized by painful mottled fingertips, ulcerations, or splinter hemorrhages. Raynaud's disease presents as a triphasic color change (white, blue, and then red) in the hands and fingers following an inciting event such as cold exposure or emotional stress. The fingers first appear pallid or white, then cyanotic or blue, and lastly hyperemic or red as circulation is restored. In cases of TOS with axillo-subclavian venous thrombosis or **Paget-Schroetter syndrome,** the arm appears acutely cyanotic and swollen due to venous obstruction.

B. **Palpation.** Normally, upper extremity pulses can be palpated at three locations: the upper medial arm in the groove between the biceps and triceps muscles (axillary and proximal brachial artery); the antecubital fossa just medial to the biceps tendon (brachial artery); and the wrist over the distal radius (radial) or distal ulna (ulnar). In young women with absent upper extremity pulses, **Takayasu's disease** (pulseless disease) should be suspected.

Skin temperature also can be assessed by palpation, especially using the more sensitive back of the examining hand or fingers. The level of skin temperature demarcation (warm to cool) in the acutely ischemic limb is just distal to the level of the arterial occlusion.

Arterial aneurysms of the upper extremities are detectable if they occur in regions where the pulse is accessible to palpation. While larger subclavian and axillary artery aneurysms may be palpable above or below the clavicle or in the axilla, smaller aneurysms in these locations may go undetected. Aneurysms of the brachial artery are most commonly pseudoaneurysms due to the artery having been accessed during an arteriogram. Aneurysms of the ulnar artery can occur in laborers as a result of repetitive trauma to the artery, which is in close proximity to the hamate bone in the wrist (**hypothenar hammer syndrome**).

Several bedside tests are available to provide information related to the diagnosis of TOS. **Adson's test** is performed by having the patient rotate the head toward the tested arm and letting the head tilt backward (to extend the neck) while the examiner extends the patient's arm. A positive test is indicated by reduction in or disappearance of the radial pulse. This test may be positive in as much as 10% to 20% of the normal population. During the elevated arm stress test (**EAST test**), the arms and hands are raised to the level of the head, and the hands are repeatedly opened and closed for 3 minutes. Symptoms of numbness, pain, or weakness on the affected side suggest neurogenic or arterial TOS. Neither of these tests in and of itself is diagnostic. Rather, findings from these provocative maneuvers should be used in conjunction with other findings from the history, physical exam, and other testing when considering the diagnosis of TOS.

C. **Auscultation.** Auscultation of upper extremity arteries should include comparison of blood pressure in both arms and examination of the supraclavicular fossa for bruit. A difference in arm pressures of more than 10 mm Hg indicates a hemodynamically significant innominate, subclavian, or axillary artery stenosis on the side with the diminished pressure. **The arm with the higher blood pressure is the more accurate systemic blood pressure,** which may be disappointing to some patients with previously undiagnosed hypertension. Because collateral flow to the arm is extensive, a proximal subclavian stenosis may still be present with a palpable pulse at the wrist. If the patient has symptoms suggesting arm claudication, the arm should be exercised for 2 to 5 minutes and the brachial pressures rechecked. With this provocative maneuver, the brachial pressure will decrease if a significant arterial stenosis exists. With TOS, some patients develop an infraclavicular bruit with passive abduction and elevation of the arm overhead.

IV. **ABDOMEN.** Most vascular pathology in the abdomen is asymptomatic and the history may not provide insight into the diagnosis. The majority of patients with **abdominal aortic aneurysms** (AAAs) are asymptomatic (Chapter 14). The acute onset of severe back or abdominal pain in a patient with a known AAA is considered a ruptured aneurysm until proven otherwise. Patients with **chronic mesenteric ischemia** relate a subtle triad of postprandial pain, weight loss, and sitophobia (fear of food) (Chapter 16). **Acute mesenteric ischemia** causes diffuse abdominal "pain out of proportion" to examination. Poorly controlled hypertension in association with worsening renal function may be evidence of **renal artery stenosis.** Occlusive aortoiliac disease can manifest as bilateral hip and buttock claudication, absent femoral pulses, and impotence (**Leriche's syndrome**). In patients with prior aortic surgery, it is important to determine the original pathology for which the operation was performed (e.g., occlusive or aneurysmal disease). Ulcerated aortoiliac atherosclerosis, which embolizes to the distal lower extremity circulation, is often associated with an abdominal bruit and painful blue toe syndrome. Sudden, bilateral leg pain, coldness, paresthesias, and paralysis are caused by **acute aortic occlusion** from (a) thrombosis of an existing aneurysm, (b) progression of severe occlusive disease, (c) a saddle embolus from the heart, or (d) an aortic dissection.

A. **Inspection.** Inspection of the abdomen is the most limited part of the examination of the abdominal aorta and its branches. The normal aortic pulsation usually is not visible. However, a large abdominal aortic aneurysm may be seen pulsating against the anterior abdominal wall, especially in thin patients.

B. **Palpation.** Although its sensitivity is limited in larger patients, palpation of the abdomen should be a part of the routine physical exam. Certain anatomic features related to the aorta and iliac arteries should be considered when one palpates the abdomen. The aorta bifurcates into the common iliac arteries at about the level of the umbilicus and, in order to assess the infrarenal aortic segment, one must palpate deeply above this surface landmark. Having the patient bend the knees, while exhaling slowly, relaxes the abdominal musculature and facilitates the exam. It should also be remembered that, unless the patient is obese, an aortic pulse should normally be palpable above the umbilicus, especially if the abdominal wall is relaxed. The normal aorta is approximately the width of the patient's thumb or 2 cm in diameter.

An aortic aneurysm should be suspected when the aortic pulse feels expansile and larger than 4 cm. Elderly patients may have a tortuous, anteriorly displaced aorta that can be mistaken for an aneurysm. Because the sensitivity of palpation is limited, an aortic ultrasound should be ordered as an easy, noninvasive test in patients in whom there are questions about aortic diameter. In addition to size, other characteristics of an aneurysm may be identified by palpation. If the enlarged aorta extends high to the xiphoid or costal margins, a suprarenal or thoracoabdominal aortic aneurysm should be suspected. Aneurysm tenderness is a sign indicating impending rupture, aneurysm leak, or the presence of an **inflammatory aneurysm**. Because of the location of the iliac arteries deep within the pelvis, aneurysms in this location are often not palpable. Occasionally, a large **internal iliac artery aneurysm** may be palpable on digital rectal examination.

C. **Auscultation.** Auscultation commonly reveals bruits when significant occlusive or aneurysmal disease of the aorta or its branches is present. Aortoiliac occlusive disease causes bruits in the middle and lower abdomen and the femoral region. Bruits secondary to isolated renal artery stenosis are faint and localized in the upper abdominal quadrants lateral to the midline. Mesenteric artery occlusive disease may be associated with epigastric bruits.

Asymptomatic bruits are an occasional incidental finding on abdominal examination of young adults, especially thin women. If the patient is not hypertensive and does not have intestinal angina or leg claudication, these bruits may be considered benign. Conversely, pathologic cervical and abdominal bruits may be present in young women with symptomatic **fibromuscular dysplasia** affecting the carotid and/or renal arteries.

V. **LOWER EXTREMITIES.** Evaluation of leg circulation may seem overwhelming at first with a large number of possible diagnoses to consider. To simplify and organize the process, an initial priority is to **categorize the temporal presentation into either acute or chronic lower extremity ischemia.** This determination allows the examiner to focus on a limited number of diagnoses and to understand the urgency of the problem. Clinical decision-making in the setting of acute ischemia is based on the status of the limb, while chronic lower extremity ischemia is further broken down into two subcategories: **claudication** and **critical ischemia.** The question, "does this process fall into the acute or chronic category?" should be asked in every instance in which the clinician is called to evaluate lower extremity circulation. If the process is chronic, the next question should be, "does this condition represent claudication or critical ischemia?" Nearly all patients with lower extremity arterial disease fall into one of these categories and, once the determination is made, the diagnostic and management process becomes more focused and clear (Chapter 13).

A. **Acute Lower Extremity Ischemia.** Acute lower extremity ischemia presents as sudden onset of symptoms. Because the arterial occlusion occurs suddenly without time to develop collateral circulation, there is limited ability to compensate and the limb may be quite ischemic. Acute extremity ischemia classically manifests the **5 Ps: pulselessness, pain, pallor, paresthesia,** and **poikilothermia.**

B. **Chronic Lower Extremity Ischemia: Asymptomatic.** Some patients with diminished or even absent lower extremity pressures or pulses may not have symptoms. Persons with a sedentary lifestyle may not be active enough to experience the symptoms of occlusive disease. The significance of asymptomatic peripheral arterial disease (PAD) relates more to the cardiac risk of the patient over time than it does to the well-being of the leg(s) (Chapters 7 and 13).

C. **Chronic Lower Extremity Ischemia: Claudication.** Claudication is leg pain that occurs with ambulation as a result of poor blood flow to a muscle group distal or beyond an arterial stenosis. This symptom often occurs at a fixed and reproducible walking distance or level of exertion and resolves when the patient stops the activity (e.g., stops walking). It is important to determine whether or not the patient's symptoms of claudication are **lifestyle limiting.** Occupational or recreational restrictions may occur as a result of exertional leg pain in some, while others may be aware of the symptoms but not limited in their daily activities. The relatively benign natural history of claudication is important to communicate to patients. With risk factor modification and adherence to an exercise program, claudication remains stable or improves in 50% of patients with only 25% requiring intervention and fewer than 5% progressing to extremity amputation.

D. **Chronic Lower Extremity Ischemia: Critical Ischemia.** Critical lower extremity ischemia—also referred to as "limb threatening"—represents the minority of patients with leg ischemia and may present in two forms: **ischemic rest pain or tissue loss** (e.g., ischemic ulcers or ischemic gangrene). These patients have severe arterial disease affecting multiple levels in the lower extremity and are at risk for amputation without revascularization. Ischemic rest pain typically is described as a burning pain on the dorsum of the foot or in the toes. This pain becomes most noticeable at night or with the leg elevated, and may be relieved by dangling the limb to enlist the help of gravity to improve perfusion.

The differential diagnosis of lower extremity ischemia is extensive, and includes neurogenic and musculoskeletal conditions. Discomfort in the leg(s) that is positional or occurs without exertion is suggestive of **lumbar disk disease** or **spinal stenosis**, and commonly occurs in those with concomitant back pain. These conditions often occur with prolonged standing and cause leg weakness and numbness relieved by change of position (e.g., leaning forward). **Osteoarthritis of the hip and knee joints** commonly occurs in the elderly and can be distinguished from vascular disease by the location and nature of the pain.

Symptoms of **diabetic neuropathy** such as paresthesia, burning pain, and numbness that affect the foot and toes may mimic ischemic rest pain. Symptoms of neuropathy are bilateral and may also involve the fingertips, while ischemic rest pain is commonly unilateral and limited to the forefoot and toes. **Nighttime leg cramps** and **restless leg syndrome** are often misinterpreted as "rest pain" because they technically occur at rest. However, symptoms from these conditions occur in the thigh and calf muscles and not in the distribution of ischemic rest pain. **Neuropathic ulcers** of the foot or toes occur in patients without protective sensation in these areas. These ulcers commonly arise in diabetic patients prone to infection as a result of poorly fitting shoes that cause foot trauma. Importantly, not all neuropathic ulcers are ischemic, as ulceration of the foot or toe may be present in patients with normal lower extremity perfusion.

A. **Inspection.** Inspection of the leg and foot may reveal important signs of acute and chronic arterial insufficiency. Acute insufficiency will produce definite changes of pallor followed by cyanosis or skin mottling. In addition, muscle weakness or paralysis, especially of the foot dorsiflexors (anterior compartment), may become obvious and is an ominous sign. After 24 hours of acute ischemia, the leg swells, the skin may blister, and the foot becomes fixed and rigid.

Claudication may have no findings on inspection other than mild muscle atrophy and/or hair loss on the leg or foot. However, critical lower extremity ischemia is associated with **elevation pallor** and **dependent rubor** of the forefoot. Additionally, skin breakdown in the toes or forefoot tissue may occur and nonhealing ulcers will appear. Neuropathic ulcers generally appear on pressure points of the foot and over the plantar aspect of the metatarsal heads and may occur in patients with a normal lower extremity pulse exam. Dry gangrene with black tissue or wet gangrene with draining purulence and foul odor can develop as ischemic wounds progress.

B. **Palpation.** Pulses are normally palpable in four locations on each lower extremity. The femoral pulse is palpated just below the inguinal ligament, equidistant from the pubic tubercle, and the anterior superior iliac spine. In obese patients, external rotation of the hip may facilitate palpation of the artery. The popliteal pulse is more difficult to feel as it lies in the popliteal space. With the patient supine and the knee slightly flexed, the examiner should hook the fingertips of the hands around the medial and lateral knee tendons and press the fingertips firmly into the popliteal space. The pulse lies slightly lateral of midline. The dorsalis pedis is a terminal branch of the anterior tibial artery and is found in the mid-dorsum of the foot between the first and second metatarsals. The posterior tibial is found behind the medial malleolus, while the peroneal artery terminates at the ankle and is not palpable on physical exam.

Grading of pulses is subjective, and a simple method is to describe the pulses as *normal, diminished, or absent and symmetric versus asymmetric* in relation to the other side. One grading system used to describe the relative strength or normalcy of pulses is 0, absent; 1+, diminished; 2+, normal; and 3+, prominent, suggesting local aneurysm. The prudent examiner should hesitate to describe a 1+ pulse as it can be easy to mistake one's own pulse or involuntary foot twitches for the patient's pulse. If a pulse is not definitively palpable, further assessment with a continuous wave Doppler should be pursued. Doppler signals should be qualified as triphasic, biphasic, or monophasic with the triphasic signal considered normal. In the absence of a palpable pulse, biphasic and monophasic signals correlate with moderate and severe arterial occlusive disease, respectively. In severe cases of acute lower extremity ischemia or chronic critical ischemia, the only Doppler signal in the foot may be a soft continuous venous signal.

Palpation is also helpful in the assessment of acute extremity ischemia (Chapter 13). Skin coldness and the level of temperature demarcation can be detected by palpation with the back of the examiner's hand and fingers. Acute ischemia also may be associated with tenderness and tenseness of the calf muscles, especially the anterior compartment. In addition, acute ischemia may cause sensory nerve damage, detectable by pinprick sensory examination or testing of proprioception in the toes.

C. **Auscultation.** Auscultation of lower extremity arteries is most useful in the femoral area, where bruits indicate local femoral artery disease or more proximal aortoiliac disease with bruits transmitted to the groin. If there is a question about the presence of a femoral bruit, walking the patient for 25 to 50 steps at the bedside often will increase lower extremity flow enough to increase the severity of the bruit. Auscultation is also important when an arteriovenous fistula is suspected, which generally has a characteristic continuous to-and-fro bruit.

Selected Readings

Cournot M, Boccalon H, Cambou JP, et al. Accuracy of the screening physical examination to identify subclinical atherosclerosis and peripheral arterial disease in asymptomatic bruits. *J Vasc Surg.* 2007;46(6):1215-1221.

The presence of femoral bruits or abnormal pulse exam predicts PAD, whereas a carotid bruit does not predict degree of stenosis.

Fields WS, Lemak NA. Joint study of extracranial arterial occlusion. VII. Subclavian steal—a review of 168 cases. *JAMA.* 1972;222(9):1139-1143.

Early case series examined patients with subclavian steal, including original descriptions of symptoms and etiology.

Lederle FA, Simel DL. Does this patient have abdominal aortic aneurysm? *JAMA.* 1999;281(1):77-82.

Proper abdominal palpation for aneurysm is a worthwhile skill, particularly in identifying AAAs > 5 cm in diameter.

Muluk SC, Muluk VS, Kelley ME, et al. Outcome events in patients with claudication: a 15-year study of 2777 patients. *J Vasc Surg.* 2001;33:251-258.

Large contemporary study of natural history of claudication confirms low risk of amputation and high risk of mortality over time.

Wennberg PW. Approach to the patient with peripheral arterial disease. *Circulation.* 2013;128(20):2241-2250.

Excellent overview of arterial examination, differential and work-up from the Mayo Clinic.

4

History and Physical Examination of the Venous System

Atherosclerotic arterial disease is a systemic, pathologic process that affects multiple vascular beds. In contrast, venous disease is usually localized to one or two anatomic areas, such as an extremity.

I. **UPPER EXTREMITIES**. The most common venous conditions to affect the upper extremities are superficial and deep venous thrombosis (DVT). **Superficial** venous thrombosis can result from intravenous access, which causes endothelial damage, local vein thrombosis, and subsequent inflammation of a peripheral vein (e.g., cephalic or basilic vein). This condition rarely progresses to DVT and is most often self-limited, requiring local treatment in the form of warm compresses applied directly to the affected vein.

Acute or chronic thrombosis of the axillary, subclavian, or innominate veins is the upper extremity equivalent of **deep venous thrombosis (DVT)** and represents a serious condition. The clinician should assess for a history of prior central venous catheter or peripherally inserted central catheter (PICC lines), as these are a risk factor for the development of central venous thrombosis. The chief complaint in most cases is arm swelling. A diffuse aching pain frequently accompanies the swelling and is worse with use or dependency of the arm.

Paget-Schroetter syndrome is synonymous with **effort thrombosis**, and refers to the development of axillary and/or subclavian vein thrombosis in the setting of repetitive upper extremity exercise. Usually, this form of axillo-subclavian vein thrombosis occurs acutely as a result of thoracic outlet syndrome, in which the subclavian vein is compressed between the subclavius muscle, clavicle, and first rib (Fig. 4.1). Chronic compression of the axillary or subclavian vein in these circumstances results in underlying endothelial injury and is a contributing factor to the thrombosis. Chronic arm swelling may also be the result of lymphatic obstruction, which usually is associated with a previous operation (e.g., node dissection for breast cancer), infection, or irradiation that involved the axillary lymph nodes.

Another cause of acute arm swelling is placement of a hemodialysis fistula or graft in the arm that has an unrecognized central venous stenosis or occlusion (e.g., subclavian or innominate vein; Chapter 20). In such cases, completing the arterial-venous circuit for dialysis increases venous flow and pressure, which exacerbates a previously asymptomatic central venous stenosis. This scenario is analogous to an overflowing sink (the arm) that results from turning a faucet on high (the high-flow fistula) in the setting of a clog in the drain (central venous stenosis).

A. **Inspection.** The examiner should inspect the arms for scars from previous indwelling venous lines or procedures and note limb size discrepancy, edema, discoloration, deformity (e.g., clavicular fracture), or venous collaterals. Subclavian vein thrombosis causes swelling of the entire arm and hand and will often result in superficial venous collateral

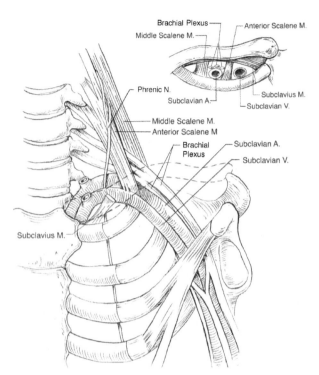

FIGURE 4.1 The thoracic outlet is a complex anatomic area with potential neurovascular compromise. The larger illustration depicts the left shoulder with associated neurovascular and bony structures of this area. The smaller inset depicts a view of the right thoracic outlet through a transaxillary view (i.e., the right arm raised). Note the important relationship of the subclavian vein and artery to the anterior scalene muscle, first rib, and clavicle.

formation across the shoulder region. Acutely, the arm may appear bluish or cyanotic, although rarely does subclavian-axillary venous thrombosis result in phlegmasia or venous gangrene. Patients in whom upper extremity venous thrombosis leads to phlegmasia often have an underlying malignancy or hypercoagulable condition such as heparin-induced thrombocytopenia and thrombosis. Following upper extremity DVT, the arm generally does not develop venous stasis dermatitis that accompanies postthrombotic syndrome in the lower extremities. Chest and shoulder collateral veins and associated arm edema are often seen in patients with end-stage renal disease with central venous obstruction (subclavian and innominate veins) from long-term indwelling dialysis catheters.

B. **Palpation.** The palpable cord associated with superficial venous thrombosis of the arm is typically pink, warm, and tender. Fluctuance or purulent drainage from the cord upon palpation suggests the diagnosis of **suppurative** or **infected thrombophlebitis,** which may require operative drainage. The internal and external jugular veins are occasionally palpable if inflamed or thrombosed, while the axillary and subclavian veins are not palpable because they lie deep to the clavicle. Arm edema, if present, should be described as pitting or nonpitting. A palpable thrill over any area of the upper extremity suggests the presence of an arteriovenous fistula.

C. **Auscultation.** Normally, venous sounds are not audible with a stethoscope. If arm swelling follows a penetrating injury or operation of the arm, listening over the scar or entrance wound may reveal a bruit caused by an arteriovenous fistula.

II. **LOWER EXTREMITIES.** Acute venous conditions of the lower extremities are generally thrombotic in nature, that is superficial or deep venous thrombosis. Unlike many vascular ailments, the history and physical examination alone are limited in making the diagnosis of DVT. In fact, only 50% of patients who are initially thought to have DVT by history and physical will have a positive duplex ultrasound. Some cases of lower extremity DVT, especially those in the calf veins, may be silent or nearly asymptomatic, presenting with only subtle leg swelling. In rare instances, the first sign of lower extremity DVT can be pulmonary embolus. DVT can lead to chronic leg swelling and ulceration months or years after diagnosis, referred to as **postthrombotic syndrome.**

Chronic venous insufficiency (CVI) covers a spectrum of venous disease ranging from varicose veins to advanced changes with leg edema, stasis dermatitis, and ulceration. Reflux within the superficial and/or deep venous system leads to physical changes due to ongoing venous hypertension in the leg. Chronic deep venous obstruction also contributes a pathologic role in many patients with advanced CVI. Physical exam is the initial method of evaluating chronic venous insufficiency, which causes visible changes on the surface of the leg.

A. **Inspection** of most limbs with acute DVT reveals normal color or a slightly cyanotic appearance. Extremity swelling is the most common sign and usually is limited to the lower leg, although thrombosis of the more proximal iliac and femoral venous circulations can lead to thigh and even buttock edema. **Phlegmasia alba dolens** (turgid, white, painful leg) or **phlegmasia cerulea dolens** (edematous, cyanotic, and painful leg) can be seen in cases of severe proximal vein thrombosis (Chapter 2). In these instances, the degree of swelling should be documented by measurement of calf and thigh diameters at a distance above or below a bony landmark to allow close and accurate serial examination of the leg.

Inspection also helps with the differential diagnosis of acute leg pain and swelling. Superficial venous thrombosis often is evidenced by a localized erythematous streak along the course of the vein, usually a tributary or the great saphenous vein. A break in the skin with surrounding erythema and induration suggests cellulitis. A localized ecchymosis over the thigh or calf may indicate that the leg pain is caused by a muscle contusion or hematoma. Diffuse, nonpainful leg edema with a thick "pigskin" appearance (peau d'orange) is typical of lymphedema.

Inspection for chronic venous insufficiency should be done with both legs exposed from the groin to the feet. Important findings may be recognized by comparing the abnormal to the normal extremity and, when possible, the patient should stand so that the veins fill. We prefer that the patient stand on a step while the examiner sits on a chair or stool. If good overhead lighting is not available for illumination of all aspects of the leg, an adjustable lamp is useful. The entire leg should be examined as the patient turns 360 degrees.

Varicose veins are dilated, saccular, and compressible unless thrombosed. Some healthy, thin patients may have prominent superficial veins that may be incorrectly thought to be varicose. Varicose veins most commonly involve the great saphenous vein on the medial side of the leg and tributaries often course around the upper calf to appear on the posteromedial aspect of the leg. Branches of the anterior accessory saphenous vein occur on the anterolateral aspect of the thigh. Tributaries of the small saphenous appear on the posterior calf from the knee to the ankle.

A localized bulge of saphenous vein immediately distal to the sapheno-femoral junction may occasionally be detected in the groin, which may be mistaken for an inguinal hernia, but is actually a **saphena varix**. A rare congenital pattern of varicosities is present in **Klippel-Trenaunay syndrome**, which is a triad of capillary hemangiomas (port-wine stains), limb hypertrophy, and varicose veins. Importantly, these patients may have persistent lateral embryologic veins and absent or abnormal deep venous systems.

    Deep venous insufficiency or obstruction, sometimes as a result of postthrombotic syndrome, is associated with specific changes in the appearance of the leg. Hyperpigmentation results from hemosiderin deposition occurring at the medial malleolus. **Lipodermatosclerosis** is a more severe manifestation of chronic venous hypertension, with the development of thickened and contracted skin and subcutaneous fat around the ankle. Stasis dermatitis may be complicated by skin ulceration, classically on the medial lower leg at the site of the perforating vein. **Venous ulcers** are usually shallow, with apparently healthy granulation tissue that bleeds with manipulation. It is important when inspecting a venous ulcer to regularly measure the dimensions and depth, and to assess surrounding skin integrity, as well as the quality of granulation tissue. The onset of a new odor or change in color, or erythema of the surrounding skin, suggests infection of the ulcer or even an epidermoid skin cancer. It is important to note that these cutaneous changes of the leg may also occur with chronic, severe superficial venous insufficiency as well. Large abdominal and pubic varicosities can appear as collateral pathways due to chronic inferior vena cava occlusion.

    Chronic diffuse lower limb swelling without stasis dermatitis may be caused by iliac vein obstruction or lymphedema. Compression of the left common iliac vein by the right common iliac artery (**May-Thurner syndrome**) can result in venous intimal fibroplasia, obstruction, and progressive left leg swelling. Venous edema most often resolves with bed rest and worsens with dependency. In contrast, primary or secondary lymphedema can result in chronic leg swelling that typically has a "pigskin" appearance and does not resolve with bed rest at night. Pelvic malignancies can obstruct lymphatics or compress iliac veins, and are in the differential of unilateral leg edema. Lipedema, the deposition of fat in the lower extremity, can easily be confused with other causes of edema, but characteristically spares the feet. Bilateral pitting lower extremity edema can also result from right heart failure, valvular heart disease, and nephrotic syndrome, and should prompt a search for other signs of systemic disease (e.g., rales, S3 gallop, hepatojugular reflux).

B. **Palpation** for calf tenderness may be present in acute DVT, but is not specific. Such tenderness may occur with muscle strain, contusion, or hematoma. Forceful dorsiflexion of the foot elicits calf pain in 35% of patients with acute DVT (**Homans' sign**). However, this test is also positive with muscular strains and lumbosacral disorders.

    Palpation can distinguish soft and compressible varicosities from those that are firm and thrombosed. Tenderness, heat, and induration over a firm varicosity define superficial venous thrombosis. The examiner should palpate for fascial defects on the medial aspect of the calf. These may represent sites of deep, incompetent perforating veins or saphenous tributaries emerging from the superficial fascia.

    Palpation may help determine the cause of leg swelling. Occasionally, chronic venous obstruction is secondary to extrinsic compression by a pelvic, femoral, or popliteal mass, and so these regions should also be examined for aneurysms or tumors. The inability to tent the skin over the interdigital webs (**Stemmer's sign**) is characteristic of lymphedema.

TABLE 4.1	Bedside Tests for Chronic Venous Insufficiency		
Name of Test	**Objective**	**Technique**	**Findings**
Trendelenburg test	Differentiates between superficial or deep venous reflux in patients with varicose veins	1. Elevate the patient's leg in the supine position in order to empty the varicosities. 2. Compress the SFJ while the patient stands.	1. Filling of varicosities despite SFJ compression suggests deep vein and perforator reflux. 2. Rapid filling of varicosities after release of compression indicates GSV reflux.
Perthes' test	Checks for obstruction of the deep veins	1. Have the patient stand to fill the varicosities and then apply a soft rubber tourniquet the midthigh. 2. The patient then ambulates or performs repetitive calf muscle contractions (tiptoe maneuvers).	1. The varicosities should collapse if the deep and perforating veins are competent. 2. If the veins remain distended, the deep and perforating veins are incompetent. 3. If the varicosities become more distended or painful, deep venous obstruction is present.
Tap test	To identify connections between varicose segments	1. Have the patient stand to fill the varicosities. 2. Percuss over a varicosity, while using the other hand to feel for an impulse from the vein at a lower level.	The impulse should be felt if the intervening segment is open and incompetent.

Note: Several bedside tests may be of interest to the venous scholar.
SFJ, saphenofemoral junction; GSV, great saphenous vein.

Several bedside tests can help the examiner better understand the underlying pathophysiology of lower extremity varicosities (Table 4.1). These tests are infrequently performed because of the excellent specificity and widespread availability of venous duplex testing.

C. **Auscultation.** Except in the cases of arteriovenous fistula in which an audible bruit may be present, a stethoscope does not provide much information about superficial or deep venous flow. In contrast, a continuous wave Doppler unit is a helpful adjunct in the bedside examination of lower extremity veins. While holding the continuous wave Doppler over the vein of interest, normal respiratory variation of the Doppler signal should be present if the vein is patent with normal flow. Additionally, if patent, flow through the vein will be audibly increased (augmentation) if the examiner's other hand squeezes the leg distally. With release of distal compression, flow will cease as competent valves snap shut. If the vein is incompetent, prolonged flow will be heard after release. Although continuous wave Doppler is quite a useful adjunct, it does not provide images or velocity measurements of flow. Duplex ultrasound, which combines B-mode imaging and pulsed wave Doppler, should be used frequently in the evaluation of symptomatic venous disease to allow more detailed examination of venous anatomy and provide useful physiologic information.

Selected Readings

Gloviczki P, Comerota AJ, Dalsing MC, et al. The care of patients with varicose veins and associated chronic venous diseases: clinical practice guidelines of the Society for Vascular Surgery and the American Venous Forum. *J Vasc Surg.* 2011;53 (5 suppl):2S-48S.
Comprehensive guidelines for treatment of chronic venous insufficiency with heavy emphasis on superficial insufficiency. Pages 9-10S highlight some valuable physical exam findings.
Krishnan S, Nicholls SC. Chronic venous insufficiency: clinical assessment and patient selection. *Semin Intervent Radiol.* 2005;22(3):169-177.
Concise review of venous physical examination and diagnostic testing for chronic venous insufficiency.
Marston WA. Evaluation of varicose veins: what do the clinical signs and symptoms reveal about the underlying disease and need for intervention? *Semin Vasc Surg.* 2010;23(2):78-84.
Classic patterns of venous insufficiency are in illustrated in color photographs.

Noninvasive Vascular Testing

This chapter summarizes the principles of selecting, performing, and interpreting noninvasive studies for conditions affecting different aspects of the arterial and venous system. It is worth emphasizing that noninvasive vascular tests supplement, but do not replace a thorough history and physical examination (Chapters 3 and 4). The safety and ease of use of this type of testing is attractive to patients and the professionals who order them, and the results often help determine the need for additional and more invasive studies or procedures. Noninvasive tests also provide a useful baseline measure before a treatment plan is implemented, as well as an assessment of the outcome after the treatment is completed. The temptation to order noninvasive vascular tests without first conducting a history and physical should be resisted as unnecessary studies can lead to unnecessary procedures and add to the cost of patient care.

I. **THE VASCULAR LABORATORY**. The laboratory should be in a quiet area and located for convenient use by both inpatients and outpatients. A medical sonographer or registered vascular technologist (RVT) usually performs the tests, which are then reviewed by a physician who is ideally a Registered Physician in Vascular Interpretation (RPVI). The setup in a vascular laboratory may be basic or sophisticated, depending on the clinical demand. Consistency and quality assurance should be the goal of vascular laboratories, the top tier of which are accredited by meeting standards set by the **Intersocietal Accreditation Commission (IAC) Vascular Testing Section**.

II. **INSTRUMENTATION**. The following is a list of equipment for the noninvasive vascular laboratory that is sufficient for the evaluation of most arterial and venous conditions.

A. **Continuous wave Doppler** system. The **Doppler effect** states that flow velocity is proportional to the frequency shift in sound waves transmitted from and reflected back to crystals within the Doppler probe by blood in motion (Fig. 5.1). To make this assessment, a Doppler probe is placed over the blood vessel and coupled to the skin with an acoustic gel. Nonacoustic skin lubricants lack the proper electrolyte content, often fail to couple the probe and the skin and, in some cases, can damage the probe crystal. Sound waves transmitted by the Doppler crystal strike moving blood cells and are reflected back to the probe while an amplifier filters sound in order to emit an audible flow signal that is proportional to the velocity of the blood. Like palpable pulses, audible Doppler signals can be qualified or graded with regard to strength and phasicity.

In a normal elastic peripheral arterial vessel, the Doppler signal is **triphasic** with three audible components, corresponding to the forward flow of systole, early reversed flow, and later forward flow of diastole. In a low-resistance arterial vessel, such as the internal carotid, celiac artery, or the common femoral after exercise, flow normally remains continuously forward or antegrade with a systolic and diastolic component. Without reversal of flow in diastole, there are only two components of an arterial

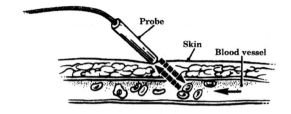

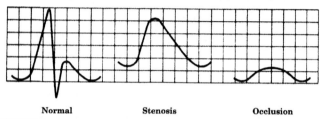

Normal   **Stenosis**   **Occlusion**

FIGURE 5.1 Doppler arterial examination. The Doppler probe is coupled to the skin with acoustic gel and angled toward the direction of arterial flow. The normal Doppler arterial signal is triphasic. Stenosis and occlusion cause diminished monophasic signals.

signal (**biphasic**). With increasing degrees of flow-limiting stenosis, the Doppler wave morphology becomes weak, lower pitched, and **monophasic**.

In practice, a continuous wave Doppler probe (range, 5 to 10 MHz) is most commonly used for performing noninvasive tests such as segmental pressures. A handheld version of the continuous wave Doppler is also a valuable tool to quickly assess arterial and venous flow. The other type of Doppler commonly used in the vascular lab is referred to as **pulsed Doppler.** Housed together, the two modalities of brightness mode or B-mode ultrasound and pulsed Doppler comprise the **duplex ultrasound unit.** Within this machine, pulsed Doppler differs from continuous wave in two ways: (a) it emits bursts or pulses of sound waves, and (b) a select portion of flow within a given vessel can be selected with the B-mode image for pulsed Doppler sampling. This technique provides more accurate measurement of frequency (velocity) of flow through different anatomic aspects of the vessel. The velocity pattern correlates with the degree of stenosis, in that higher velocities suggest a greater degree of luminal narrowing. Although continuous wave Doppler can also analyze velocity patterns, it receives information from all aspects of the vessel and may also receive signals from adjacent arteries or veins making detailed, objective interpretation difficult and less specific than duplex.

B. **Plethysmography** uses the principle of volume change associated with blood flow in a body region (i.e., an extremity) to make assessment of perfusion. Air (APG) and photoplethysmography (PPG) are the most common types to be used in today's more comprehensive vascular labs. The basic tools for APG are a blood pressure cuff, inflated to optimize contact with the leg, a transducer, and recording instrument. PPG uses a probe to emit infrared light into the superficial skin layers and a photoelectric detector to measure the reflected light. The amount of light absorbed depends on the blood volume in the skin. A waveform is transduced and recorded during normal conditions and then during and following inflation of an occlusive cuff. Baseline measurements and changes during and following cuff inflation correspond to different degrees of blood flow in the segment of extremity being examined.

C. Mentioned previously, **duplex** combines real-time, B-mode ultrasound to provide black and white (gray scale) images of the vessel and **pulsed wave Doppler** to sample flow velocity in select areas of a given vessel. The angle of insonation should be kept close to 60 degrees, as this provides the best return signal for spectral analysis and velocity measurement. With pulsed wave Doppler technology, not only is the velocity converted into an audible flow pattern but also visually into a flow spectrum showing velocity over time and a color flow pattern.

Spectral analysis pertains to the visual representation of the different velocities of blood cells traveling in the vessel within the sampling volume and provides insight into the degree of narrowing (**i.e., stenosis**) as well as the degree of uniform (**laminar**) versus chaotic (**turbulent**) flow. The duplex parameters used for to assess the severity of a vessel stenosis are (a) spectral width during systole, (b) peak systolic velocity (PSV), and (c) end diastolic velocity. A normal spectrum (Fig. 5.2) reading sampled from a vessel with no focal stenosis consists of a low PSV (e.g., <125 cm/s in the internal carotid), a uniform band of frequencies, representing velocities, during systole and a clear space or window beneath the velocity measurement. In this case, blood cells are traveling the same velocity (i.e., laminar flow) with limited turbulence. With a small degree of stenosis, turbulence can be detected, resulting in **spectral broadening** during the deceleration phase of systole. Further stenosis results in more spectral broadening until the window beneath the systolic peak is "whited out" and filled with many different velocity measures (i.e., blood cells traveling at many different velocities). As the stenosis increases, spectral broadening is accompanied

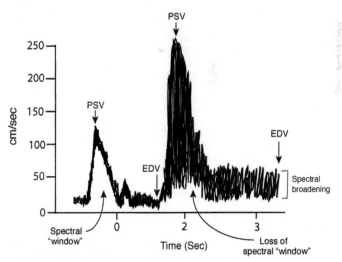

FIGURE 5.2 Arterial spectrum analysis. The Doppler spectrum analysis allows classification of the degree of stenosis. The most common parameters used for this classification are spectral broadening (with loss of the normal "spectral window"), elevation in peak systolic velocity (PSV; normal <120 cm/s), and elevation in end diastolic velocity (EDV).

by an increase in the PSV. With the highest degrees of luminal narrowing or stenosis (i.e., high grade or critical), the end diastolic velocity measure is elevated as the pressure drop across the stenosis increases. Spectral broadening in these cases reflects the many different velocities of cells within the vessel resulting from turbulent flow.

The third Doppler mode used within the duplex machine is referred to as color flow imaging, which is helpful in detecting the direction of flow within the vessel. In this case, red indicates flow toward and blue flow away from the transducer. Higher velocities move toward white in the color spectrum. Laminar flow is uniform in color while a stenosis results in a bright "flow jet" of color and a mosaic distal to the stenosis reflective of turbulent flow. Color flow is particularly useful for tracing tortuous vessels and identifying areas of vessel ulceration. The term power Doppler refers to a visual representation of flow with directionality removed and is also useful to see the anatomy of the blood vessel.

D. **A treadmill** at low speeds of 1.5 to 2.5 miles per hour at a 10% to 12.5% grade is used to perform lower extremity noninvasive tests during and immediately following exercise.

E. **Transcutaneous oximetry** requires a transcutaneous electrode probe and calibrated instrument for measuring oxygen tension on the skin, which is used as a surrogate marker for blood flow.

F. **Blood pressure cuffs** of various sizes, including miniature cuffs for digital pressures in the fingers and or toes.

III. **ASSESSING LOWER EXTREMITY ARTERIAL OCCLUSIVE DISEASE.** Noninvasive lab evaluation of the lower extremities is useful in the setting of functional ischemia, or claudication (tiring or pain in the extremity with walking), as well as more severe critical leg ischemia (ischemic rest pain or tissue loss). Noninvasive testing documents the severity of occlusive disease, provides a baseline for follow-up, and can help predict potential for tissue healing. Testing can sometimes help clarify whether leg pain is related to peripheral vascular disease or nonvascular etiologies in patients with atypical symptoms. However, no combination of vascular tests can serve as a substitute for a thorough history and physical exam.

A. **Ankle-brachial index** (ABI) provides useful information about lower extremity perfusion and is a great adjunct to the basic physical exam. This test can be performed at the bedside with a handheld Doppler and a manual blood pressure cuff. The Doppler probe is placed over an arterial signal at the foot, typically the dorsalis pedis or the posterior tibial artery (Fig. 5.3). A blood pressure cuff on the calf is inflated until the arterial signal occludes or disappears. As the cuff is deflated, the pressure at which the signal is again audible is recorded. The test should be performed with the patient in the supine position and the greater of the two pressures at the foot selected as the numerator in the ABI equation. Next, the pressure of each arm is recorded in a similar manner and used as the ABI denominator. If there is more than a 10-mm Hg difference between arm pressures, the higher pressure should be selected as the denominator, keeping in mind that a diminished arm pressure could indicate a subclavian artery stenosis. Normally, the pressure in the leg is slightly higher than that in the arm, due to a higher resistance in the lower extremities and the **normal ABI is ≥1.0**.

When performed in the noninvasive lab, ABIs may be combined with a plethysmograph for something referred to as pulse volume recordings or PVRs. In this setting, ABI measurements provide more complete and standardized data that can be used as part of the clinical assessment of patients with lower extremity occlusive disease. ABIs should also be performed following an open or catheter-based revascularization to confirm improvement and establish a new baseline. A change in an ABI value of more than 0.15 is considered a significant change in perfusion.

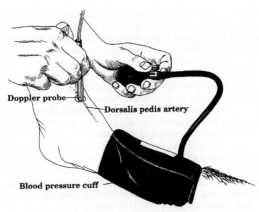

Doppler probe

Dorsalis pedis artery

Blood pressure cuff

FIGURE 5.3 Measurement of ankle blood pressure with a standard blood pressure cuff and a handheld continuous wave Doppler unit. This ankle pressure can be compared to the brachial (arm) blood pressure to calculate the ankle-brachial index (ABI).

For simplicity sake, lower extremity circulation can be considered in three different anatomic levels: aortoiliac, femoropopliteal, and tibial (Chapter 13). In limbs with one level of arterial occlusive disease, the ABI is usually 0.5 to 0.85, while an index of less than 0.5 indicates multilevel disease. ABIs may be falsely elevated or noncompressible in those with long-standing diabetes or severe chronic kidney disease. Patients with these conditions may develop **medial calcinosis** of the tibial vessels, which renders them difficult or impossible to compress with a manual blood pressure cuff. In these cases, the Doppler signal in the foot will not occlude despite inflating the cuff to pressures that are well above the systolic blood pressure and painful for the patient. In such instances, the ABI calculation should not be pursued but simply be documented as **noncompressible**. In this situation, combining PVRs with ABIs can provide more complete information. Table 5.1 lists common scenarios found in association with several categories of ABIs. However, it should be remembered that some patients with abnormal ABIs do not fall in these categories and more than two-thirds of patients with reduced ABIs are asymptomatic, as a result of well-developed collateral perfusion or just a sedentary lifestyle.

B. **Toe pressures** are useful in those with medial calcinosis and noncompressible ABIs, as the digital vessels of the toes are often spared from this process. To obtain toe pressures, a 2-cm cuff is applied to the great toe, and a PPG sensor is placed on the tip because the area is too small to assess with

TABLE 5.1	Categories of Clinical Severity for the Ankle-Brachial Index (ABI)
ABI Measurement	**Clinical Correlation**
1.2–2.0 or greater	Medial calcinosis or noncompressible
0.95–1.2	Normal
0.5–0.95	Claudication
0.2–0.5	Rest pain
0.0–0.2	Tissue loss or gangrene

a standard Doppler. The greatest value of toe pressures may be in their ability to predict healing of ischemic foot ulcers or toe and foot amputation sites. A toe-brachial index of less than 0.7 is abnormal and an absolute toe pressure of less than 30 mm Hg suggests insufficient perfusion to heal a wound of any type

C. **Pulse volume recording (PVR)** is a form of APG, developed by Raines and Darling at Massachusetts General Hospital, in which lower extremity pulsatility is used as an indirect measure of arterial flow. In order to perform the test, an air-filled blood pressure cuff of appropriate size is placed on the lower extremity, usually on the thigh, calf, and/or ankle then inflated to a baseline pressure of about 65 mm Hg. The cuff is attached to the plethysmograph, and small fluctuations in limb volume as a result of pressure changes are then recorded as arterial contours. The contour provides qualitative information about the arterial flow, corresponding to the direct intra-arterial pressure waveform recording at that level.

Characterized by a sharp upstroke (**anacrotic slope**), distinct pulse peak, and rapid decline (**catacrotic slope**), the normal PVR tracing becomes progressively flattened and prolonged with increasing stenosis (Fig. 5.4). PVRs can be quantified by amount of chart deflection, but labs often use different scales. The greatest emphasis is placed simply on qualitative wave morphology. A severely attenuated or flat PVR tracing at the ankle correlates with poor wound healing. PVRs are particularly useful when combined with ABIs or segmental pressures to provide a more complete picture of limb blood flow. For example, patients with medial calcinosis may have falsely elevated ABIs, such that the PVRs provide a better estimate about the severity of disease (Fig. 5.5). Further, patients with severe abnormalities in vessel Doppler signals may have relatively preserved PVR waveforms providing information on collateralization. The PVR can also be helpful in evaluating the young patient whose claudication may be due to **popliteal artery entrapment** by the medial head of the

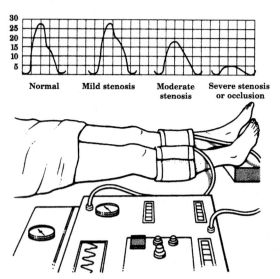

FIGURE 5.4 Pulse volume recordings. The normal pulse volume recording becomes progressively flattened and prolonged with increasing arterial stenosis.

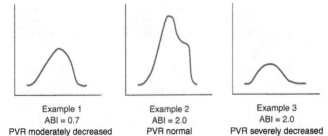

Example 1	Example 2	Example 3
ABI = 0.7	ABI = 2.0	ABI = 2.0
PVR moderately decreased	PVR normal	PVR severely decreased

FIGURE 5.5 Ankle-brachial index (ABI) and pulse volume recording (PVR) are complementary, as shown in these examples. In example 1, the ABI of 0.7 is decreased with a correspondingly dampened PVR waveform, suggesting more proximal peripheral arterial occlusive disease (PAOD). In example 2, the ABI of 2.0 is well above the normal range indicating incompressible tibial vessels due to medial calcinosis. However, the PVR in this example is normal suggesting no significant PAOD. In example 3, the ABI is 2.0 in conjunction with a severely dampened PVR, consistent with both medial calcinosis and severe PAOD.

gastrocnemius muscle. Such patients usually have normal ankle PVR tracings at rest but with active plantar flexion or passive dorsiflexion of the foot, the gastrocnemius contracts and compresses the popliteal artery so that the real-time PVR tracing flattens.

D. **Segmental pressures** can be useful in patients with abnormal ABIs to better approximate the level and degree of arterial obstruction. Measurements are obtained by the same technique as ABIs, except that blood pressure cuffs are placed at the thigh, upper calf, and ankle. The Doppler probe is always placed over the best arterial signal at the ankle level. Two standard 10 to 12 cm cuffs can be used on the upper and lower thigh. Alternatively, a single large cuff (18 to 20 cm diameter) can be placed as proximal as possible on the thigh. In general, the larger thigh-to-cuff ratio will result in higher pressures in the thigh than in the ankle, so that the normal thigh-brachial index is 1.3 to 1.5.

Some decrease in pressure between the proximal thigh and the ankle is normal, but a pressure decrease of 15 to 30 mm Hg between adjacent segments suggests an intervening arterial stenosis. Segmental pressures should also be compared at the same level between legs, as a lack of symmetry implies arterial disease in the leg with lower pressures. Figure 5.6 provides examples of arterial occlusive disease at various anatomic levels.

PVRs are usually combined with segmental pressures at each level to improve accuracy, especially in patients with falsely elevated pressures from calcified tibial vessels. Segmental PVR tracings normally show augmentation from the thigh to the calf, caused by differences in cuff volume and a high ratio of well-vascularized calf muscle. Therefore, the calf PVR should have a slightly greater amplitude than that of the thigh. If it does not, a superficial femoral artery lesion should be suspected. Disease in the common or proximal superficial femoral artery can mimic aortoiliac disease by causing a decrease in the thigh pressure, particularly if a single large cuff is used on the thigh. Simple palpation of the femoral pulse can also distinguish between aortoiliac and superficial femoral artery occlusion. Segmental pressures can also be misleading when collateral blood flow is so well developed that a significant gradient is not present across an occluded segment. These limitations of segmental leg pressures emphasize that results must be combined with findings on physical exam for accurate detection of the occlusive lesions.

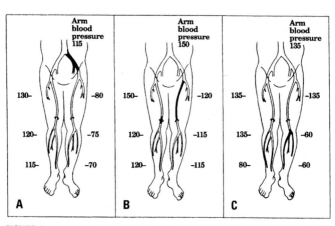

FIGURE 5.6 Segmental leg pressures. **(A)** Segmental leg pressures in a normal lower extremity (*right*) and one with isolated left iliac artery occlusion (*left*). **(B)** Segmental leg pressures with a distal occlusion of the superficial femoral artery (SFA) at Hunter's canal (*right*), compared to proximal occlusion of the SFA (*left*). **(C)** Segmental leg pressures with distal tibial artery occlusions (*right*) and tibial disease extending into the proximal popliteal artery (*left*).

E. **Exercise or treadmill ABIs** can unmask the presence of arterial occlusive disease in a select group of patients with ambulatory leg pain. Treadmill ABIs are useful in patients with symptoms of exertional pain that have normal, palpable pulses and only mildly decreased ABIs at rest. In these cases, a mild arterial stenosis does not result in a measurable pressure decrement while the patient is sitting at rest. *Remember: his or her symptoms are with ambulation.*

Under normal flow conditions (i.e., no arterial stenosis), the treadmill ABI will increase slightly and remain elevated for a few minutes following ambulation as flow into the extremity increases with exertion. However, in patients with a proximal arterial stenosis, vasodilation of the leg musculature distal to that narrowing results in an increase in velocity of blood across the stenosis as the body attempts to supply the leg with blood. This phenomenon results in a decrease in pressure distal to the stenosis with a corresponding decreased ABI and a delay in return to baseline. Insight into this basic concept of hemodynamics is provided in part by **Bernoulli's principle**, which states that with increased velocity across a fixed stenosis, there is loss of kinetic energy distal to the stenosis and a necessary decrease in pressure (Chapter 1 and Table 1.1).

When checking exercise ABIs measures are first performed at rest and then the patient is asked to walk at a rate of 2 mph at a 5 to 10 degrees incline for 5 minutes or until the leg pain becomes significant. The ankle pressures and ABI are recorded immediately after exercise and for 5 to 10 minutes postexercise. As noted, with normal arterial perfusion, there will be an increase. In those with a drop, the time to return to baseline, or latency, can be another feature suggesting the severity of the stenosis. In addition to measurement of ABIs after exercise, recording of the time to onset of leg pain, recovery from the pain, and the location of pain is important, as it defines the overall effect on the patient. At the same time, the general cardiac and respiratory reserve of the patient can be observed. Exercise should be terminated if the patient complains of chest pain, dyspnea, or dizziness.

Exercise ABIs may be most helpful if there is confusion about whether leg symptoms are caused by arterial occlusive disease or a musculoskeletal or neurologic condition such as **spinal stenosis**. Normal treadmill pressures in these cases effectively exclude arterial occlusive disease and point to a musculoskeletal or neurologic condition. There is no additional diagnostic value in performing treadmill ABIs if a patient has obvious arterial occlusive disease, typical claudication, and reduced ABIs at rest.

F. **Transcutaneous oximetry** ($TcPO_2$) provides local measurement of skin oxygen tension, which indirectly reflects arterial perfusion in the foot. The principle of $TcPO_2$ involves heat application (45°C) to the skin, which produces hyperemia and oxygen excess. Since oxygen diffuses along a concentration gradient from the capillaries to the tissues, it can diffuse across the skin where it is measured by a modified **Clark platinum oxygen electrode.** Local vasodilation allows for $TcPO_2$ to accurately approximate arterial Po_2.

The transcutaneous electrode is applied to the skin at various levels on the lower extremity. A normal $TcPO_2$ reading exceeds 55 mm Hg, but levels of less than 30 mm Hg suggest arterial ischemia. Critical ischemia manifest by ischemic tissue loss or rest pain is associated with forefoot $TcPO_2$ levels of 0 to 10 mm Hg. $TcPO_2$ can also help predict healing of ischemic foot ulcers, with levels greater than 20 mm Hg necessary for healing. $TcPO_2$ is generally only accurate if local infection has been controlled and edema in the foot has been minimized.

$TcPO_2$ can be particularly useful in evaluating patients with long-standing diabetes and/or peripheral neuropathy, in whom the origins of resting foot or toe pain or ulcerations may be unclear. In such cases, ABIs will often be noncompressible as a result of medial arterial calcinosis, and in these cases, the $TcPO_2$ provides a measure of perfusion that may help distinguish whether the pain or ulceration is the result of arterial insufficiency or severe neuropathy (Tables 5.2 and 5.3).

G. **Duplex ultrasound** is an accurate noninvasive method for evaluating lower extremity circulation and can be used to create a "road map" of arterial disease. Duplex provides visual information about plaque morphology as well as physiologic information about the speed and flow of blood within the vessel. Together, this information can help characterize and quantify degrees of stenosis. Arterial occlusion is identified by absence of color-flow imaging, and collaterals may be visualized proximal and distal to an occlusion or stenosis. A jet on color-flow image suggests a stenosis,

TABLE 5.2	Criteria for Ischemic Rest Pain		
Noninvasive Study	Unlikely	Probable	Likely
Ankle pressure (mm Hg)			
Nondiabetic	>55	35–55	<35
Diabetic	>80	55–80	<55
Ankle PVR category	Normal	Moderately decreased	Severely decreased or flat
$TcPO_2$ (torr)	>40	10–20	0–10

Note: The higher ankle pressure criterion in diabetics is due to false pressure elevation secondary to decreased compressibility due to medial calcinosis.
PVR, pulse volume recording; $TcPO_2$, transcutaneous oxygen tension.

TABLE 5.3	Criteria for Healing Ischemic Foot Lesions		
Noninvasive Study	Unlikely	Probable	Likely
Ankle Pressure (mm Hg)			
Nondiabetic	<55	55–65	>65
Diabetic	<80	80–90	>90
Ankle PVR category	Severely decreased or flat	Moderately decreased	Normal
TcPO₂ (torr)	<20	40–50	>50
Toe pressure (mm Hg)	<30	30–50	>50

Note: The higher ankle pressure criterion in diabetics is due to false pressure elevation secondary to decreased compressibility due to medial calcinosis.
PVR, pulse volume recording; Tc_{PO_2}, transcutaneous oxygen tension.

and velocities are then measured using pulsed Doppler proximal to, at the stenosis, and distal to the stenosis. The **systolic velocity ratio (SVR)** is calculated by dividing the PSV at or within the stenosis by the PSV proximal to the stenosis. An SVR of greater than 2.5 or an absolute PSV greater than 200 cm/s correlates with a greater than 50% stenosis. However, there are limitations to arterial duplex as a complete exam is time-consuming and its accuracy depends on the qualifications and experience of the sonographer. Obesity and overlying bowel gas limit visualization of the aorta, visceral, and iliac vessels, and the tibial vessels can be difficult to image if they are calcified or if there is an overlying skin disorder or edema.

Surveillance duplex following lower extremity revascularization can identify an "at risk" or failing vascular reconstruction (open or endovascular) otherwise not detected by history and physical. In these instances, early or preemptive identification of renarrowing following a revascularization procedure may help to preserve the **primary patency** of that intervention. Recurrent leg symptoms and/or a significant decrease in the ABI (0.15 or more) detects a failing bypass in only 50% of cases. **A technical defect, myointimal hyperplasia,** and **recurrent atherosclerosis** are the main causes of renarrowing or restenoses following revascularization procedure. Regardless of the cause, renarrowing of the reconstructed vessel or bypass graft threatens the durability and primary patency of the revascularization and predisposes it to acute thrombosis. Identification of an "at-risk" vascular reconstruction (open or endovascular) prior its thrombosis and failure allows for a preemptive intervention on, and salvage of the narrowed segment. Following this type of preemptive intervention, the reconstructed vascular segment or bypass graft is said to have **assisted primary patency** (i.e., its patency was assisted or maintained before it failed). The favorable limb salvage rates associated with **assisted primary patency** compared to a failed or thrombosed vascular segment, or one that has been reopened after it has failed (referred to as **secondary patency**), is the main reason behind performing surveillance duplex and other noninvasive vascular testing after a vascular reconstruction has been performed.

Duplex criteria have been developed to identify the "at-risk" arterial reconstruction and include a segment or bypass graft with a focal *PSV of greater than 300 cm/s, a systolic velocity ratio of greater than 3.5 at the* renarrowed location or stenosis, or *low velocities throughout the entirety of the segment or graft (<40 to 45 cm/s)*. It is common practice to reassess or surveille a vascular reconstruction (bypass or endovascular intervention) every 3 months in the first year after procedure, and every 6 to 12 months thereafter.

IV. **THE RENAL ARTERIES** can also be evaluated for stenosis in the noninvasive vascular laboratory by duplex ultrasound. Testing should be considered for patients with resistant hypertension and/or progressive chronic kidney disease (Chapter 15). A lower frequency duplex probe (2 to 3 MHz) is used for deeper penetration of the abdomen and visualization of the renal vessels. Evaluation can be limited by obesity and overlying bowel gas and is dependant upon the qualifications and experience of the vascular technologist. Inadequate visualization of the renal arteries may occur in 5% to 15% of studies, and the presence of multiple or accessory renal arteries decreases the sensitivity of the examination.

PSV is measured in the renal artery and compared against PSV in the aorta (**renal-aortic ratio, or RAR**). General criteria for a greater than 60% stenosis of the renal artery are **PSV greater than 200 cm/s and RAR of greater than 3.5**, although these numbers can vary between different vascular labs. Atherosclerotic renal artery disease usually occurs at the renal orifices, whereas **fibromuscular dysplasia** often affects the midsegments of the renal arteries (Chapter 15). Although renal artery duplex has a high level of accuracy, a negative test does not definitively rule out the presence of a significant stenosis. Ultimately, the clinician's pretest probability of disease is the most important factor in determining who should undergo further testing with magnetic resonance arteriography (MRA), computed tomographic arteriography (CTA), or arteriography.

V. **MESENTERIC ARTERIAL OCCLUSIVE DISEASE** involving the **superior mesenteric artery (SMA)** and **celiac** vessels may also be assessed with duplex ultrasound. Chronic mesenteric ischemia is characterized by *postprandial pain, weight loss, and sitophobia (food fear)*, whereas patients with acute mesenteric ischemia have intense abdominal pain that is initially out of proportion to the exam and may eventually lead to peritonitis (Chapter 16). Unlike patients with chronic mesenteric ischemia, those with acute ischemia are often better served with immediate CTA, standard catheter-directed arteriography, or laparotomy (Chapter 16).

Duplex of the mesenteric vessels should be conducted with the patient having fasted for 8 to 10 hours prior to the exam. Patients with chronic mesenteric ischemia are almost always quite thin, which facilitates a fairly detailed duplex evaluation of the superior mesenteric and celiac arteries (and their branches). **Generally, a peak systolic velocity of greater than 275 cm/s in the SMA and a velocity of more than 200 cm/s in the celiac artery are predictive of greater than 70% stenoses in these vessels**. As for other anatomic locations (i.e., carotid, femoral, aortoiliac), duplex criteria for significant mesenteric stenoses differ slightly among different vascular labs. As in the case of the renals, atherosclerosis usually affects the orifices of the superior mesenteric and celiac arteries. As such, duplex can occasionally identify retrograde flow in the gastroduodenal or common hepatic arteries as a hallmark sign suggestive of severe celiac artery stenosis. The inferior mesenteric artery (IMA) should be examined for patency or occlusion. Isolated disease of the IMA in the absence of SMA or celiac disease does not result in CMI, but can be associated with ischemic colitis when inadequate collateral flow is present (Chapter 16). When there is a high index of suspicion for CMI, an inadequate or negative duplex study should be followed by further imaging such as CTA, MRA, or angiography.

VI. **NONINVASIVE VASCULAR TESTING OF THE UPPER EXTREMITIES** is quite useful for a variety of conditions that affect the circulation of the arms and hands. As with the feet and toes, PPG can be used to assess digital blood flow in the hands and fingers with the probe placed on the fingertips to record arterial waveforms. A qualitative examination of waveform morphology is helpful on its own, and can be combined with digital pressure measurements if desired. **Raynaud's syndrome** causes an intense transient vasospasm of the digital vessels and is most often diagnosed clinically (Chapter 17). Patients with vasospastic Raynaud's will have normal digital pressures, and PPGs may be normal or have a "peaked pulse" pattern as a result of increased distal resistance. A number of nonatherosclerotic conditions (e.g., Buerger's disease, autoimmune disease, repetitive vibratory trauma) can cause actual occlusion of the forearm and digital arteries. Severe chronic kidney disease and long-standing diabetes can also lead to calcification and obstruction of the distal arteries and decreased digital pressures and dampened PPG waveforms in the affected fingers.

A small percentage of patients with upper extremity hemodialysis access develop a condition referred to as **upper extremity vascular steal** (Chapter 20). In such cases, either too large of arterial inflow or an arterial stenosis (e.g., in the axillary or brachial artery) *proximal* to the fistula results in blood preferentially flowing into the low-resistance venous system of the fistula effectively "stealing" from the hand. Depending on the severity, and the amount of flow "stolen" by the arteriovenous fistula, the patient may experience pain, coolness, cyanosis, and even tissue loss in the affected hand. In these cases, finger PPGs hand will be dampened in comparison with the other hand and will often reverse or return to normal with manual compression of the arteriovenous fistula. Persistently abnormal PPGs with fistula compression imply arterial occlusive disease of the forearm and hand *distal* to the arteriovenous connection.

Thoracic outlet syndrome (TOS) that results in arterial compromise is less common than neurogenic or venous TOS. Arterial compression at the thoracic outlet can result in stenosis, aneurysm, or even thrombosis of the subclavian artery. Provocative maneuvers such as hyperabduction and external rotation of the arm can result in diminished digital blood pressures and PPGs (Chapters 3 and 17). Duplex can also reveal a thrombosed subclavian artery or aneurysm. The noninvasive lab findings should be correlated with clinical symptoms and additional workup such as CTA or angiography to make the diagnosis of arterial TOS.

Arterial occlusive disease in the upper extremity can be identified with careful assessment of pulses in brachial, radial, and ulnar arteries and comparison of blood pressure measurements between the two arms. A difference of more than 10 mm Hg between the arms suggests a proximal arterial stenosis, an occurrence that is *more frequent in the left subclavian than in the right*. Duplex can be used to diagnose arterial disease in the upper extremity in a manner similar to the lower. This test is used less commonly in the upper extremities due to a lower prevalence of atherosclerotic disease in the arms compared to the legs. Additionally, disease of the subclavian artery is difficult to detect because of the location of the artery within the chest and behind the clavicle. A proximal subclavian artery stenosis can result in a condition referred to as **subclavian steal syndrome**. In such cases, exertion of the arm results in vasodilation of the distal musculature with a subsequent increase in velocity across the proximal stenosis. This increased velocity across a fixed stenosis results in a decrement in distal pressure and reversal of flow in the vertebral artery, which is distal to the subclavian stenosis. Abnormal retrograde or bidirectional flow in the vertebral artery can be detected on duplex at baseline and is a sign of proximal subclavian artery occlusive disease.

VII. CAROTID ARTERIAL DISEASE

A. **Duplex ultrasound** is the test of choice for the initial evaluation of extra-cranial carotid disease. Developed in the mid-1980s, duplex allowed accurate, inexpensive, and noninvasive evaluation of the carotid arteries. Although contrast arteriography was and is still useful in a small number of cases, it is invasive and carries an associated risk of causing stroke. Contrast arteriography also introduces risk related to the use of contrast agents and at the femoral artery puncture or access site. CTA and MRA have improved substantially, yet both of these imaging modalities require administration of contrast agent and are relatively expensive compared to duplex. Currently, the most common reasons for carotid duplex are the presence of a cervical bruit or the history of neurologic symptoms such as a transient ischemic attack or stroke (Chapter 12).

Similar to the use of duplex in other vascular distributions, B-mode imaging is combined with pulsed Doppler to provide a visual image and physiologic evaluation of the common, internal, and external carotid arteries. Using the B-mode image, the Doppler signal is positioned in the center of blood flow within the vessel at an optimal **angle of insonation** to allow (a) *spectral analysis* and (b) *measurement of velocities*. The first indication of an abnormal flow disturbance is turbulence, which may not initially be reflected by elevated velocities but instead by **spectral broadening**, which has been discussed previously (Fig. 5.2). As the amount of disease worsens and a stenosis develops, velocities become elevated, first the peak systolic and eventually the end diastolic velocity. In cases of the most severe stenosis, there may only be a trickle of flow through the vessel (i.e., a preocclusive stenosis) or even a complete carotid artery occlusion (Fig. 5.7; Table 5.4).

In addition to spectral analysis and velocity measurement, carotid plaque morphology and color-flow analysis from duplex provide useful information. Carotid plaques may be characterized as smooth, irregular, or ulcerated, and the degree of calcification also noted. A heterogeneous or mixed plaque contains a combination of echolucent and echodense signals and can indicate pending intraplaque hemorrhage. Color-flow analysis not only identifies areas of turbulence but is also useful for mapping tortuosity of the vessel.

Carotid stenoses were originally categorized using duplex criteria developed by Dr. Eugene Strandness and a group at the University of Washington in Seattle. The criteria were defined or validated by comparing thousands of duplex ultrasounds to the "gold standard" of the day, carotid arteriography. Specifically, spectral analysis and velocity

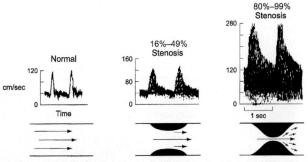

FIGURE 5.7 Internal carotid artery Doppler spectrum patterns. (The criteria are summarized in Table 5.4.) The percentage refers to the degree of stenosis.

TABLE 5.4	Criteria for Carotid Artery Disease Based on Duplex Ultrasonography[a]		
ICA Stenosis	PSV	EDV	Ratio ICA/CCA
1%–39%	<115 cm/s	<40 cm/s	<1.8
40%–59%	<130 cm/s	>40 cm/s	<1.8
60%–79%	>130 cm/s	>40 cm/s	>1.8
80%–99%	>250 cm/s	>100 cm/s	>3.7
Occluded	No ICA signal	No ICA signal	—

Note: The echogenic characteristics of the carotid plaque should be noted to be homogeneous (uniform echo pattern) or heterogeneous (complex echo pattern).
CCA, common carotid artery; EDV, end diastolic volume; ICA, internal carotid artery; PSV, peak systolic velocity.
[a]Duplex ultrasound criteria for grading the severity of cervical carotid occlusive disease may vary from one vascular laboratory to another, and requires ongoing internal validation and quality review. The criteria in the table are a representative example from one of our existing vascular laboratories.

measurements were compared to the relationship between the greatest point of narrowing versus the estimated normal diameter of the carotid bulb on arteriography (degree of stenosis). Specific spectral patterns and velocity ranges were then correlated with increasing degrees of carotid narrowing, and criteria were established for a range of duplex findings from A (normal carotid with no disease) to D+ (high-grade, preocclusive stenosis) (Table 5.4).

Growing experience has confirmed that carotid duplex is accurate, especially in the mid to high range of stenosis (50% to 99%) where its sensitivity and specificity are over 95%. In some instances, duplex may have limitations in differentiating a very high-grade stenosis from internal carotid occlusion. In such cases, flow beyond the stenosis may be so sluggish or limited that it is not detected or recognized by the sonographer and the findings are interpreted as occlusion. Depending on the clinical setting, additional diagnostic studies may be necessary to differentiate stenosis versus occlusion in these cases. Today, that usually means MRA or CTA, and rarely arteriography.

Duplex also provides useful information about the vertebral arteries in patients with nonlateralizing, posterior cerebral symptoms such as dizziness, vertigo, blurred vision, and ataxia (Chapter 12). In most instances, the proximal vertebral artery (i.e., the V_1 segment) can be studied directly and flow-limiting stenosis visualized and quantified with duplex. Indirect assessment of the vertebral is also made by determining the direction of flow (antegrade, retrograde, or bidirectional), which may indicate proximal occlusive disease of the subclavian or innominate arteries (i.e., subclavian steal). The more distal vertebral segments (V_2 to V_4) are surrounded by the vertebral bodies and cannot generally be assessed by duplex.

In most cases, carotid duplex is the only imaging modality necessary for surveillance prior to endarterectomy. Additional imaging is only needed when duplex cannot provide complete information because of clinical factors related to the patient's presentation, anatomy, or technical factors related to performance of the duplex (Chapter 12). In such instances, other noninvasive studies such as CTA and MRA complement duplex by providing images of the proximal and distal carotid circulations and of the brain. Contrast arteriography carries a low but finite risk of stroke and access site complications (1% to 2%) and is typically reserved for cases when duplex, CTA, and MRA are unable to provide complete information.

Limitations of duplex exist in its inability to examine the proximal, intrathoracic vessels (aortic arch and supra-aortic trunk) and the distal cervical and intracranial carotid circulation. Additionally, the quality and reliability of duplex is directly related to the qualifications and experience of the vascular sonographer. As such, additional imaging may be indicated depending on the experience level of a given vascular lab, as well as in cases of an anatomically high or distal carotid bifurcation, which precludes fully visualizing the carotid bulb and internal carotid artery with duplex. Additional imaging may also be necessary if the end of the stenosis is not appreciated or there is suspicion of tandem stenoses in the aortic arch, proximal common, or distal intracranial carotid arteries. Lastly, duplex may overestimate the degree of disease or stenosis in the carotid that is contralateral to a complete carotid artery occlusion (i.e., the other carotid artery is occluded). This phenomenon is thought to occur as velocities increase throughout the patent carotid artery as a compensatory mechanism to maintain cerebral perfusion. Some choose to pursue additional imaging (e.g., CTA) of the carotid circulation in this clinical scenario.

B. **Transcranial Doppler** (TCD) is a less commonly used noninvasive method to assess the intracranial circulation. TCD devices emit pulses of ultrasound from a 2 MHz probe through bony "windows" to the intracranial arteries. By placing the probe superior to the zygomatic arch, one can insonate the distal internal carotid siphon, anterior cerebral artery A1 segment, middle cerebral artery M1 segment, and posterior cerebral artery P1 and P2 segments. The ophthalmic artery and a portion of the internal carotid siphon may be assessed with the transorbital approach, and the suboccipital window is used to insonate the distal intracranial segment of the vertebrobasilar system.

A variety of clinical applications have been described for TCD that can be of use to the vascular specialist. The intracranial circulation can be assessed for collateral flow patterns in cases with severe bilateral carotid artery stenosis or occlusion. During carotid endarterectomy, TCD may be used to monitor for microembolic events, and intracranial vasospasm and stenosis or occlusions can also be detected. However, the total impact of TCD on the current evaluation of cerebrovascular disease remains relatively small compared to the role of extracranial carotid duplex ultrasonography.

VIII. **MRA AND CTA.** These noninvasive tests are typically performed in the radiology department, outside of a traditional vascular laboratory. As has been discussed, these modalities, in combination with duplex, provide a definitive diagnosis of vascular pathology without standard arteriography in most cases. In preparation for vascular and endovascular interventions, MRA and CTA are widely used as adjunctive diagnostic and planning studies or sometimes as the sole imaging modality. The choice whether or not to utilize this technology, and if so which kind, depends largely on the availability and quality of these studies at a particular institution.

Magnetic resonance imaging (MRI) relies on the principle that hydrogen nuclei (protons), when subjected to a magnetic field, align themselves in the direction of the field's poles. However, bursts of radio waves of appropriate frequency will alter this alignment (excitation). Following each radio frequency burst, the protons realign themselves with the magnetic field. This realignment (relaxation) is associated with the emission of a faint radio signal. A computer translates these signals into an image of the scanned area, which reveals varying densities of protons that correlate with different tissues (e.g., soft tissue and bone).

The physics of MRI are well suited for imaging vascular disease. In rapidly moving blood, the hydrogen nuclei do not line up in the applied magnetic field and thus produce little or no signal when stimulated by a radio frequency burst. The result is a natural contrast between the blood and the vessel wall. Several techniques of MRI have evolved in order to optimize resolution of blood vessels, but the use of contrast-enhanced MRA is most popular. Gadolinium is a heavy metal analog that is injected intravenously to enhance the clarity of MR arterial images.

Spiral or helical CT scanners have the ability to collect a volume of data by continuously rotating 360 degrees over the entire area of interest. Three-dimensional and center vessel reconstructions can be created based upon coronal, sagittal, and axial images. Visualization of the vasculature is enhanced by the use of 100 to 150 cc of contrast for a typical CTA. Nonionic contrast is preferable due to decreased pain with injection and lower risk of contrast nephropathy in patients with kidney disease.

All of the major vascular beds can be imaged by CTA or MRA. Imaging of intracranial vessels and parenchymal disease with either modality provides high-quality images and visually appealing three-dimensional reconstructions. MRI is generally thought to be superior to CT in evaluating cerebral edema, and has the potential to accurately stage strokes and to determine the optimal time for any cerebrovascular operation in such patients. Mesenteric or renal artery stenoses can also be visualized by either modality with sensitivity and specificity approaching that of invasive angiography. The timing of the contrast bolus and thickness of the data acquisition is key to providing good visualization of these vessels. These imaging studies are also very useful with the coexistence of an aortic aneurysm, dissection, or other abdominal pathology. Although small abdominal aortic aneurysms are followed with ultrasound, enlarging or larger aneurysms are usually imaged with CTA (Chapter 14). The greatest experience with preoperative planning and postoperative surveillance for endovascular aneurysm repair has been with CTA and not MRA although critical assessment of MR and duplex technology for surveillance is ongoing.

Lower extremity arterial occlusive disease is frequently evaluated by CTA or MRA (Chapter 13). Images similar to arteriography can be created with postprocessing techniques. By and large, arteriography is considered the gold standard prior to lower extremity bypass. However, some authors have found that high-quality MRA can identify obscure distal target vessels not seen on angiography. MRA may be obscured by venous artifact, if timing is not optimal. A particular strength of MR is the ability to simultaneously visualize muscular and tendinous structures. For example, popliteal artery entrapment from surrounding musculature can be diagnosed with positional stress. MR has also shown great promise in diagnosing venous thrombosis and obstruction, and is of the most value in areas inaccessible by ultrasound such as the abdominal, pelvic, and innominate veins. Protocols have been developed for the CT diagnosis of DVT, which can be combined with lung scan to detect pulmonary thromboembolus (Chapter 19).

Certain limitations exist that are specific to each MRA and CTA, the major one being cost. In addition, patients with metallic life-support systems (e.g., pacemakers) are excluded from MRI since the magnet creates problems with their function and some intracranial arterial aneurysm clips preclude accurate MRI. Finally, some patients become quite claustrophobic during MRI and are unable to tolerate its completion. CTA involves exposure to ionizing radiation, and iodinated contrast can cause allergic reactions and anaphylaxis, albeit uncommonly. Of even greater concern is the potential damage to the kidneys caused by the contrast agents used during CTA (contrast nephropathy), particularly in the elderly and in those with existing diabetes mellitus or renal insufficiency. An advantage of MRA has been that the use of gadolinium-based contrast does not have such a strong propensity to contrast nephropathy. However, the US Food and Drug Administration has issued warnings regarding reports of nephrogenic systemic fibrosis after gadolinium injection in patients with severe renal insufficiency. Vascular specialists can therefore no longer rely on MRA as a diagnostic tool in this subgroup of renal patients. CTA can be limited by the presence of vessel wall calcification that can obscure the lumen, whereas calcium does not cause artifact on MRA. More so than CTA, MRA is more difficult to interpret in areas with prior metallic stents, which can cause a loss of signal within the stent. Therefore, stents may give the false appearance of a stenosis or occlusion, although nitinol stents produce fewer artifacts. MRA also has a greater tendency to overestimate native artery stenosis. Some authors also caution that less expensive but effective methods of vascular imaging such as duplex ultrasound must not be abandoned during the current rapid proliferation of these diagnostic modalities.

IX. **VENOUS DISEASE.** Symptoms of venous disease are nonspecific, and therefore can be difficult to diagnose by physical examination alone (Chapters 2 and 4). The indications to assess for venous reflux may include leg swelling, varicose veins, and venous ulceration. The clinical signs of DVT are notoriously insensitive, and patients may in fact be entirely asymptomatic. Accurate diagnosis of venous diseases in the noninvasive vascular laboratory is therefore essential in establishing a diagnosis and can be potentially lifesaving in the setting of DVT. Although the diagnosis of DVT by venography is primarily of historical interest, contemporary treatment with **catheter-directed thrombolysis** has witnessed a resurgence of this procedure.

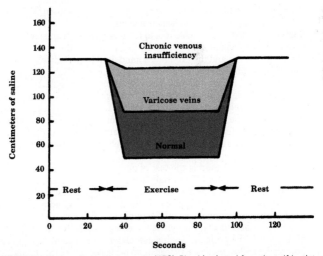

FIGURE 5.8 Venous air plethysmography (APG). Blood is ejected from the calf by tiptoe maneuvers. A recording cuff on the calf measures the residual volume (RV) at the nadir. Patients with no reflux have a low RV, due to efficient calf muscle ejection. Chronic deep venous insufficiency is associated with the highest RV due to pooling of blood in the calf. Superficial reflux from varicose veins results in an intermediate RV.

TABLE 5.5	Duplex Criteria for Acute Deep Venous Thrombosis

Noncompressible, enlarged vein in transverse plane
Visualization of thrombus
No flow by color imaging
Failure to dilate with Valsalva maneuver[a]
Lack of respiratory phasicity

[a]Applies to femoral vein.

A. **Venous insufficiency (reflux)** can be measured physiologically using air plethysmography or APG. With this technique, a recording pneumatic cuff is gently inflated on the leg to assess the relative amount of blood volume in the leg with various maneuvers. Next, to empty the leg of venous blood, the patient can perform toe raises that will contract the calf muscles and empty the venous system. Then, the patient stands without actively contracting the calf muscles on that leg (so that the calf muscles do not eject venous blood). The subsequent venous refill volume that occurs into the calf over time is determined by assessing small changes in the inflated pneumatic cuff. Patients with venous reflux will have shorter refill times (i.e., rapid venous refill into the leg). Deep venous reflux will have a more profound effect than superficial reflux. This technique can be modified to assess for chronic venous outflow obstruction. In this maneuver, a separate thigh cuff is then inflated to 60 to 80 mm Hg to occlude the venous outflow. Arterial flow continues to fill the calf over several minutes. The thigh cuff is then released. The recording calf cuff measures the venous outflow, which will be much slower in limbs with more proximal venous outflow obstruction (Fig. 5.8). Because it measures the physiologic function of the lower extremity venous system, APG is not helpful in determining the presence of acute DVT.

B. **Duplex ultrasound** is a valuable tool in the diagnosis of venous reflux and thrombosis. Venous reflux should be assessed with the patient in the standing position and the examiner's hand used to periodically squeeze the calf to augment venous flow toward the heart. When compression from the hand is then released, the vein of interest should be interrogated with duplex. Reflux will result in prolonged retrograde flow toward the foot and prolonged **valve closure times** (>1.0 seconds). Using a pneumatic cuff on the calf that can be inflated and rapidly deflated helps to standardize the test, while freeing up the examiner's hands. The Valsalva maneuver can also be used to assess for reflux at the saphenofemoral junction.

Duplex ultrasound is the test of choice for suspected acute DVT (Table 5.5 and Chapter 19). Normally, a vein should be entirely compressible by the ultrasound probe. The compression test is best performed in the transverse view (vein appears circular). In the longitudinal axis, the probe can unintentionally be off the midline, which can falsely lead the examiner to believe that the vein is not compressible. Incompressibility of the vein is the principal finding associated with thrombosis. Lack of flow on color-flow mode also suggests an occlusion. Fresh thrombus may be very echolucent, so that its presence in a vein may be difficult to visualize. Acutely, the vein is enlarged also. Over time, thrombus becomes echogenic (white) and chronically may show evidence of recanalization (wall thickening, irregular flow lumen) and venous contraction. Central veins, such as the iliac and subclavian veins, are more difficult to directly evaluate with duplex and compression maneuvers, because of their location. Indirect parameters such as phasicity of flow must be examined to assess patency of more central veins. The absence of normal femoral vein dilation with Valsalva maneuver can occur in the presence of iliac vein thrombosis and normal respiratory variation in flow, referred to as phasicity, may also be absent with flow continuous.

Selected Readings

AbuRahma AF, Srivastava M, Stone PA, et al. Critical appraisal of the carotid duplex consensus criteria in diagnosis of carotid artery stenosis. *J Vasc Surg.* 2011;53:53-60.

AbuRahma AF, Stone PA, Srivastava M, et al. Mesenteric/celiac duplex ultrasound interpretation criteria revisited. *J Vasc Surg.* 2012;55(2):428-436.e6; discussion 435-436. doi: 10.1016/j.jvs.2011.08.052.

Fleming SH, Davis RP, Craven TE, Deonanan JK, Godshall CJ, Hansen KJ. Accuracy of duplex sonography scans after renal artery stenting. *J Vasc Surg.* 2010;52(4):953-957; discussion 958. doi: 10.1016/j.jvs.2010.04.055.

Hariri N, Russell T, Kasper G, Lurie F. Shear rate is a better marker of symptomatic ischemic cerebrovascular events than velocity or diameter in severe carotid artery stenosis. *J Vasc Surg.* 2018. pii: S0741-5214(18)30995-9. doi: 10.1016/j.jvs.2018.04.036.

Kim AH, Augustin G, Shevitz A, et al. Carotid Consensus Panel duplex criteria can replace modified University of Washington criteria without affecting accuracy. *Vasc Med.* 2018;23(2):126-133. doi: 10.1177/1358863X17751655.

Norgren L, Hiatt WR, Dormandy JA, Nehler MR, Harris KA, Fowkes FGR. Inter-society consensus for the management of peripheral arterial disease (TASC II). *J Vasc Surg.* 2007;45(suppl):5-67.

Rose SC. Noninvasive vascular laboratory for evaluation of peripheral arterial occlusive disease. Part I. Hemodynamic principles and tools of the trade. *J Vasc Interv Radiol.* 2000;11:1107-1114.

Rose SC. Noninvasive vascular laboratory for evaluation of peripheral arterial occlusive disease. Part II. Clinical applications: chronic, usually atherosclerotic, lower extremity ischemia. *J Vasc Interv Radiol.* 2000;11:1257-1275.

Rose SC. Noninvasive vascular laboratory for evaluation of peripheral arterial occlusive disease. Part III. Clinical applications: nonatherosclerotic lower extremity arterial disease and upper extremity arterial disease. *J Vasc Interv Radiol.* 2001;12:11-18.

Stone PA, Glomski A, Thompson SN, Adams E. Toe pressures are superior to duplex parameters in predicting wound healing following toe and foot amputations. *Ann Vasc Surg.* 2018;46:147-154. doi: 10.1016/j.avsg.2017.08.012.

US Preventive Services Task Force; Curry SJ, Krist AH, Owens DK, et al. Screening for peripheral artery disease and cardiovascular disease risk assessment with the ankle-brachial index: US Preventive Services Task Force recommendation statement. *JAMA.* 2018;320(2):177-183. doi: 10.1001/jama.2018.8357.

Wang Z, Hasan R, Firwana B, et al. A systematic review and meta-analysis of tests to predict wound healing in diabetic foot. *J Vasc Surg.* 2016;63(2 suppl):29S-36S. e1-2. doi: 10.1016/j.jvs.2015.10.004.

Zierler RE, Jordan WD, Lal BK, et al. The Society for Vascular Surgery practice guidelines on follow-up after vascular surgery arterial procedures. *J Vasc Surg.* 2018;68(1):256-284. doi: 10.1016/j.jvs.2018.04.018.

6

Risk Factors
and Risk Modifications

As patients age, the number of medical conditions that can adversely affect their health and operative risk increases. Many of these medical conditions are risk factors for atherosclerosis that increase the risk of coronary artery disease and peripheral vascular disease (e.g., lower extremity occlusive and cerebrovascular disease) (Fig. 6.1). When these factors are controlled, the risk of vascular disease progression and adverse perioperative events are reduced. However, when risk factors are not controlled, they work in concert in the development of vascular disease and increase the risk of adverse perioperative events. This chapter focuses on some of these cardiovascular risk factors and on counseling patients about how to minimize cardiovascular events around the time of vascular interventions. Specific pathways that

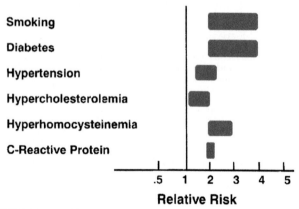

FIGURE 6.1 Range of independent impact of each atherosclerotic risk factor in the development of lower extremity vascular disease. Smoking indicates comparison versus former smoking. (From Hirsch AT, Haskal ZJ, Hertzer NR, et al.; for the writing committee. ACC/AHA 2005 guidelines for the management of patients with peripheral arterial disease [lower extremity, renal, mesenteric, and abdominal aortic]: a collaborative report from the AAVS/SVS/SCAI/SVMB/SIR and the ACC/AHA task force on practice guidelines. *J Am Coll Cardiol.* 2005;e1-e192, with permission.)

can be used to stratify periprocedural risk once a specific vascular intervention is planned are addressed in Chapter 7.

I. **TOBACCO ABUSE**. Cigarette smoking is an independent predictor of vascular disease, failure of vascular interventions, and adverse perioperative events. While cigarette smoking is associated with the development of coronary artery disease, there is evidence that its negative effects are more concentrated on the cerebrovascular and lower extremity circulations. Smoking increases the risk of stroke at least twofold and the risk of lower extremity occlusive disease four- to sixfold (two times it negative impact on the coronary circulation). Continued tobacco use is responsible for vascular disease progression, while smoking cessation mitigates these effects. Studies have shown that the risk of death, myocardial infarction (MI), amputation, and bypass graft failure are all lower in those who have stopped smoking compared with active smokers. The precise mechanisms of smoking's harmful effects on the heart and blood vessels are not fully understood, due in part to the fact that the chemical milieu produced by the burning of tobacco produces thousands of chemical by-products. It is generally accepted, however, that nicotine is the stimulant and addictive component of tobacco. Despite its addictive property, nicotine does not appear to participate in the adverse effects of smoking on the vascular system. In contrast, oxidizing agents in tobacco are known to cause vasoconstriction, hypertension, and endothelial dysfunction, which, in addition to inhibition of prostacyclin, cause a relative hypercoagulable state. The effect of these oxidizing substances in cigarette smoke leads to augmented lipid deposition, platelet aggregation, and smooth muscle cell dysfunction. Collectively, these harmful effects stimulate the formation of new atherosclerotic lesions and cause existing lesions to be less stable and more prone to thrombosis.

Convincing smokers to quit is not easy, as most are affected by a stubborn chemical addiction. Studies show that techniques available to help patients stop smoking are not likely to succeed unless the patient desires to stop and is willing to commit to a multifaceted cessation plan. Patients who can be made to understand the negative impact of continued smoking to their condition and those who have good motivation and support mechanisms generally will stop. Unfortunately, not all patients have this combination of understanding, motivation, and support as only 40% of men and 30% of women who quit smoking remain free of tobacco use 1 year later.

Most studies of smoking cessation pharmacotherapy have focused on nicotine as the addictive element in tobacco. Nicotine replacement therapy comes in several forms, including transdermal patches, gum, nasal spray, inhalers, and sticks meant to simulate cigarettes. A newer nicotinic receptor agonist based on the structure of cytosine, called varenicline (Chantix Pfizer, Inc., New York, NY), has shown effectiveness in helping individuals quit smoking. The antidepressant bupropion (Wellbutrin and Zyban, GlaxoSmithKline, Brentford, Middlesex, UK) has also been used with some success to reduce symptoms of withdrawal and achieve smoking cessation. Combination therapy consisting of bupropion and nicotine replacement has been shown in some studies to improve cessation rates compared to either therapy alone (Fig. 6.2). Interestingly, a new nicotine vaccine is being evaluated that in theory turns the body's immune system against the chemical before it is able to reach the brain and cause addictive effects. Most studies have found that the effectiveness of any of these medications in assisting with smoking cessation is increased if they combined with formal counseling and/or psychotherapy

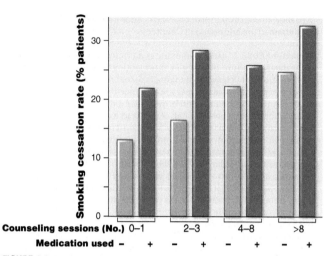

FIGURE 6.2 Abstinence from smoking based upon cessation therapy used at 6 and 12 months. (From Jorenby DE, Leischow SJ, Nides MA, et al. A controlled trial of sustained-release bupropion, a nicotine patch or both for smoking cessation. *N Engl J Med.* 1999;340:685-691, with permission.)

sessions. Regardless of the method used, the best long-term results to date report cessation rates of only 20% to 25%, although evidence suggests rates may be higher with the newer nicotine receptor agonists.

II. **HYPERTENSION.** The management and control of hypertension mitigates the development and progression of peripheral arterial disease and the risk of adverse periprocedural cardiac events such as stroke, MI, and cardiovascular death. The risk of each of these is two to four times higher in hypertensive patients compared with patients with normal blood pressure. Traditional guidelines have set systolic blood pressure of 140 mm Hg or lower and diastolic pressure of 90 mm Hg or lower as "normal" target numbers. More recent information suggests that lower target numbers of 130/80 or lower are beneficial in patients with diabetes, renal insufficiency, and certain forms of heart disease.

Three common categories of antihypertensive medications are **beta-receptor blockers, calcium channel blockers,** and medications that alter the renin-angiotensin system, either through **inhibition of the angiotensin-converting enzyme (ACE inhibitors)** or through **angiotensin receptor blockade (ARBs).** Beta-blockers and ACE inhibitors have been shown to reduce the incidence of MI and cardiovascular death in those with coronary disease, and ACE inhibitors have been shown to reduce these same adverse outcomes in patients with peripheral arterial disease. While the effectiveness of beta-blocker therapy in reducing periprocedural cardiovascular complications has been largely dismissed, use to reduce long-term cardiac events in those with known coronary artery disease remains a pillar. Thus, it is a part of most vascular patients' medical management.

Medications that block the renin-angiotensin-aldosterone system are effective at lowering blood pressure and they also have favorable effects on arterial wall and myocardial cell remodeling. The specifics of these effects are not well defined and represent an important area of research; however, these medications in particular may favorably modify the cardiovascular system through a mechanism that is independent of their effects on blood pressure.

The central acting medication **clonidine** and the direct vasodilator **hydralazine** are also useful in treating more significant degrees of hypertension and diuretics such as **hydrochlorothiazide** and **Lasix** (furosemide) can be used alone or in combination with one of the other antihypertensive agents. Importantly, improvements in blood pressure control can also be realized by healthy lifestyle modifications, such as an improved diet, weight loss, and initiation of an exercise program. If blood pressure measurements remain elevated and refractory despite months of treatment with multiple agents, renal artery occlusive disease (e.g., renovascular hypertension) should be considered as a possible etiology.

III. **HYPERLIPIDEMIA.** Control of high serum lipids may slow the progression of atherosclerosis. In particular, **statin medications** or hydroxymethylglutaryl (HMG)-CoA reductase inhibitors not only control cholesterol but also appear to halt atherogenesis and may even lead to plaque regression. This class of medications also have helpful effects on the vascular endothelium and smooth muscle cells and antithrombotic properties. The use of statin medications has been shown to reduce all types of cardiovascular events. In the **Scandinavian Simvastatin Trial**, drug therapy for hypercholesterolemia was associated with a 38% reduction in the development or worsening of claudication. The **Heart Protection Study** revealed reductions in coronary events, strokes, and peripheral intervention requirements in those with and without diagnosed peripheral vascular diseases using simvastatin (Zocor, Merck & Co., Inc., West Point, PA) (Fig. 6.3). Retrospective reviews have noted a reduction in carotid endarterectomy restenosis and improved durability in those taking lipid-lowering agents.

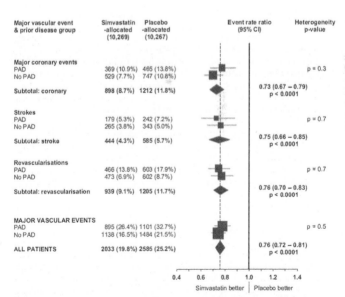

FIGURE 6.3 The effects of simvastatin use in those with and without peripheral vascular disease on the major cardiovascular end points of coronary events, stroke, and revascularization requirements. (From Heart Protection Study Collaborative Group. Randomized trial of the effects of cholesterol-lowering with simvastatin on peripheral vascular and other major vascular outcomes in 20,536 people with peripheral arterial disease and other high-risk conditions. *J Vasc Surg.* 2007;45:645-654, with permission.)

In addition to cholesterol, the **main components of a serum lipid profile are low-density lipoprotein (LDL), high-density lipoprotein (HDL), and triglycerides.** Normal cholesterol levels are defined as less than 200 mg/dL, while 200 to 240 mg/dL is borderline, and greater than 240 mg/dL is considered high. LDL is often referred to as the "bad cholesterol" and levels greater than 160 mg/dL are considered high and need reduction, ideally to less than 100 mg/dL. In those at highest risk for a cardiovascular event, it is recommended to reduce the LDL level to 70 mg/dL. Most guidelines suggest that levels of the "good cholesterol," HDL be between 40 and 60 mg/dL. Levels of HDL below 40 mg/dL are associated with the development of cardiovascular disease, while levels greater than 60 mg/dL are considered protective against this condition. Triglycerides should be below 150 mg/dL, which can be achieved with the use of fibric and nicotinic acid derivatives such as **gemfibrozil** and **niacin.** Cholesterol may also be lowered by the bile acid–sequestering resins **cholestyramine** and **colestipol** as well as niacin.

As a rule, serum measurements of cholesterol and triglycerides should be determined after a 12-hour fast. A low-fat (35% of calories), low-cholesterol (<300 mg daily) diet remains the cornerstone of treatment of hyperlipidemia, and when combined with regular exercise is much more effective. Regular aerobic exercise has been shown to be especially effective in increasing HDL levels. Importantly, alcohol may exacerbate hypertriglyceridemia and elimination of alcohol intake should be an initial step in managing this potentially harmful condition. Although past recommendations called for a 3-month trial of diet management before medications were added, it is now common for statins to be started earlier, particularly as the understanding of the benefits of this class of medications evolves.

The **side effects of statin therapy** are uncommon but can be significant in some individuals. These include hepatic toxicity and severe migrating myositis (i.e., muscle pains) which causes pain and soreness in the large muscle groups of the extremities and core. Therefore, patients receiving statins must be evaluated on a routine basis by the prescribing physician and his or her care team and have liver function and creatinine kinase levels monitored during statin therapy. Resolution of the myositis in patients experiencing this side effect often takes several weeks to fully resolve.

IV. **DIABETES MELLITUS.** Diabetes has both macrovascular and microvascular effects. It is an independent predictor for stroke and lower extremity occlusive disease. The need for amputation in diabetics with lower extremity arterial occlusive disease is approximately 10 times that of nondiabetics. While tight glycemic control is important in preventing microvascular events, such as nephropathy, retinopathy, and neuropathy, it remains unclear if this reduces cardiovascular events. It appears likely that diabetics with intensive glucose control do have lower rates of claudication and need for revascularization and foot or extremity amputation. While there is limited evidence, rigorous glucose control actually reduces atherosclerosis, it may aid in preventing or clearing and healing soft tissue infections in patients with this condition. The **American Diabetes Association** recommends maintaining a **glycosylated hemoglobin (A1C)** of less than 7% in diabetics with peripheral vascular disease. Meticulous foot care to include appropriate protective measures such as appropriately fitting shoes, moisturizing skin care, and daily inspection is critical to avoid development of calluses and ulcers, which may lead to infection, necrosis, sepsis, and amputation.

V. **ANTIPLATELET THERAPY.** Antiplatelet medications reduce the incidence of cardiovascular events in patients with peripheral vascular disease. It is important to understand that this benefit is not necessarily related to improved leg symptoms or walking distance in those with claudication, but instead to a reduction in life-threatening stroke and or myocardial infarction. As an example, the **Antithrombotic Trialists' Collaboration** meta-analysis showed a lower rate of MI, stroke, and vascular death in patients with peripheral vascular disease who took antiplatelet therapy. This reduction was between 20% and 30% in those with intermittent claudication and those who had undergone peripheral bypass grafts or peripheral angioplasty. Antiplatelet therapy also reduces subsequent cardiovascular events in those with asymptomatic cerebrovascular disease and other atherogenic risk factors. Similarly, the use of antiplatelet therapy after a stroke or a prior carotid endarterectomy has been shown to provide stroke risk reduction.

Most studies on the effectiveness of antiplatelet therapy have focused on the use of **aspirin**, which competitively inhibits the **cyclooxygenase enzyme** within the platelet. Inhibition of cyclooxygenase blocks the production of **prostaglandin** and **thromboxane A2 (TXA2)** from arachidonic acid. The detrimental effect of TXA$_2$ comes from its activation of the **GP IIb/IIIa binding site** on the platelet, which allows fibrinogen to bind, which causes platelets to aggregate or clump together. By inhibiting cyclooxygenase and ultimately TXA$_2$, aspirin prevents platelet aggregation. The antiplatelet effect of aspirin lasts for about 72 hours and can be achieved with 81 mg per day, which has a lower bleeding risk than the 325 mg dose.

Clopidogrel (Plavix, Sanofi-Aventis/Bristol-Myers Squibb Company, New York, NY) is another antiplatelet medication (75 mg daily) that works as a noncompetitive inhibitor of the **adenosine diphosphate (ADP) receptor** on platelets. The effect of clopidogrel on this receptor is irreversible and lasts for the duration of the platelet, which is about 7 to 10 days. Binding of ADP to its platelet receptor is necessary for activation of the same GP IIb/IIIa receptor triggered by TXA$_2$. The IIb/IIIa receptor is important as the binding site for fibrinogen, which initiates platelet aggregation. Both low- and high-affinity ADP receptors are present on platelets, and the active metabolite of clopidogrel also inhibits the low-affinity ADP receptor. Through these actions on the ADP binding sites and ultimately the GP IIb/IIIa receptor, clopidogrel provides a more thorough or stronger antiplatelet effect than aspirin in most patients.

Results from the **Clopidogrel versus Aspirin in Patients at Risk of Ischemic Events (CAPRIE)** trial were reported. In individuals with previous MI or stroke, or in those with diagnosed peripheral vascular disease, clopidogrel reduced cardiovascular events by 8.7% (5.32% vs 5.83% per year) compared with aspirin. In those with peripheral vascular disease, the benefit with clopidogrel was greater, with the risk of vascular death, stroke, or MI reduced by almost 24% (3.71% vs 4.86% per year) at 3 years. The findings of CAPRIE were in favor of clopidogrel, and many who treat those with peripheral vascular disease use this medication as first-line therapy based on these data. However, the absolute risk reduction with clopidogrel in CAPRIE was small, and aspirin remains an established and less expensive antiplatelet therapy. These findings are relevant when considering a medication that will be taken for many years; some providers prefer using aspirin as the initial therapy and use clopidogrel as an effective alternative. Combination therapy with aspirin and clopidogrel is somewhat controversial and no studies have shown benefit of dual- versus single-agent treatment. Benefit from dual antiplatelet therapy has been difficult to demonstrate in clinical studies because of the increased risk of bleeding associated with the combination of these agents.

While the question of which antiplatelet medication to use may not have a single answer that applies to all patients, guidelines exist to assist the provider in this area. There is a consensus based on several clinical trials that some form of antiplatelet therapy, either aspirin or clopidogrel, is indicated in patients with peripheral vascular disease to reduce the long-term cardiovascular event rate including cardiovascular death (class/level of evidence 1A) (see Table 7.2). Because aspirin has been around the longest, it has the benefit of having demonstrated its effectiveness in more than one controlled study. The use of aspirin is therefore supported by class/level 1A evidence, which denotes the consensus on efficacy (class 1) supported by multiple randomized controlled trials (level A). In contrast, clopidogrel was more recently introduced and has only been shown to be effective in one trial (CAPRIE). Use of clopidogrel in this setting is therefore supported by class/level 1B evidence, indicating the consensus on efficacy (class 1) supported by one randomized controlled trial (level B).

Other medications with differing mechanisms providing antiplatelet effects are also available. These include **picotamide**, a thromboxane synthase inhibitor, that directly inhibits the production of TXA_2 and **cilostazol** (Pletal, Otsuka America Pharmaceutical, Inc., Rockville, MD) and **dipyridamole** (Persantine Boehringer Ingelheim Pharmaceuticals, Gaithersburg, MD), which inhibit the phosphodiesterase enzyme within platelets. Dipyridamole, which may have a unique role in preventing secondary stroke, also stimulates prostacyclin synthesis and potentiates the platelet inhibitory actions of prostacyclin. However, some of these effects may not occur at therapeutic levels of the drug; hence, the mechanism of action of dipyridamole remains somewhat poorly defined.

VI. **HYPERHOMOCYSTEINEMIA.** High serum levels of the amino acid **homocysteine** are associated with an increased risk of arterial occlusive disease. This condition carries an independent two- to threefold increased risk for developing lower extremity occlusive disease, intermittent claudication, coronary artery disease, and stroke. Increased homocysteine levels are found in 30% to 50% of those with cardiovascular disease, and evidence suggests that hyperhomocysteinemia also promotes progression of peripheral arterial disease. Finally, this condition places those with peripheral arterial disease at a three- to fourfold increase in vascular morbidity and mortality compared to those with normal levels of the amino acid.

The causes of hyperhomocysteinemia may include either a genetic alteration in the enzymes responsible for its metabolism, or deficiencies in vitamin B_{12} and folate, which are cofactors in this process. B-complex vitamins, cobalamin (B_{12}), pyridoxine (B_6), and folic acid have all been noted to reduce plasma levels of homocysteine and have been targeted as potential therapies for this risk factor. However, there is as of yet no correlation between reducing amino acid levels and reducing cardiovascular events. In fact, a trend indicating a reciprocal effect has been noted. Studies are ongoing and more information should be available in the coming years.

VII. **C-REACTIVE PROTEIN AND FIBRINOGEN.** An association has been noted between elevated plasma levels of the inflammatory markers **C-reactive protein** and **fibrinogen** and vascular disease. Specifically, increased levels of these markers have been identified in patients with lower extremity occlusive disease, coronary artery disease, and stroke. This relationship is thought to be an association and not causative, meaning these molecules do not cause vascular disease but are simply markers of the immune-mediated process of atherosclerosis. The role of these molecules in identifying and treating vascular disease is not fully understood, and there are no recommendations as to their use in clinical practice.

VIII. **OBESITY.** While obesity may not be, in and of itself, a risk factor for the development of peripheral vascular disease, it does make management of the condition difficult. Obesity leads to, or exacerbates, degenerative joint disease and diabetes mellitus and limits respiratory capacity and exercise programs for those with lower extremity occlusive disease. Obesity makes endovascular access to the femoral arteries and operative exposure in the groin, abdomen, and retroperitoneum more difficult, and it is a risk factor for periprocedural complications such as pneumonia, venous thrombosis, and pulmonary embolism. Obesity increases wound complication rates, including those overlying femoral artery exposures in the groin. Because of these complicating factors, many surgeons and interventionalists encourage, if not require, patients to engage in a weight loss program and show substantial progress before performing an elective vascular procedure.

Patients who are 20 to 40 pounds above ideal weight are considered moderately obese. Morbidly obese patients (100 pounds overweight) seldom can be expected to lose substantial weight before elective surgery. Therefore, the benefits of elective abdominal or extremity vascular procedures in these patients must be carefully considered in the context of higher risks of periprocedural complications. Occasionally, providers point out that preoperative weight loss may be unsafe, and that insistence on weight loss may discourage patients from returning for treatment. This line of reasoning points to the importance of formal dietary consultation in some patients to avoid any disadvantages of unhealthy weight loss before a procedure is performed. In the authors' experience, safe weight reduction can be accomplished in the majority of moderately obese patients who require an elective procedure. Ideally, the patient's weight should be brought to within 10% of ideal body weight. In some cases, this concerted effort may serve as a life-altering event in which the weight reduction becomes not just necessary for the procedure but is continued throughout the patient's life. If successful, weight reduction improves not only a patient's peripheral vascular health but also their overall well-being. The following guidelines for periprocedural weight reduction are effective.

A. The **importance of preoperative weight reduction** as a means to facilitate a safe and complication-free procedure must be explained to the patient. We emphasize that elective surgery can almost always be postponed until this discussion has been had and some degree of weight loss has been achieved.

B. A **definite time** period to achieve a weight loss goal is proposed and a tentative surgery date is proposed. Most moderately obese patients will benefit from losing 10 to 30 pounds. To ensure safe, gradual weight reduction, we recommend consultation with a dietician and loss of no more than 1 to 2 pounds per week. For some patients, this means delaying their procedure for 3 to 6 months to allow progress toward their goal. We have also found it important to recheck patients during this time period to ensure they are making progress and not having worsening of their vascular symptoms or problems with the weight reduction program.

C. **Alcoholic beverages** are a commonly overlooked source of calories, and this fact should be emphasized to patients who drink regularly. For some patients, reducing or eliminating alcohol intake prior to the procedure will have benefits beyond just caloric intake.

D. Most patients find it very difficult to lose weight and **stop smoking** at the same time. Consequently, it is recommended to allow some chronic smokers to continue some smoking while they diet. An agreement can be made with the patient that smoking will stop when the patient is hospitalized for elective surgery. Some may question this relatively late discontinuance of smoking; however, in the authors' experience, this approach usually results in successful weight reduction and has not led to increased pulmonary morbidity.

IX. **EXERCISE.** Regular exercise is important for the patient's overall cardio-vascular condition, pulmonary function, and reduction of excess weight. Exercise has positive benefits on the patient's blood pressure, lipid profile, and insulin sensitivity as well. Regular lower extremity exercise in the form of a **structured or supervised walking program** is important in those with peripheral vascular disease. Walking increases skeletal muscle's metabolic adaptation to ischemia and may enhance collateral blood flow, resulting in stabilization or improvement of claudication. A variety of walking programs can be initiated in patients with vascular disease; however, a simple program that has helped the majority of the authors' patients emphasizes the following four concepts:

A. **Dedicated Walking Time.** Patients establish a defined period of walking above and beyond that which they perform as part of normal daily activities. Patients who do not have time or the capacity to commit to a daily walking program should be reassured that dedicating a period of time to mild or moderate exercise every other day or three to four times per week can also be very beneficial.

B. **Walking Instructions.** Patients are instructed to walk at a comfortable pace and stop for a brief rest whenever leg pain (e.g., claudication) becomes significant. If patients experience no leg pain, they should continue walking for the 30 to 45 minutes set aside for the program. In bad weather, patients may use a treadmill or stationary exercise bicycle or walk inside (i.e., in a shopping mall). The walk-rest routine should be continued until the patient has performed at least 30 minutes walking (not including the rest periods). It is helpful to inform patients that as the leg adapts, the frequency and duration of rests will decrease.

C. **Recording Walking Time, Length, and Weight Loss.** Patients should be encouraged to record their walking program, including time and distance, on a calendar or in a journal. Patients who are obese should combine this with daily or weekly weight measurements, as success with walking often goes hand in hand with weight loss. Recording their effort holds the patient accountable and offers a means to see successes over time. After 6 to 8 weeks, most patients can double or triple their comfortable walking distance and may also achieve weight loss.

D. **Supervision and Follow-Up.** A follow-up visit with a provider or a phone call from one of the patient's vascular team during this period is critical to provide encouragement and supervision of this important endeavor.

Selected Readings

Brott TG, Halperin JL, Abbara S, et al. 2011 ASA/ACCF/AHA/AANN/AANS/ACR/ASNR/CNS/SAIP/SCAI/SIR/SNIS/SVM/SVS Guideline on the management of patients with extracranial carotid and vertebral artery disease. *Circulation.* 2011;124:e54-e130.

CAPRIE Steering Committee. A randomized blinded trial of clopidogrel versus aspirin in patients at risk of ischaemic events. *Lancet.* 1996;348:1329-1339.

Conte MS, Pomposelli FB, Clair DG, et al. Society for Vascular Surgery practice guidelines for atherosclerotic occlusive disease of the lower extremities: management of asymptomatic disease and claudication. *J Vasc Surg.* 2015;61:2S-41S.

Gerhard-Herman MD, Gornik HL, Barrett C. et al. 2016 AHA/ACC Guidelines on the management of patients with lower extremity peripheral artery disease: a report from the American College of Cardiology/American Heart Association task force on Clinical Practice Guidelines. *Circulation.* 2017;135:e726-e779.

Heart Protection Study Collaborative Group. Randomized trial of the effects of cholesterol-lowering with simvastatin on peripheral vascular and other major vascular outcomes in 20,536 people with peripheral arterial disease and other high-risk conditions. *J Vasc Surg.* 2007;45:645-654.

Norgren L, Hiatt WR, Dormandy JA, et al., Inter-society consensus for the management of peripheral arterial disease (TASC II). *J Vasc Surg.* 2007;45(suppl S):S5-S61.

Perioperative Risk Stratification and Clinical Guidelines

Most patients with manifestations of peripheral vascular disease requiring intervention have existing cardiac, pulmonary, and/or kidney diseases that increase their risk of periprocedural morbidity and mortality. Preoperative preparation must include an accurate assessment of the patient's risk related to these vital organ systems, taking into account the indication for the procedure, the type of anesthetic required, and optimization of coexisting medical conditions. This chapter focuses on assessing and reducing periprocedural cardiac risk according to evidence-based guidelines. Additionally, this chapter discusses the significance of coexisting carotid occlusive and chronic kidney disease and optimizing pulmonary function. Finally, new directions in the perioperative management of diabetes mellitus are outlined.

I. **PERIOPERATIVE CARDIAC RISK.** A key factor in achieving excellent results from elective vascular surgery, open or endovascular, is accurate assessment of anesthetic risk. Although clinical sense and experience contribute a great deal to an initial impression of anesthetic risk, more objective data also assist with assessment of operative risk. Historically, preoperative physical condition was correlated with anesthetic morbidity and mortality using the American Society of Anesthesiologists (ASA) classification. This grading system refers only to a patient's overall physical condition and does not consider the type of anesthesia, extent of operation, or experience of the surgeon. There are five levels of ASA classification, with 1 indicating a healthy individual and 5 noting extreme coexisting medical conditions. The letter "e" is added to indicate an emergency procedure. In 1977, Goldman developed a more involved scoring system to evaluate perioperative cardiac risk from 1,000 patients having undergone general surgical procedures. When this system was applied prospectively to 99 patients undergoing elective aortic surgery, the **rates of cardiac complications were higher than those in the original study of general surgical procedures.** This finding was among the first reporting the high incidence of significant coronary artery disease (CAD) in patients undergoing vascular procedures.

A. **Evidence-Based Algorithm.** MI is the leading cause of death following vascular procedures, occurring in 3% to 6% of elective cases. Additionally, some degree of myocardial ischemia is present following 20% to 40% of vascular procedures, depending upon how aggressively the diagnosis is pursued. Hertzer and colleagues of the Cleveland Clinic defined the prevalence of CAD in vascular patients, demonstrating **that severe but correctable CAD existed in nearly one-third of patients presenting for surgical treatment of peripheral vascular disease** (abdominal aortic aneurysm, 32%; cerebrovascular disease, 26%; arteriosclerosis of the lower limbs, 28%). Severe, correctable CAD was present in about 50% of patients with angina pectoris and 30% with a previous myocardial infarction.

Following this seminal report came more than two decades of study aimed at reducing cardiac morbidity and mortality around the time of peripheral vascular intervention. Much of this effort focused on identifying those with silent but correctable coronary disease prior to the planned procedure; the assumption being that in such individuals, coronary angiography followed by revascularization would reduce perioperative risk and increase survival. While this approach emphasizing coronary revascularization was beneficial in subsets of patients, such as in the **Coronary Artery Surgery study (CASS)**, it is not applicable to all those undergoing vascular procedures. In fact, more recent publication of the **Coronary Artery Revascularization Prophylaxis (CARP)** trial showed that among patients with stable cardiac symptoms, preoperative coronary revascularization does not improve short- or long-term survival. Findings from the CARP study and others like it have resulted in more balanced recommendations that propose a more selective role of preoperative coronary revascularization while emphasizing periprocedural medical therapy (e.g., beta-blockers, statins, and ACE inhibitors). The following paragraphs outline the contemporary guidelines on perioperative cardiac risk assessment.

1. **Eagle and associates identified key clinical markers of increased cardiac risk in patients undergoing vascular operations (Eagle criteria):** (a) angina pectoris, (b) prior MI, (c) congestive heart failure, (d) diabetes mellitus, and (e) age greater than 70 years. The risk for a perioperative cardiac event increases with the number of criteria present (Table 7.1). With three or more, the risk of a perioperative cardiac event is 30%, with 77% of these patients having severe CAD on coronary angiography. Although the Eagle criteria are largely of historical importance, they provide a very good and concise listing of key clinical factors to be considered prior to elective vascular procedures.

2. In 1996, the **American College of Cardiology and American Heart Association published guidelines for preoperative cardiac evaluation.** These guidelines were revised in 2002, 2007, and again in 2014 to provide a framework for considering cardiac risk associated with noncardiac surgery. Three prominent themes from the updated guidelines include the following:

   Preoperative coronary intervention is rarely necessary unless otherwise indicated independent of the planned procedure.

   Preoperative evaluation is not performed to "give clearance to operate," but instead should provide an assessment of the patient's medical condition and present a risk profile that can be used to make treatment decisions.

TABLE 7.1 Original Eagle Criteria

Clinical Criteria	Number of Criteria Present/% Risk for Cardiac Event
Angina pectoris	
Prior myocardial infarction	0 criteria/2% risk
Congestive heart failure	1 or 2/10% risk
Diabetes mellitus	3 or more/30% risk
Age >70 years	

(From Eagle KA, Coley CM, Newell JB, et al. Combining clinical and thallium data optimizes preoperative assessment of cardiac risk before major vascular surgery. *Ann Int Med.* 1989;110:859-866, with permission.)

No preoperative testing should be performed unless it is likely to influence patient treatment (e.g., if it will actually change the perioperative management).

Additionally, starting in 2007, guidelines were converted from tabular format to listing of recommendations written in sentences to express more complete thought. Also, a clearer explanation of the clinical evidence supporting each guideline is provided using **levels of evidence and classification of recommendations** (Table 7.2). Specifically, levels of clinical evidence A, B, or C are cross-referenced with classification of recommendations (I, IIa, IIb, and III) to give the provider an estimate of the certainty and size of each guideline. For example, level A evidence indicates the strongest estimate of certainty coming from evaluation of several patient groups with a consistency of direction and magnitude of effect. Level A evidence is supported by more than one randomized clinical trial or a meta-analysis, while level B evidence stems from a single randomized trial or several nonrandomized trials. It is important to note that guidelines supported by level B or C evidence are not necessarily weak. Some clinical questions are not well suited for clinical trials, or the optimal time to perform such a trial may have passed. In some cases the clinical consensus in favor of a test or therapy is so strong that there is no need for investment to initiate a trial to prove the point. In such instances **classification of recommendations** is useful, as it provides a broader perspective than just the published or hard evidence for or against a given test or therapy (Table 7.2). Armed with this basic understanding of levels of evidence and classification of recommendations, the provider can proceed in taking the patient's medical history and perform a review of systems, focusing on three areas that relate directly to the cardiac evaluation algorithm in the contemporary guidelines (Fig. 7.1):

TABLE 7.2	Levels of Clinical Evidence and Classification of Recommendations
Levels	
Level A	Evidence from multiple randomized trials or metaanalyses
Level B	Evidence from single randomized trial or nonrandomized studies
Level C	Evidence from retrospective or case studies or from expert opinion
Classification	
Class I	Treatment or procedure is useful or effective (i.e., benefit far outweighs the risk, and treatment *should* be performed)
Class IIa	Recommendation in favor or treatment or procedure being useful or effective (i.e., benefit outweighs the risk, and *it is reasonable* to perform treatment)
Class IIb	Usefulness or effectiveness less well established (i.e., benefit is equal to or greater than the risk, and the procedure or treatment may be considered)
Class III	Treatment or procedure is not useful and may be harmful (i.e., risk outweighs the benefits, and treatment should not be performed)

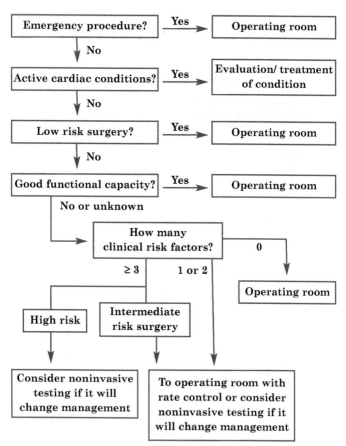

FIGURE 7.1 American Heart Association 2014 guidelines for preoperative cardiac evaluation.

1. Identification of **active cardiac conditions** (Table 7.3)
2. Identification of **estimated perioperative risk** for major adverse cardiovascular events (Table 7.3)
3. Evaluation of the patient's **functional capacity** (Table 7.4)

Active cardiac conditions represent conditions that, if present, should be thoroughly evaluated and treated *before* noncardiac surgery, even if it means a delay in or cancellation of a nonemergent case (Fig. 7.1). These conditions include unstable coronary syndromes, decompensated heart failure, significant arrhythmias, and severe valvular disease. This guideline represents a class I recommendation supported by level B evidence. The patient should also be evaluated to estimate perioperative cardiac risk. This is done most commonly by recognizing the presence of the six risk factors in the Revised Cardiac Risk Index (RCRI). These include history of ischemic heart disease, compensated heart failure, cerebrovascular disease, diabetes mellitus, renal insufficiency, and planned intrathoracic/abdominal

Clinical Assessment of Cardiac Risk

Active cardiac conditions (should be evaluated and treated before surgery)
Unstable coronary syndromes (myocardial infarction within 30 days, unstable or severe angina)
Decompensated congestive heart failure
Significant arrhythmias (high-grade atrioventricular block, symptomatic ventricular arrhythmias supraventricular arrhythmias with uncontrolled ventricular rate, newly recognized ventricular tachycardia and symptomatic bradycardia)
Severe valvular disease

Revised Cardiac Risk Index (6-factors)
History of ischemic heart disease
Compensated or prior congestive heart failure
History of cerebrovascular disease (TIA or CVA)
Diabetes mellitus (Insulin-dependent)
Renal insufficiency (Cr ≥ 2.0 mg/dL)
Intrathoracic, intra-abdominal, or suprainguinal vascular surgery

or suprainguinal vascular surgery (Table 7.3). This is simply the original Eagle criteria along with high-risk operations. Other risk calculators are now also recognized and include those from investigations of the American College of Surgeons and Society for Vascular Surgery quality databases. These RCRI factors are used in the final step of the cardiac evaluation and care algorithm in managing patients undergoing a high-risk surgery who have an unknown or poor functional capacity (Fig. 7.1).

Estimation of **functional capacity** is also critical and can be accomplished by simply interviewing the patient about his or her living situation and daily activities. Functional capacity is expressed in

Estimated Energy Requirements for Various Activities

1 MET
Sitting at rest
Eat, dress, or use the toilet
Walk indoors around the house

4 METs
Light work around the house
Walk a block or two on level ground (at 4 mph pace)
Climb flight of stairs or walk on slight incline
Brisk walk on level ground
Heavy work around the house
Moderate recreational activities (golf, bowling, dancing)

Greater than 10 METs
Strenuous sports (swimming, tennis, jogging)

MET, metabolic equivalent.

metabolic equivalents (METs) and has been shown to correlate well with oxygen uptake by formal treadmill testing (Table 7.4). In patients who have moderate or better functionality (>4 METs) without symptoms, preoperative management is unlikely to be changed based on additional cardiac testing. In contrast, cardiac risk is increased in persons who are unable to meet a 4-MET demand, such as performing daily activities, and these patients may benefit from preoperative cardiac testing depending upon the magnitude of the planned procedure (Fig. 7.1). Once the provider has established the presence or absence of active cardiac conditions and the estimated risk of cardiovascular events, and assessed the patient's functional status, he or she can move to the **cardiac evaluation and care algorithm** to determine the need for and appropriateness of preoperative cardiac testing. This five-step approach provided as part of the contemporary 2014 guidelines, is as follows:

Step 1. *Is the planned procedure an emergency?* If so then the patient should proceed to the operating room (class I recommendation with level C evidence). In these cases, the situation does not allow for further cardiac assessment, and recommendations will focus on perioperative optimization with medications and monitoring and surveillance for cardiac events in the postoperative period. If the procedure is not emergent then the provider should proceed to the next step.

Step 2. *Does the patient have active cardiac conditions?* If so then these should be evaluated and treated prior to the planned procedure (class I recommendation with level B evidence). Consideration of proceeding with the operation may be given after these conditions have been evaluated and treated. If the patient does not have any identifiable active cardiac conditions, the provider should proceed to the next step.

Step 3. *What is the estimated risk based on combined clinical/surgical risk?* This step now combines the prior guidelines risk stratification by procedure risk, then by clinical risk factors. The updated RCRI added the risk of intrathoracic/abdominal or suprainguinal vascular operations. Yet, clinical judgment may be required for procedures previously considered "intermediate" risk. A list of procedures considered low, intermediate, and high risk is provided in Table 7.5 Does the patient have 0-1 RCRI predictors? If so then the patient with no active cardiac conditions should proceed to the planned surgery (class I recommendation with level B evidence). If the patient has ≥2 RCRI predictors, the provider should proceed to the next step.

Step 4. *Does the patient have moderate or better functional capacity (≥4 METs)?* If so then the patient with no active cardiac conditions and good functional capacity can proceed with surgery without additional cardiac testing (class I recommendation with level B evidence). If the patient has poor or unknown functional capacity (Table 7.4), the provider should proceed to the final step in the algorithm (Fig. 7.1).

Step 5. *Will further testing affect the extent or type of surgery or the perioperative care?* If the patient has poor or unknown functional capacity and no active cardiac conditions, and investigation of coronary perfusion will affect the magnitude of surgery offered, then noninvasive testing is recommended (class IIa recommendation with level B evidence). **This is particularly pertinent to vascular procedures as open, anatomic revascularization might be tempered to extraanatomic, hybrid, or endovascular procedures with less risk.**

TABLE 7.5	Estimates of Risk for Various Procedures

Low Risk
Diagnostic angiography
Basic extremity endovascular procedures

Intermediate Risk
Open carotid endarterectomy
Carotid artery stenting
Endovascular aneurysm repair
Open extremity bypass (femoral popliteal bypass)
Open extraanatomic bypass (axillobifemoral bypass)

High Risk
Open aortic reconstruction for aneurysm disease
Open aortic reconstruction for occlusive disease (aortobifemoral bypass)
Other major vascular surgery

It is noteworthy that two studies have failed to show a difference in outcome between patients who underwent additional cardiac testing versus those who proceeded to the operating room with optimal medical management in this situation. Yet, as noted, in patients with elevated risk with over two RCRI predictors, and poor functional capacity, additional cardiac testing is recommended if it will change the patient's management (class IIa recommendation with level B evidence). In patients with abnormal cardiac stress testing, coronary catheterization and revascularization should be considered and recommended accordingly (class I recommendation with level A evidence). As most vascular procedures are at least intermediate in risk, and options in operative approach many, combining clinical and procedural risk in Step #4 simplifies the approach to cardiac assessment for those undergoing vascular procedures. By definition, if a patient has undergone **previous** coronary revascularization, he or she has a history of ischemic heart disease, which is the first of the six RCRI risk factors. In such instances, if the revascularization was in the previous 5 years and the patient is asymptomatic with good functional status, then noninvasive cardiac testing is not recommended. If the revascularization is more than 5 years or if the patient is undergoing a high-risk vascular operation, then noninvasive cardiac testing should be considered if it will change the patient's perioperative management.

B. **Noninvasive cardiac testing** refers to those methods used to identify areas of myocardium at risk for ischemia and infarction during times of stress. The goal of these tests in relation to vascular patients who may be undergoing an invasive procedure is to recognize those who are asymptomatic and may be at high risk of adverse cardiac outcomes from otherwise undetected coronary disease. Generally, if such tests are positive, patients then undergo invasive coronary angiography to define the anatomy of the coronary arteries, which allows treatment either by percutaneous (**percutaneous transluminal coronary angioplasty**) or open surgical (**coronary artery bypass grafting; CABG**) means. Findings on cardiac testing may also allow for more intensive perioperative monitoring, safer anesthetic techniques, or even changing the operative plan from a high-risk open vascular operation to a less invasive intermediate-risk alternative (e.g., endovascular vs open; or extraanatomic bypass vs open aortic reconstruction). For simplicity's sake, noninvasive cardiac stress testing can be thought of in three main categories: **exercise stress testing, dobutamine stress echocardiography**, and **radionuclide myocardial perfusion**.

1. **Resting and exercise electrocardiogram (ECG) testing.** The resting 12-lead ECG provides good information relating to both perioperative events and long-term morbidity and mortality in patients with known CAD. An existing Q wave provides an estimate of left ventricular function, perioperative cardiac complications, and long-term mortality. The presence of either left ventricular hypertrophy or ST-segment depression on a preoperative 12-lead ECG has also been shown to predict adverse perioperative events. The 2014 guidelines suggest that preoperative resting 12-lead ECG is reasonable in patients who are undergoing vascular surgical procedures (class IIa recommendation, level B evidence). Generally, the ECG should be obtained within 30 days of the planned procedure.

   The use of a treadmill in combination with the 12-lead ECG (exercise stress ECG) provides much more information about a patient's functional capacity and risk of perioperative coronary events. Exercise ECG was pioneered by **Robert A. Bruce** while at the University of Washington in the early 1960s. Bruce is widely held as the "father of exercise cardiology" and the so-called **Bruce protocol** used during this test bears his name. This protocol has been extensively validated and consists of seven stages, each lasting 3 minutes resulting in 21 minutes of exercise for the complete test. During stage 1, the patient walks at 1.7 mph at a 10% incline; the speed and incline are increased for subsequent stages. There is a modified Bruce protocol that is commonly used in patients whose functional capacity does not allow completion of the full 21 minutes. **The goal during the protocol is for the patient to reach 85% of maximum predicted heart rate, which is roughly 220 (210 for women) minus the patient's age.** In clinical practice, patients rarely complete the entire 21-minute protocol, as most are unaccustomed to exercise. However, completion of 9 to 12 minutes of the protocol is adequate, providing that the patient reaches the 85% predicted maximum heart rate. The ability of the patient to reach this goal maximum heart rate is in itself a good prognostic sign. **Horizontal or downsloping ST-segment depression (≥2 mm) is the most reliable indicator of myocardial ischemia during the test.**

   The sensitivity of exercise ECG for detecting myocardial ischemia depends upon the extent of coronary occlusive disease. It has been shown that as many as 50% of patients with single vessel coronary disease who have good functional capacity will have a normal exercise ECG. In contrast, the sensitivity and specificity have been shown to be as high as 86% and 53%, respectively, in patients with multivessel disease. Exercise ECG is not appropriate for all patients and should not be performed in those with unstable angina, recent MI, or those with poorly controlled heart failure.

2. **Dobutamine stress echocardiography (DSE)** combines two-dimensional echocardiography with infusion of the pharmacologic agent, dobutamine, and has become an important tool to evaluate preoperative cardiac function in patients who are not candidates for exercise ECG. Echocardiography itself is a standard noninvasive ultrasound imaging modality of the heart, which is able to assess not only the structural components, such as the chambers and valves, but also the function and contractility of the myocardium (e.g., wall motion).

Even the resting or nonstress component of this exam is useful, as resting left ventricular ejection fraction and/or diastolic function have been shown to be important factors in estimating perioperative risk. Infusion of the β_1-receptor agonist dobutamine increases myocardial contractility and heart rate and therefore myocardial stress and oxygen demand. During this "stress" phase of the test, significant coronary artery occlusive lesions can be identified by regional wall abnormalities in the distribution of the affected coronary vessels. Simply put, the myocardium can be visualized as failing in areas where blood flow is restricted during stress. The negative predictive value of DSE has been shown consistently to be above 95%, meaning that patients with a normal exam have extremely low rates of perioperative myocardial events. Increasing experience with DSE has lead to its preference over radionuclide myocardial perfusion imaging in some centers, with studies suggesting that it has twice the sensitivity of other testing modalities. DSE is limited in certain patients in whom echocardiography does not provide good images of the heart. Additionally, dobutamine should not be used as a stressor in patients with serious arrhythmias, severe hypertension, or hypotension.

3. **Radionuclide myocardial perfusion imaging** is the third main category of preoperative cardiac testing methods. This modality uses nuclear medicine technology to assess the heart at rest and during stress induced by infusion of a pharmacologic agent. During a follow-up image or scan of the heart, hours after the baseline and stress images, this technique examines the heart muscle in the "recovered" or post–stress phase. Radionuclide perfusion imaging is accomplished by injection of a radionuclide or tracer into the patient, which is preferentially taken up by the myocardium. The tracer, usually technetium-99m sestamibi or thallium-201, emits small amounts of gamma rays detectable by a gamma camera or imager. Baseline images of the heart are obtained after injection of the tracer, which allows assessment of myocardial perfusion and determination of ejection fraction. A pharmacologic stressor, typically dipyridamole, adenosine, regadenoson, or dobutamine, is then administered to increase cardiac contractility and heart rate. Images are obtained during stress, and areas of myocardium that are malperfused or that fail during stress can be imaged and mapped. Four to six hours following the stress images, a scan is repeated to assess the areas of myocardium where the perfusion defects were visible. If the areas have returned to normal, the ischemia is termed **reversible ischemia** and attributed to a fixed coronary occlusive lesion or stenosis. These areas of myocardium in which reversible ischemia (RI) can be demonstrated are at risk and are felt to be critical during the perioperative period. If the areas remain without perfusion in the delayed imaging phase, the ischemia is termed **irreversible ischemia** and attributed to an area of the myocardium destroyed by a previous infarction. Areas of irreversible ischemia are not at risk and are felt to be less important during the acute perioperative period. Radionuclide perfusion imaging with stress has a high sensitivity (90% to 95%) for detecting patients at risk for perioperative cardiac events. The risk using this modality appears to be directly proportional to the amount of myocardium at risk, as reflected by the extent of reversible ischemia or RI. Body habitus, arrhythmias, and cardiomyopathies can limit nuclear stress testing. Rarely, false-negative results can occur in patients with ischemia in all coronary territories, as the tracer is equally diminished across zones. This is called "balanced ischemia."

To summarize, all the three categories of noninvasive cardiac testing are useful in identifying vascular patients at risk for perioperative cardiac events, and each has strengths and weaknesses. However, these tests should be used selectively in appropriate patients and only in instances where their findings will result in tangible changes in perioperative management (Fig. 7.1). In general, patients should be considered for coronary angiography only if they have active cardiac conditions or poor functional status, two or more RCRI predictors, and evidence of ischemia during noninvasive cardiac testing. As far as which test to employ, the experience and expertise of an institution's cardiac laboratory in this area plays an important role and may ultimately be as important as the particular type of test ordered.

C. Preoperative Coronary Revascularization. Following this selective approach, only about 5% of patients with peripheral vascular disease will undergo preoperative coronary angiography and some type of coronary revascularization, either open (e.g., CABG) or percutaneous (e.g., percutaneous coronary intervention [PCI]). Although revascularization prior to vascular procedures in patients with coronary disease seems inherently reasonable, the pathophysiology of perioperative cardiac morbidity limits its effectiveness. Specifically, a number of studies have shown that mild, nonobstructive coronary lesions may be just as important in causing myocardial infarction as high-grade stenoses or occlusions seen on coronary angiography. This fact stems from the dynamics of the atherosclerotic plaque, which is often independent of degree of stenosis. Even in sites of milder stenosis, an atherosclerotic plaque may become "unstable" and rupture, causing platelet aggregation and coronary thrombosis. This phenomenon suggests that preoperative revascularization may not reduce perioperative ischemic complications in all patients. This fact combined with the risks associated with coronary angiography, and revascularization has resulted in recent studies that support a very selective application of coronary revascularization to certain groups of patients.

An early publication from the CASS, which looked at outcomes in patients with both peripheral vascular and coronary occlusive disease, demonstrated short- and long-term benefits in those who received CABG prior to vascular intervention. Although favorable from the standpoint of preoperative revascularization, subgroup analysis suggested that the benefits were mostly limited to patients with three-vessel CAD and were inversely related to ejection fraction. This study and others like it, showing benefit of preoperative revascularization, have mostly been retrospective analyses; not until publication of the **CARP trial** has there been a randomized, prospective study comparing preoperative revascularization (CABG or PCI) versus no revascularization in vascular patients.

In CARP, roughly 500 patients were randomized to either coronary revascularization (n = 258; 141 PCI and 99 CABG) or no revascularization (n = 252). The study enrolled patients undergoing open aortic surgery or open lower-extremity revascularization for severe claudication or critical ischemia. Importantly, the study did not randomize the highest risk patients with left main coronary stenosis (>50%), severe aortic valve stenosis, or depressed ejection fraction (<20%). Conclusions from CARP found that among patients with stable cardiac symptoms, coronary artery revascularization prior to major elective vascular procedures can be done safely (1.7% mortality). However, preoperative revascularization does delay (median time 54 days), and in some cases prevents, the vascular operation (13% of coronary revascularization group did not undergo intended vascular operation). Finally, coronary artery revascularization in stable patients does not provide short-term benefit or improve long-term survival. Later, CARP registry and cohort subanalyses from all patients screened for enrollment, found that only in those with left main CAD, which was 4.6% of the group, did a statistical survival benefit occur with prevascular surgery coronary revascularization. CABG appeared to protect perioperative outcomes over PCI. Finally, recent prospective randomized trials from Europe have suggested in those undergoing aortic or carotid operations, preoperative coronary assessment and revascularization when indicated improved long-term survival and reduced cardiac morbidity.

The lack of clear benefit of preoperative revascularization is undoubtedly due in part to an increase in the use of beta-blockers, antiplatelet agents, ACE inhibitors, and statin medications. Emerging evidence is fairly clear that optimization of such medical therapy in the perioperative and long-term postoperative period decreases cardiovascular morbidity and mortality. It should be noted that despite the excellent findings of the CARP trial, the overall risk of early cardiac morbidity (8.4% early MI) and late mortality (23% mortality at 27 months) was still significant. **Although the clinical evidence relating to coronary revascularization prior to vascular procedures may seem conflicting or even confusing, adherence to the AHA/ACC guidelines offers the clinician the best opportunity to make solid, evidence-based decisions and provide optimal care.**

D. **Cardiac conduction abnormalities** must also be recognized and defined before any vascular procedure is performed. As was previously noted, current guidelines suggest that preoperative resting 12-lead ECG is reasonable in patients with no clinical risk factors who are undergoing vascular surgical procedures (class IIa recommendation, level B evidence). Performance of a resting 12-lead ECG within 30 days of the procedure will identify many of these conduction abnormalities. First-degree atrioventricular block, right or left bundle-branch block, and bifascicular or trifascicular blocks are usually chronic and seldom progress to complete heart block. Thus, temporary pacing is usually not required for these conduction disturbances. In contrast, patients with second-degree, Mobitz type II, or third-degree atrioventricular block should be evaluated for perioperative pacing support, as these disturbances are more serious and prone to progress to complete heart block. Whether such pacing is temporary or permanent largely depends upon the discretion of the cardiology and anesthesia consultants. Permanent pacemakers are usually required for complete heart block or intermittent complete heart block.

Patients with **implanted cardiac pacemakers** present unique challenges during vascular procedures, as electrocautery may adversely affect the pulse generator. To prevent this possibility, the rate of the pacemaker can be converted to a fixed-rate prior to the operation. Complexities involving the operation of pacemakers mandate that the vascular specialist consult with a cardiologist familiar with electrophysiology in order to establish a safe, yet rational, perioperative management plan.

II. **COEXISTING CAROTID OCCLUSIVE DISEASE.** This is present in 10% to 20% of patients with vascular disease of the aorta and/or extremities. Most often, this disease is asymptomatic and detected by the presence of a cervical bruit. In these instances, evaluation with duplex ultrasound is appropriate and has already been performed in many instances. Although the presence of coexisting carotid occlusive disease often raises concerns regarding an increased risk of periprocedural stroke, there is little evidence confirming this correlation, especially in asymptomatic patients. Furthermore, there is no clinical evidence that preemptive repair of carotid stenoses decreases the perioperative risk of stroke associated with vascular procedures. Even if the patient is found to have a high-grade asymptomatic carotid stenosis (>80%), the authors' recommended practice is generally to proceed with the planned aortic or extremity procedure. The carotid disease is then managed on its own merit in the weeks and months that follow.

Exceptions to this practice include **symptomatic carotid stenoses**, which should be repaired prior to other planned vascular procedures. Additionally, an asymptomatic high-grade lesion in the setting of a contralateral carotid occlusion may be considered for repair depending upon its appearance on duplex ultrasound and the planned vascular procedure. Finally, bilateral preocclusive lesions are often managed with this same consideration of preemptive repair; however, there are limited clinical data to guide the clinician in these cases. In some instances, patients with large or symptomatic aneurysms or limb-threatening ischemia of the leg must have these problems addressed urgently and sometimes accept a small but finite risk of perioperative stroke associated with the carotid disease.

III. **COEXISTING PULMONARY DISEASE**. This disease is a leading cause of postoperative morbidity and mortality, with many studies showing that pulmonary complications are at least as common as cardiac complications. Complicating this scenario is the fact that most patients undergoing vascular operation have some degree of chronic lung disease from smoking.

A. The initial **history and physical examination** will identify the patients at highest risk of pulmonary problems. They often are dyspneic at rest or with minimal exertion or exhibit chronic cough and sputum production. Other more advanced findings include a hyperinflated chest with distant breath sounds and use of accessory neck and abdominal muscles to assist with breathing. Patients with a component of reactive airway or bronchospasm may have wheezing. A simple bedside assessment of the degree of airway obstructive disease can be made by having the patient take a deep inspiration and then expire as quickly as possible while the examiner listens with a stethoscope. Normal complete expiratory time is less than 3 seconds; however, for patients with obstructive lung disease, this time is often 4 to 8 seconds. This simple bedside test also can be used to monitor clinical improvement during bronchodilator therapy.

B. A preprocedural **chest x-ray** (anterior-posterior and lateral projections) can provide insight into the chronicity and severity of obstructive lung disease and assess for evidence of lung cancer such as pulmonary nodules or effusions. Chest x-rays also provide a crude estimate of heart size and can be used to follow interstitial lung disease or identify blebs. The authors' practice is to have a new chest x-ray within a month of a procedure performed on active smokers and to insist that one has been performed within the prior 6 months in all others undergoing vascular operation.

C. **Pulmonary function testing** and measurement of **arterial blood gases** need not be routine but are indicated for patients in whom significant pulmonary disease is suspected. One of the most reliable predictors of high pulmonary risk is the forced expiratory volume at 1 second (FEV_1). Significant postoperative pulmonary complications can be expected in patients with an FEV_1 of less than 15 mL/kg or less than 1 L. If the FEV_1 is less than 70% of that predicted, the spirometry should be repeated after administration of an inhaled bronchodilator. An increase of at least 15% in FEV_1 indicates that preoperative bronchodilator therapy may enhance pulmonary function. This improvement may be especially important for the patient who has marginal lung function and requires elective surgery. Although measurement of arterial blood gases should not be routine, baseline values may help in patients with severe chronic obstructive pulmonary disease (COPD). For example, an elevated $PaCO_2$ (>45 mm Hg) is associated with increased perioperative pulmonary risk.

TABLE 7.6	Pulmonary Risk Reduction Strategies

Preoperative
Smoking cessation for at least 8 weeks
Treat airflow obstruction in patients with COPD or asthma (beta-agonist inhalers)
Antibiotic and delay elective surgery if respiratory infection is present
Patient education regarding lung expansion

Intraoperative
Limit duration of surgery to <3 hours
Use of epidural anesthesia
Substitute less invasive procedures when possible

Postoperative
Deep-breathing exercises or incentive spirometry
Continuous positive airway pressure if mechanically ventilated
Epidural anesthesia

COPD, chronic obstructive pulmonary disease.
(Adapted from Smetana GW. Preoperative pulmonary evaluation. *N Engl J Med*. 1999;340:937-944.)

D. Optimizing or improving pulmonary function (Table 7.6) in patients with chronic lung disease before the planned procedure can decrease the incidence of postoperative respiratory complications at least twofold. Preoperative preparation may require that the patient stop smoking, that antibiotics for bronchitis and bronchodilators be administered, and that the patient be instructed in deep breathing.

1. **Smoking cessation** for 8 weeks before any planned vascular procedure is ideal so that cilia regeneration within the lining of the lungs can occur and chronic cough (e.g., bronchorrhea) can resolve. Complete cessation is often difficult for many patients who are anxious before hospitalization, although most can be convinced to reduce cigarette consumption to some degree, which is also useful. A reasonable request is to reduce smoking to half a pack (10 cigarettes) per day, with a commitment to stop when admitted to the hospital. Often the planned vascular procedure can be used as a reason to initiate a formal smoking cessation program, which can be of significant help in the perioperative period as well as in the long term for the patient.

2. **Respiratory infections** in patients with COPD are most often caused by *Streptococcus* or *Haemophilus* species, and some type of penicillin antibiotic (e.g., ampicillin or amoxicillin) is effective treatment. Importantly, any respiratory infection must be adequately treated before elective surgery, even if this means delaying the procedure.

3. **Bronchodilators** remain the cornerstone of therapy for patients with COPD, and now are often combined with an inhaled form of steroid. However, we often find that vascular patients with known pulmonary disease are not receiving optimum doses of inhaled bronchodilators or may not be receiving the inhaled steroid component when they are being evaluated for a procedure. If the patient's reactive airway component is known to be significant, the inhaler regimen should be optimized preoperatively, in some instances by use of a nebulizer for a few days. Also, for patients with significant reactive airway disease, a short but high dose of oral steroids may be necessary in the perioperative period to improve (at least temporarily) the patient's pulmonary mechanics.

4. **Deep breathing maneuvers** with the incentive spirometer have been shown to decrease the incidence of pulmonary complications after open vascular procedures. Furthermore, the effectiveness of this adjunct has been shown to improve if the patient receives preoperative instruction, as opposed to waiting until the postoperative period to teach the method. The practice of sending the spirometer home with the patient days before the procedure is even advocated by some. In these instances, the patient can become familiar with the breathing technique and can initiate pulmonary exercises prior to the planned procedure. Avoiding perioperative pulmonary complications is multifactorial and includes nursing instruction, patient motivation, and early postoperative ambulation and adequate pain control.

IV. **COEXISTING KIDNEY DISEASE.** Kidney disease is commonly present in vascular patients and has been shown to be associated with a higher risk of periprocedural cardiac events. The relevance of renal dysfunction in the perioperative period is underscored by its inclusion as one of the clinical risk factors (Table 7.3). Preexisting renal disease (serum creatinine ≥2.0 mg/mL) has also been shown to be a risk factor for postoperative renal dysfunction and increased overall morbidity and mortality. **Estimated creatinine clearance,** which is a more accurate assessment of renal function, provides an approximation of glomerular filtration and has also been used to predict periprocedural morbidity and mortality. This method takes into account patient age and weight as well as serum creatinine levels in the following formula: **Estimated creatinine clearance = (140 − age [y] × weight [kg]) / (72 × serum creatinine [mg/dL])** *(multiply by 0.85 for women).* The normal range of estimated creatinine clearance is 55 to 145 mL/min/1.73 m^2 in men and 50 to 135 mL/min/1.73 m^2 in women.

A measure of renal function (either serum creatinine or creatinine clearance) should be checked routinely in vascular patients prior to any open or endovascular intervention. The authors' routine includes an assessment of renal function within 30 days of any vascular procedure. Depending upon the degree of renal dysfunction, protective measures may be taken or alterations made in the operative plan to account for this condition. One of the simplest adjuncts in patients with chronic renal disease is preprocedural hydration with crystalloid to establish a urine output of 0.5 to 1 cc/kg. Generally, this requires gentle hydration with 1 to 2 L of crystalloid in the hours before the planned procedure. Other specific renal protective strategies employed prior to and during endovascular procedures to minimize the harmful effects of contrast agents are discussed in Chapter 9.

V. **DIABETES MELLITUS.** This is the most common metabolic condition to occur in vascular patients, and its presence should increase suspicion for CAD. Additionally, perioperative cardiac events have been shown to occur more frequently in those with diabetes, and it too has been included as one of the clinical risk factors in the ACC/AHA guidelines (Table 7.3). Diabetes can be particularly difficult to manage in the perioperative period, when oral intake is varied and physiologic stress is high, resulting in a state of insulin resistance from increased levels of glucagon, epinephrine, and cortisol. Nonetheless, **hyperglycemia has been shown to be an independent risk factor for cardiovascular events, and the severity of hyperglycemia has been shown to be directly proportional to mortality during myocardial infarction.** In the perioperative period, blood glucose levels are typically managed with frequent blood sugar measurements and use of adjusted doses or infusions of short-acting insulin. Although blood sugar ranges of 150 to 250 mg/dL used to be acceptable, more recent evidence strongly supports a more aggressive approach in the perioperative period, using continuous intravenous insulin infusion to maintain blood glucose levels between 100 and 150 mg/dL. Specifically, the **American College of Endocrinology has provided a position statement recommending that preprocedural glucose concentrations should be less than 110 mg/dL, with maximal glucose not to exceed 180 mg/dL in hospitalized patients and that concentrations should be less than 110 mg/dL in patients in the intensive care unit.** While these strict ranges may not be achievable in all patients, this position statement emphasizes the importance of emerging clinical evidence in this area.

The **preoperative management** of the diabetic patient depends on the timing of the vascular procedure and whether the patient's usual therapy consists of insulin, an oral hypoglycemic, or both. The complicating factor is the fact that patients are kept without food or drink (e.g., nothing per mouth) prior to their procedure predisposing them to hypoglycemia. Patients who are insulin dependent and scheduled for their procedure early in the day (before 9 A.M.) should not take their insulin dose in the morning. They may be asked to bring their insulin with them if they are a morning admission. The blood sugar level is checked upon arrival and if greater than 100 mg/dL, the patient should receive one-half the usual intermediate-acting insulin dose. If the blood sugar is less than 100 mg/dL, the patient should receive a dextrose-containing solution once an intravenous line is established. Insulin-dependent patients who are scheduled for a procedure later in the day should be asked to take one-half the usual dose of intermediate-acting insulin instead of the full dose in the morning with whatever is allowed to be taken by mouth. Patients taking oral hypoglycemic agents should be advised not to take the oral agents in the morning of the vascular procedure.

The so-called brittle diabetic can have wide variations in blood sugar levels despite frequent glucose monitoring; in these patients, levels are optimally controlled with a continuous intravenous insulin drip. An infusion of 1 to 4 units of regular insulin per hour generally results in good control. In the acute postoperative period, various sliding scales of intravenous infusion rates (units/hour) exist, which allow the infusion of insulin to change according to blood glucose levels. **However, rare, severe, and sustained hypoglycemia can cause significant neurologic damage and is a particular risk related to the use of continuous insulin infusions.** To avoid inadvertent rapid insulin infusion, we recommend mixing only 10 units of regular insulin in 250 mL of D5W or D5NS and infusing at a rate of 25 to 100 mL/h (1 to 4 units) using an infusion pump. One should also infuse a dextrose-containing solution when using an insulin drip and have an ampule of high-concentration dextrose nearby for use should the patient become hypoglycemic.

Selected Readings

Beattie WS, Abdelnaem E, Wijeysundera DN, Buckley DN. A meta-analysis comparison of preoperative stress echocardiography and nuclear scintigraphy imaging. *Anesth Analg.* 2006;102:8-16.

Eagle KA, Rihal CS, Mickel MC, Holmes DR, Foster ED, Gersh BJ. Cardiac risk of non-cardiac surgery: influence of coronary disease and type of surgery in 3368 operations. CASS investigators and University of Michigan Heart Care Program. Coronary artery surgery study. *Circulation.* 1997;96:1882-1887.

Fleisher LA, Fleischmann KE, Auerbach AD, et al. 2014 ACC/AHA guideline on perioperative cardiovascular evaluation and management of patients undergoing noncardiac surgery. *J Am Coll Cardiol.* 2014;64:e77-e137.

Garcia S, Moritz TE, Ward HB, et al. Usefulness of revascularization of patients with multivessel coronary artery disease before elective vascular surgery for abdominal aortic and peripheral occlusive disease. *Am J Cardiol.* 2008;102:809-813.

Illuminati G, Schneider F, Greco C, et al. Long-term results of a randomized controlled trial analyzing the role of systematic pre-operative coronary angiography before elective carotid endarterectomy in patients with asymptomatic coronary artery disease. *Eur J Vasc Endovasc Surg.* 2015;49:366-374.

McFalls E, Ward H, Moritz T, et al. Coronary artery revascularization before elective major vascular surgery. *N Engl J Med.* 2004;351:2795-2804.

McFalls EO, Ward HB, Moritz TE, et al. Clinical factors associated with long-term mortality following vascular surgery: outcomes from the coronary artery revascularization prophylaxis (CARP) trail. *J Vasc Surg.* 2007;46:694-700.

Moghissi ES, Korytkowski MT, DiNardo M, et al. American Association of Clinical Endocrinologists and American Diabetes Association Consensus statement on inpatient glycemic control. *Diabetes Care.* 2009;32:1119-1131.

Monaco M, Stassano P, Di Tommaso L, et al. Systematic strategy of prophylactic coronary angiography improves long-term outcome after major vascular surgery in medium-to high-risk patients. *J Am Coll Cardiol.* 2009;54:989-996.

O'Neil-Callahan K, Katsimalis G, Tepper M, et al. Statins decrease perioperative cardiac complications in patients undergoing noncardiac vascular surgery. The statins for risk reduction in surgery (StaRRS) study. *J Am Coll Cardiol.* 2005;45:336-342.

Rihal CS, Eagle KA, Mickel MC, Foster ED, Sopko G, Gersh BJ. Surgical therapy for coronary artery disease among patients with combined coronary artery and peripheral vascular disease. Coronary Artery Surgery study (CASS) registry. *Circulation.* 1995;91:46-53.

Ward HB, Kelly RF, Thottapurathu L, et al. Coronary artery bypass grafting is superior to percutaneous coronary intervention in prevention of perioperative myocardial infarctions during subsequent vascular surgery. *Ann Thorac Surg.* 2006;82:795-801.

Perioperative Planning and Care of the Vascular Patient

Optimal care of the vascular patient in the operating room or endovascular suite requires a thorough understanding and awareness of details related to **monitoring**, patient **preparation and positioning**, and **anesthesia**. Attention to each of these areas ensures the best chance for a safe, technically successful procedure with the lowest risk of morbidity and mortality. Each vascular procedure, whether it is an open aneurysm repair in the operating room or a percutaneous lower extremity arteriogram in the imaging suite, requires a well thought-out and communicated plan. Optimal patient identification, planned procedure, and preparation and positioning should be accomplished through a "final time-out" or **operating room or endovascular suite briefing**. This step is important to ensure that all members of the care team are aware of the patient, the procedure, and surgical sight. The monitoring and anesthesia plans are especially relevant in transition to care of the patient in the postprocedure setting, which can be the recovery room, postanesthesia care unit (PACU), inpatient ward, or intensive care unit (ICU). This chapter emphasizes the principles of basic cardiac and respiratory monitoring, patient preparation and positioning, and anesthesia. An understanding of these should be of particular value to surgical house staff, nurses, and other vascular providers who are often the first into the operating room or endovascular suite and the first to recognize and treat problems during the postoperative period.

Operative Plan and Anesthesia

Improved anesthetic management has been a key factor in the reduction of perioperative morbidity and mortality in vascular and endovascular surgery. The preoperative assessment of the patient and his or her comorbidities form the basis for selecting the most appropriate anesthetic. The anesthesia team must be aware of the planned procedure and its conduct. The type and depth of anesthetic varies widely among the range of vascular and endovascular procedures to be performed. Therefore, for the smooth conduct of any vascular or endovascular operation, regardless of level of complexity, communication between the vascular and anesthesia providers must begin before the start of the case and continue throughout.

Clinical examples that emphasize the need for communication include the **requirement for patients undergoing certain endovascular procedures to remain fully awake and directable** during a given procedure. In these instances, patients may need to remain still, hold their breath, or have neurologic evaluation during the procedure (e.g., during carotid arteriography or stenting). Any sedation in such cases may be too much and result in an overly sedated, noncooperative patient and a suboptimal procedure. The **effectiveness of regional anesthesia for certain extremity procedures** also needs to be discussed ahead of time to avoid placement of a peripheral nerve block or regional anesthetic that does not fully anesthetize the planned area of operation (e.g., nerve block that anesthetizes the forearm and hand when the planned operation is the upper arm and axilla). And finally, the

anesthesia team must be aware of specific aspects of the procedure, open or endovascular, that are most stressful to cardiac, cerebral, respiratory, and renal function in order to manage the patient effectively.

I. **PERIOPERATIVE PHYSIOLOGIC MONITORING.** provides clinical data critical to assessment and maintenance of cardiac, respiratory, neurologic, and renal function during and after any open or endovascular procedure. The magnitude of the procedure and the patient's medical condition determine the extent of monitoring, and it should be recognized that in some instances, the information gathered may be misleading or imprecise and may not influence the overall outcome of the patient. It is important to understand the limitations of monitoring and use only techniques and devices that will provide useful or actionable information.

A. **Basic Intravenous Access and Monitoring.** All patients should have at least one sizable (16- or 18-gauge) intravenous line as well as electrocardiographic (ECG), temperature, and blood pressure monitoring. A urinary catheter and collection system to measure urine output may be needed for operations that last longer than a few hours or endovascular interventions that require the patient to remain supine for several hours following the procedure.

B. **Pulse oximeters**, which attach to a finger or toe, are used to measure arterial oxygen saturation of hemoglobin. Pulse oximetry functions by positioning a pulsating arterial vascular bed between a two-wavelength light source and a detector. A familiar plethysmograph waveform results. Because the detected pulsatile waveform is produced from arterial blood, the amplitude of each wavelength is related to reduced versus oxidized or oxyhemoglobin and allows continuous beat-to-beat calculation of oxygen saturation. The instrument's ability to calculate saturation can be impaired by hypothermia, hypotension, and vasopressor medications. The placement of an additional pulse oximeter probe on another site in these instances is recommended (at the alternate extremity or a more central location such as ear or nose).

C. **Arterial and Central Venous Access.** More significant open vascular operations or cases in which the patient's blood pressure can be expected to be labile may require an indwelling radial artery line, and occasionally a central venous catheter. The arterial line allows easier blood sampling for measurements of arterial blood gas, hematocrit, electrolytes, and glucose, as well as continuous blood pressure tracings. The central venous line allows measurement of central venous pressure (CVP) and infusion of resuscitative fluids and medications at a more brisk rate, depending upon the size of the catheter or sheath.

D. Pulmonary capillary wedge pressure measured with a **Swan-Ganz pulmonary artery (PA) catheter** is a guide to left-sided (left atrium and left ventricle) filling pressures and even left ventricular function. The PA catheter also allows the measurement of cardiac output and mixed venous oxygen saturations (Svo_2) as an indicator of oxygen delivery and end-organ extraction. Although some anesthesia providers prefer a PA catheter in all major open vascular cases, their routine use has greatly diminished as several studies have shown that they do not improve patient outcome. As such, **selective use of PA catheters for patients with ventricular dysfunction, significant valvular disease, unstable angina, or recent myocardial infarction who require open vascular surgery on an urgent or compelling basis is recommended.** If there is question about the need for a PA catheter, the surgeon and anesthesia provider should discuss the indications in the context of the overall operative plan. Figure 8.1 illustrates the pressure tracings as the Swan-Ganz catheter is floated through the right heart to a wedge

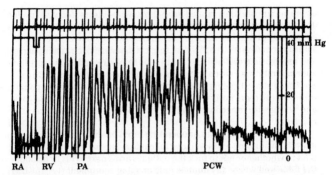

FIGURE 8.1 Swan-Ganz pulmonary catheter tracings as the catheter is advanced from the right atrium (RA) through the right ventricle (RV) and pulmonary artery (PA) to a wedged position in a pulmonary artery (PCW). The pressures shown are within normal limits. Abnormal values are discussed in the text.

position in a PA. Although there are complications related to the use of PA catheters, most of the risks are incurred in the process of obtaining central venous access.

Oximetric PA catheters allow continuous monitoring of Svo₂, which is an early indicator of change in the patient's physiologic well-being. SvO₂ may be used to assess the effectiveness of a specific intervention, with a decrease in saturation indicating worsening oxygen delivery (e.g., myocardial infarction) or increased end-organ extraction (e.g., sepsis). An SvO₂ of less than 60% indicates physiologic compromise and should prompt a reevaluation of the patient, to find the source or explanation. The SvO₂ can be followed as an early measure of treatment success such as the response to administration of an inotropic agent. Oximetric PA catheters are more expensive than the standard PA catheters and should only be placed in cases where such physiologic detail will be used. **Despite the physiologic information that this technology provides, the value of using PA catheters is debatable, as some prospective studies have shown that their use does not improve mortality.**

E. **Transesophageal echocardiography (TEE)** is another option for monitoring cardiac function in the operating room. TEE is a sensitive method to detect myocardial ischemia manifest by the development of **myocardial wall motion abnormalities** and can accurately assess left ventricular filling and function (e.g., ejection fraction).

F. **Core temperature monitoring** is important for open aortic or extremity vascular cases that last for more than 2 to 3 hours. Hypothermia (<35°C) is associated with risk for cardiac events, including ventricular tachycardia related to elevated levels of circulating catecholamines. In addition, hypothermia contributes to coagulopathy by adversely affecting the enzymes that participate in the clotting cascade. Esophageal, intravenous, or bladder temperature monitors are all generally accurate. Warming the operating room to 75°F before the patient enters and using warm air plastic drapes (Bair Hugger, Augustine Medical, Inc., Eden Prairie, MN) are helpful measures to maintain the patient's core temperature.

II. **PATIENT POSITIONING AND OPERATING ROOM BRIEFING.** Positioning the patient on the operating or endovascular table is critical and should occur as part of the **final time-out** or **operating room briefing.** This preparatory step assures that the members of the team know each other as well as the patient and the planned procedure, including its stepwise conduct. The surgical site and procedure are reviewed and critical steps and necessary equipment are anticipated among the key players in the room: **surgeon or endovascular specialist, surgical assistant(s), circulating nurse(s),** and **anesthesia provider(s).** Optimally, this briefing is led by the surgeon or endovascular specialist and occurs with all present at the same time. The operating room briefing program has been shown to serve in conjunction with the more basic and familiar "time-out" to reduce wrong patient and wrong site procedures and improve patient safety and procedural efficiency.

Once the final time-out or operating room briefing has occurred, final patient positioning and setup can take place. Special attention should be paid to whether or not to tuck the patient's arms next to his or her side on the table and where any fluoroscopic imaging equipment (i.e., the c-arm or wall-mounted imaging arm) will be positioned during the procedure. Again, anticipation and planning before the final preparation and draping are important for a safe, effective, and efficient procedure.

In addition to positioning for proper retraction and/or fluoroscopic imaging, patient positioning has been shown to be critical in avoiding pressure-related injuries to the skin and peripheral nerves in certain susceptible areas. The most common pressure-related problems in the authors' experience have been lateral heel and malleolus ulcers. These ulcers are multifactorial and often occur in patients with lower extremity ischemia who undergo longer duration procedures. Pressure-related heel ulcers can be prevented by elevating the legs on soft towels so that the heels do not rest directly on the operating table or by placing soft eggcrate padding under the heels themselves. Attention should also be paid to the lateral leg to assure no undue pressure over the fibular head leading to peroneal neuropraxia. Another potential problem occurs when the upper extremities are tucked along the sides of the patient and pressure from the edge of the operating table compresses the ulnar nerve, causing a neuropraxia. This bothersome problem can be prevented by gently wrapping the elbow region with a soft eggcrate pad to protect the ulnar nerve.

Positioning of the head, eyes, ears, and neck should also be performed with care. Patients with carotid disease or musculoskeletal conditions such as arthritis may be susceptible to injury secondary to poor positioning. Gentle positioning of the neck in the neutral position is best when possible, and the eyelids should be gently taped closed to avoid corneal abrasions. Limitations of range of motion involving the neck or extremities should be noted before patient positioning, and movement after induction of anesthesia should not involve motion beyond these limits. The risk of injury to the skin can be minimized by accounting for ECG leads, catheter connectors, or three-way stopcocks and jewelry that may be in contact with the patient's skin. In addition, the patient's skin should not be directly exposed to metal.

III. **ANESTHETIC PLAN FOR AORTIC SURGERY.** The determinants of safe anesthesia for an aortic operation (endovascular or open) include careful control of the patient's blood pressure, intravascular volume, and myocardial performance within context of the patient's baseline cardiac risk. As these patients commonly have coronary artery disease or some degree of heart failure, the onset of new tachycardia, anemia, or extremes of blood pressure as a result of the procedure can result in myocardial ischemia and infarction or a dangerous arrhythmia. Therefore, the anesthesia team must be aware of the basic sequence of the operation and each step's hemodynamic consequences. The surgeon must also be aware of organ system performance during the operation (e.g., tachycardia or oliguria), as this provides insight into the management of these systems in the postoperative period. Some of the most useful information regarding the patient's physiologic responses can be gained during the operation. Furthermore, the surgeon must understand how the anesthesia team manages the patient during critical parts of the operation and be willing to contribute information that he or she deems important.

Anesthesia options for aortic operations include use of a **regional technique (e.g., epidural or spinal), a mixed regional and general technique, or a general anesthetic technique**. The selection of anesthetic is of course influenced by type of aortic surgery—open or endovascular. All open aortic cases require a general anesthetic, which can be performed as the sole method or augmented by addition of an epidural. Endovascular aneurysm repair (EVAR) can be performed under an epidural anesthetic alone, although some surgeons prefer general anesthesia in these cases to allow for more direct control of the patients' respiratory status. Local anesthesia and conscious sedation is used for percutaneous aortic interventions and has been described as feasible for select patients undergoing EVAR.

The mixed technique is most common with open aortic cases and consists of general anesthesia and intubation supplemented with a continuous epidural anesthesia using a mixture of local anesthetics (e.g., bupivacaine) and narcotics (e.g., fentanyl). Epidural catheters are safe in vascular patients and can be used in those who will receive heparin as part of the procedure, but only after the epidural catheter has been placed (i.e., only use heparin once the epidural catheter has been placed). In these cases, the heparin is held for several hours before and after the time of catheter removal to reduce the incidence of epidural or subdural hematomas. These complications are rare, especially in instances where an atraumatic epidural puncture and catheter placement were made at the start of the anesthetic.

It is important to remember that epidural anesthesia with local anesthetics may cause peripheral vasodilation and reduced blood pressure, requiring administration of intravenous volume or vasopressors to compensate and raise the blood pressure. The use of a mix of narcotics and local anesthetics or just narcotics for the epidural in such cases usually alleviates this sometimes challenging response. The authors have also found that a continuous epidural narcotic infusion is a safe and effective method of controlling postoperative pain for 48 to 72 hours after open abdominal or lower extremity operations. It also assists in pulmonary dynamics and toilet. General endotracheal anesthesia may offer the greatest control of the hemodynamics and respiratory system for patients with significant pulmonary and cardiac disease.

A. **Unexplained hypotension** during aortic surgery (open or endovascular) must be met with a calm but rapid assessment of the patient for possible causes.

1. **Palpation of the aorta or transduction of femoral sheath pressures** should be performed to confirm the anesthesia monitor's initial indication. If there is a strong aortic pulse or normal pressures transduced through the femoral access sheaths, attention should be focused on the monitoring systems (e.g., compression or occlusion of the arterial line).

2. **Bleeding from endovascular access vessel** can occur during placement of device sheaths through the iliac vessels and even at the aortic bifurcation. The diagnosis of iliac or aortic perforation can be accomplished by performing flush aortography or retrograde angiography through the femoral sheaths. If there is a high suspicion that perforation of an access vessel is responsible for hypotension, a compliant balloon and covered stent should be quickly readied on the back table as the diagnostic maneuvers are performed.

3. **Myocardial infarction or arrhythmia** should be indicated by findings on ECG or TEE.
4. **Tension pneumothorax** resulting from preoperative central venous line placement will be accompanied by distended neck veins and high airway pressures shown on the anesthesia machine's ventilator.
5. **Cardiac tamponade** from right atrial injury during preoperative line placement will also be accompanied by distended neck veins but more normal airway pressures initially.
6. **Malignant hyperthermia** is a rare but serious complication accompanied by increases in end-tidal CO_2 and in the patient's core temperature. It may also be accompanied by mixed acidosis, increased O_2 consumption with decreased Svo_2, and rhabdomyolysis.
7. **Manipulation or withdrawal of the intestines** from the abdomen during open aortic surgery may also cause hypotension, which usually can be corrected with a fluid bolus or a one-time dose of ephedrine or a phenylephrine.
8. **Blood pressure may also decrease when the inferior vena cava is compressed or retracted** secondary to decreased venous return to the heart (preload); the surgeon should inform the anesthesia team prior to performing this maneuver.

B. **One of the most stressful steps for the myocardium** during aortic operations is occluding the aorta with a vascular clamp during open operations, or with an endovascular balloon during endovascular procedures (i.e., EVAR). This maneuver acutely increases left ventricular afterload and strain and can cause supranormal pressures in the aortic arch and cerebral circulation. Aortic occlusion, whether from a clamp or an endovascular balloon, increases blood pressure and pulmonary capillary wedge pressure, which may result in ST-segment changes or ventricular irritability on the ECG monitor. The healthy heart can tolerate these changes fairly well; however, the diseased heart is at higher risk. In the case of a severely impaired heart, the blood pressure and cardiac output may actually decrease with placement aortic occlusion. In such cases, and in an apparent paradoxical step, titration of peripheral vasodilators is necessary to reduce afterload acutely. Inotropic support should also be added if necessary to stabilize the hemodynamics. For these reasons, it is imperative that the surgical and anesthesia teams communicate regarding the timing and positioning of the aortic cross-clamp or balloon and its release.

With aortic occlusion, renal blood flow and urine output is likely to decrease, even if the aortic clamp or balloon is below the renal arteries. This effect can often be mitigated by establishing a diuresis before the aortic occlusion using hydration and on occasion, administration of intravenous mannitol (12.5 to 25 g). The preoperative central venous, pulmonary wedge pressure and left ventricular function should also be considered to confirm the patient is adequately hydrated prior to initiating this type of a diuresis. If mannitol is not effective, 10 to 20 mg of furosemide may also be given, although this decision should be discussed between the surgical and anesthesia teams before giving the medication. During any diuresis, potassium and other electrolyte levels must be carefully monitored and supplemented to prevent arrhythmias that result from their depletion.

C. **Blood loss**
1. **Significant blood loss** may occur during open aortic operations when the aneurysm sac is opened as a result of brisk back-bleeding from lumbar arteries and the inferior mesenteric artery. Here again, the anesthesia team should be made aware of this operative maneuver so they may anticipate the need for increased volume resuscitation, including administration of blood and blood products, while this maneuver is performed and these vessels are oversewn.

2. **Blood loss can be substantial** enough during open aortic cases to require transfusion. The alternative to banked blood transfusion is **autotransfusion**, which can be accomplished by use of the cell saver device set up at the beginning of the case. Dilutional coagulopathy may occur after 4 to 6 units of blood are transfused and platelets and clotting factors (fresh frozen plasma—FFP) must be given to the patient in this scenario. The use of the **thromboelastogram (TEG)** can also provide a qualitative analysis of the ability of the blood to clot, which can be used to guide specific factor replacement. Empiric transfusion of blood products in anticipation of aortic clamp removal can be performed but should be carefully considered. FFP and platelets may be especially important when the newly positioned aortic graft is opened, as any coagulopathy may result in problematic anastomotic or retroperitoneal bleeding. The threshold hemoglobin level to begin transfusion should be determined on a patient-by-patient basis depending upon the severity of underlying disease and type of operation performed. **The surgeon and anesthesia team should communicate regularly about the transfusion of blood and blood products.**

D. **Fluid Replacement.** Throughout the aortic procedure, adequate amounts of fluid, usually crystalloids such as normal saline or Ringer's lactate, should be given. Fluid replacement should be guided by indices of ventricular filling, maintenance of a good cardiac index, and adequate urine output (at least 0.5 cc/kg/h). It is not uncommon for crystalloid to be administered at rates up to 750 to 1,000 mL/h during open aortic procedures due to evaporative fluid loss from exposed bowel and associated blood loss. Because patients are prone to becoming hypothermic during long operations, crystalloids and blood products should be warmed as they are infused. In addition, hypothermia can be prevented by using a heating tent (Bair Hugger) and by increasing the operating room temperature.

E. **One of the Most Critical Times of an aortic operation is Release of the Aortic Clamp or Deflation of an Aortic Occlusion Balloon.** This maneuver rapidly decreases cardiac afterload and can lead to profound hypotension. The surgeon should prepare the anesthesia team several minutes before unclamping or balloon deflation, and the aortic occlusion should be released slowly while the surgeon views the arterial blood pressure tracing. If significant hypotension occurs, the clamp can be partially or completely reapplied or the compliant balloon reinflated while resuscitation is achieved. Hypotension can be minimized by intravascular volume loading, avoidance of myocardial depressants, and vasodilators, as well as inhalation anesthetic agents prior to clamp release or balloon deflation. In some cases, small amounts of sodium bicarbonate will be beneficial; the authors generally give intravenous calcium chloride, which increases myocardial contractility and blood pressure. **If one reverses heparin with protamine at the end of the operation, it must be administered slowly (e.g., use an initial test dose), as it can cause hypotension or bradycardia.** In rare cases, protamine may lead to severe bronchospasm and hemodynamic instability.

IV. **CAROTID ARTERY SURGERY.** Anesthesia for carotid artery interventions (open or endovascular) must be administered carefully to avoid wide variations in blood pressure and cerebral perfusion. Additionally, it is necessary to avoid oversedation in cases where patients need to be awake in order to assess their neurologic status. In addition to **general anesthesia** for carotid interventions, options include **cervical block** for awake, open carotid operations and simple **local anesthetic with mild sedation** for carotid artery stenting (CAS).

The common clinical concern during any carotid intervention is cerebral perfusion and neurologic evaluation. During both awake, open carotid operations and CAS, it is important for the patient to be communicative and directable to assess neurologic status as a marker of adequate cerebral perfusion. Too much sedation during these cases can result in the inability to determine whether the patient's decreased neurologic status is due to the anesthetic or to the carotid intervention. During carotid interventions, the surgeon must understand basic control mechanisms for cerebral blood flow, methods of monitoring cerebral perfusion, and the effects of different anesthetic agents on cerebral metabolism.

A. **Cerebral Blood Flow.** There are four major determinants of cerebral blood flow in the normal brain.

    1. **Local metabolic factors.** Accumulation of local metabolic products causes vasodilation of blood cerebral vessels as part of normal autoregulation and increases local intracerebral flow.

    2. **Arterial oxygen tension (Pao_2).** Within wide limits, Pao_2 does not significantly influence cerebral blood flow.

    3. **Arterial carbon dioxide tension ($Paco_2$)** affects cerebral blood flow throughout its physiologic range. As $Paco_2$ is decreased, cerebral blood flow decreases, and vice versa. This effect is mostly acute and diminishes with time.

    4. **Cerebral perfusion pressure** (mean arterial pressure minus intracranial pressure or venous pressure). Within wide ranges of perfusion pressure, cerebral flow is maintained in a steady state by autoregulation of the cerebral vessels.

        In diseased states, these control mechanisms are altered. Autoregulation is altered so that the acceptable mean arterial pressure is different and the point at which autoregulation becomes lost is also altered. Blood vessels in an ischemic brain are maximally vasodilated and therefore blood flow becomes a direct function of perfusion pressure (i.e., mean arterial pressure). If clamping or balloon occlusion of the carotid artery is necessary during a given procedure, having the anesthesia team work to maintain normotension to slightly elevate the patient's mean arterial pressure should optimize overall cerebral perfusion (despite the carotid clamping or balloon occlusion) via collateral routes, including the contralateral carotid and vertebral arteries.

B. **Monitoring.** There are at least three methods to assess adequate cerebral perfusion during carotid cross-clamping or balloon occlusion:

    1. Awake patient who has no neurologic changes during the operative carotid occlusion maneuver (cross-clamp or balloon occlusion)

    2. A normal electroencephalogram (EEG) that does not change with carotid operative occlusion maneuver

    3. Measurement of carotid artery stump pressures as a reflection of overall maintained cerebral perfusion

    4. These methods as well as the indications for use of a temporary vascular shunt during open carotid endarterectomy are described in greater detail in Chapter 12.

C. **Types of Anesthesia and Anesthetic Agents.** The goals of anesthesia for carotid surgery include maintaining consistent blood pressure, regulation of the patient's $Paco_2$ to maximize oxygenation to any ischemic brain, and smooth emergence from general anesthesia for neurologic examination in the operating room. **General anesthesia** during open carotid operations is preferred by some surgeons and may afford more direct control of the patient's blood pressure and the patient's airway and therefore ventilatory status. General anesthesia is also preferred by some who are leading carotid operations in a teaching setting, where the length of the operative case may be slightly longer and instructional comments made more openly. One of the most common general anesthetic techniques for carotid surgery is **balanced anesthesia** of barbiturates, nitrous oxide, narcotics, and muscle relaxants. Volatile agents and barbiturates may offer some protection against ischemia because cerebral oxygen demand is reduced.

In contrast, some surgeons prefer **local or regional anesthesia** for awake, open carotid operations as a safe technique that allows immediate detection of neurologic change when the carotid artery is clamped. This technique avoids the potential cardiodepressant effects of general anesthesia and may afford patients a quicker recovery. Studies and years of experience have shown no difference in complication rates or recovery times between the two types of anesthetic approaches used during carotid endarterectomy.

Volatile anesthetics are generally considered to be cerebral vasodilators, with halothane being the most potent and isoflurane the least. In contrast, most of the intravenous anesthetic agents lead to some degree of cerebral vasoconstriction. Any real or clinically significant effects these agents have on cerebral perfusion are difficult to predict and, as a result, the choice of one versus another type of anesthetic is less important than maintaining a normal to slightly elevated **mean arterial blood pressure** during the time of carotid clamping or balloon occlusion. The ability of either volatile or intravenous agents to suppress metabolism and provide cerebral protection occurs only at anesthetic depths that could impair hemodynamic stability. Halothane can cause hypotension and myocardial depression. Deep anesthesia with a volatile agent such as halothane may also increase intracranial pressure and promote intracerebral blood flow steal from at risk or ischemic areas. Prevention of ischemia with direct augmentation of cerebral perfusion either by increasing the mean arterial pressure or placing a temporary vascular shunt is likely more beneficial than any attempt with anesthetics to prolong the brain's tolerance to ischemia.

V. **LOWER EXTREMITY ARTERIAL RECONSTRUCTIONS.** Lower extremity arterial reconstructions can be performed using either **general anesthesia** or **regional anesthesia** alone, or **mixed general and regional anesthesia**. Simple, **local anesthesia with sedation** may also be used for percutaneous lower extremity interventions. The choice depends upon on whether the case is open or endovascular, patient comorbidities, and anesthesia and surgeon experience and preference. In our experience, continuous epidural anesthesia is an acceptable method for open femoral popliteal bypass grafting, including instances of a concomitant retrograde iliac stent placement (i.e., hybrid open and endovascular procedure). In the early postoperative period, the epidural catheter can be left in place for a limited period of time to achieve postprocedure pain relief.

The indication and appropriateness of a regional technique should be decided by the anesthesia team in consultation with the vascular providers. The surgeon should provide input on the choice of anesthetic and its potential ramifications. The individual patient's acceptance of and ability to safely have a regional anesthetic must also be considered. Factors such as dementia, risk of pulmonary aspiration, and previous back or spine injury may decrease the advisability of a regional technique. The use of regional anesthesia in patients receiving anticoagulation or antiplatelet therapy remains unsettled and decisions are often based on an individual patient's situation. Although most studies reveal low complication rates of epidural anesthesia placed in association with antiplatelet therapy or low molecular weight heparin, the risk is not zero. Because bleeding complications in this setting can lead to significant morbidity, the authors defer to their anesthesia colleagues on a case-by-case basis as to which patients are candidates for epidural anesthesia. Once an epidural catheter is in place, this same expertise is needed to determine the need to hold antiplatelet or anticoagulation medications before and around the time of catheter removal.

Anesthesia for acute lower extremity ischemia, such as in the instance of an arterial embolism, is often complicated, as these cases tend to occur in critically ill patients at high risk for general anesthesia. If necessary, exposure of the femoral artery and performance of a thromboembolectomy can be accomplished using local anesthesia. However, general anesthesia is preferred for most cases of acute lower extremity ischemia because they may require a longer time period to restore perfusion to the diseased extremity. This is especially true in cases requiring intraoperative arteriograms, arterial bypasses, or fasciotomy as part of treating the acutely ischemic lower extremity.

VI. **LOWER EXTREMITY VENOUS PROCEDURES.** The majority of lower extremity venous cases are performed using local anesthesia. Larger cases that involve removal of the great saphenous vein and or large superficial varicose veins may benefit from a regional or general anesthetic, but these cases are less common. Local tumescent anesthesia with or without an oral anxiolytic such as diazepam is all that is necessary to perform basic endovenous ablation of the saphenous vein with laser or radiofrequency. In the authors' experience, even most open venous operations, such as stab phlebectomy and high ligation and removal of the saphenous vein, can be accomplished with local anesthesia and intravenous conscious sedation. Here again, communication between the vascular provider and the person or persons providing anesthesia is essential. Communication and planning can often optimize use of local anesthetic with conscious sedation and reduce the need and therefore the small risk associated with epidural or spinal anesthesia. Patient, surgeon, and anesthesia experience and preference play a large role in the decision as to the optimal method in these cases.

Selected Readings

Brewster DC, O'Hara PJ, Darling RC, et al. Relationship of intraoperative EEG monitoring and stump pressure measurements during carotid endarterectomy. *Circulation.* 1980;62(suppl 1):I4-I7.

Bush HL Jr, Hydo LJ, Fischer E, et al. Hypothermia during elective abdominal aortic aneurysm repair: the high price of avoidable morbidity. *J Vasc Surg.* 1995;21:392-402.

Clagett GP, Valentine RJ, Jackson MR, et al. A randomized trial of intraoperative autotransfusion during aortic surgery. *J Vasc Surg.* 1999;29:22-31.

Cullen ML, Staren ML, el-Ganzouri A, et al. Continuous epidural infusion for analgesia after major abdominal operations: a randomized, prospective, double blind study. *Surgery.* 1985;98:718-728.

Ereth MH, Oliver WC Jr, Santrach PJ. Perioperative interventions to decrease transfusion of allogeneic blood products. *Mayo Clin Proc.* 1994;69:575-586.

Frank SM, Fleisher LA, Breslow MJ, et al. Perioperative maintenance of normothermia reduces the incidence of morbid cardiac events. A randomized clinical trial. *JAMA.* 1997;277:1127-1134.

Lilly MP, Gopal K. Intraoperative management. In: Cronenwett JL, Johnston KW, eds. *Rutherford's Vascular Surgery.* Philadelphia: Elsevier; 2014.

Makary MA, Mukherjee BA, Sexton JB, et al. Operating room briefings and wrong-site surgery. *J Am Coll Surg.* 2007;204(2):236-243.

Mannucci PM. Hemostatic drugs. *N Engl J Med.* 1998;339:245-253.

Massimo F, Mannucci PM. Adjunct agents for bleeding. *Curr Opin Hematol.* 2014;21:503-508.

Sandham JD, Hull RD, Brant RF, et al. A randomized, controlled trial of the use of pulmonary artery catheters in high-risk surgical patients. *N Engl J Med.* 2003;348:5-14.

Valentine RJ, Duke ML, Inman MH, et al. Effectiveness of pulmonary artery catheters in aortic surgery: a randomized trial. *J Vasc Surg.* 1998;27:203-212.

Wiklund RA, Rosenbaum SH. Anesthesiology. First of two parts. *N Engl J Med.* 1997;337:1132-1141.

Wiklund RA, Rosenbaum SH. Anesthesiology. Second of two parts. *N Engl J Med.* 1997;337:1215-1219.

Youngberg JA, Lake CL, Roizen MF, et al, eds. *Cardiac, Vascular and Thoracic Anesthesia.* Philadelphia: Churchill Livingstone; 2000.

9 Indications and Preparation for Angiography

Angiography is the direct intravascular administration of radiographic contrast agent or dye in order to gain anatomic information about a particular blood vessel or group of blood vessels. **Arteriography** is defined as angiography of the arterial system, and **venography** is angiographic imaging of the veins. Historically, angiography has mostly served a diagnostic purpose, providing a road map to guide appropriate surgical intervention. In current vascular practice, there has been a remarkable increase in the number of minimally invasive techniques to treat disease and injury from within the vessel lumen—the so-called **endovascular procedures**. As many are performed using small wires and catheters, another commonly used term for these techniques is **catheter-based procedures**. Common endovascular procedures are balloon angioplasty, stenting, stent-graft repair, embolization, and catheter-directed thrombolysis. A number of vascular specialties are trained in angiography and endovascular procedures including interventional radiology, cardiology, and vascular surgery. A more appropriate term for a physician performing endovascular procedures is a "**vascular interventionalist**" or "**endovascular specialist**."

I. **INDICATIONS.** Nearly every vessel in the body can be imaged with angiography by a motivated and skilled vascular interventionalist. However, the indications for angiography are just as important as the skills required to perform the procedure. Even the simplest angiographic procedures carry risk to the vessels being imaged and to the patient as a whole. Therefore, *angiography should not be undertaken without clear and appropriate indications.* History, physical exam, and noninvasive vascular tests are often sufficient to make the diagnosis of vascular disease (Chapters 3 to 5). The indications for extremity, cerebrovascular, renal, and mesenteric arteriography are discussed in detail in their respective chapters. In general, angiography should only be employed **when the additional anatomic information will clearly affect the clinical management of the patient.**

Informed consent for angiography includes an explanation of the indications, alternative methods of diagnosis, and potential complications. Patients should understand that angiography can be either diagnostic or therapeutic and that, in general, solely diagnostic angiograms are becoming less common given the improved imaging capability of noninvasive modalities (duplex, computed tomography angiogram [CTA], and magnetic resonance arteriography [MRA]). Additionally, endovascular treatments are often possible in the same setting as the diagnostic angiogram following the diagnostic aspect of the case. Angiography remains a preferred diagnostic modality for some specific vascular emergencies, such as acute mesenteric or limb ischemia, and can also help solve certain diagnostic dilemmas.

The objective and potential outcomes of the angiogram should be understood from the outset and explained to the patient. The patient should understand that attempts at diagnosing and/or treating the condition with noninvasive modalities have been exhausted and that angiography is necessary for clinical decision-making. We generally inform patients undergoing a lower extremity arteriogram for chronic limb ischemia of three possible outcomes of the procedure:

1. Diagnostic information leading to an endovascular therapy during the same case or at a later date
2. Diagnostic information that will provide information for the performance of an open operation at a later date
3. Diagnostic information leading to no further intervention due to disease pattern, severity, or patient condition

The decision to proceed with endovascular or surgical treatment depends on the patient's anatomy, medical comorbidities, and clinical presentation. In many cases, either endovascular or open surgical therapy may be appropriate. It is important that the patient be presented with **balanced and realistic expectations** about any procedure, its durability, the need for future interventions, and potential complications.

Endovascular procedures have proven themselves to have significant advantages in certain vascular disease and injury scenarios. As an example, endovascular aortic aneurysm repair has reduced morbidity and mortality associated with this treatment of this disease, shortened recovery times, and allowed treatment in patients who would not otherwise be suitable for open repair (Chapter 14). However, the success and rapid recovery that patients often experience with endovascular procedures should be viewed in the context of evidence supporting long-term outcomes both of the procedure and the patient (i.e., is the endovascular procedure durable and will the patient have good mid- and long-term survival?). Vascular specialists should be cautious in lowering their threshold for performing a procedure to treat vascular diseases simply because of the availability of endovascular techniques. The potential benefits of intervention should be tempered with an understanding of the natural history of the disease and life expectancy of the patient. The majority of patients with lower extremity claudication, for example, can be treated medically and with a modest walking program and will experience no worsening in their disease. Intervention, whether endovascular or surgical, should be limited to patients with progressive, lifestyle-limiting claudication or the minority who progress to critical limb ischemia.

II. PREPARATION

A. Prior to angiography, the endovascular specialist should **review the patient's history, lab work, and indications for the procedure.** Many of these procedures are performed on an outpatient basis. The informed consent forms are also reviewed, and the patient and his or her family should have the opportunity to ask "last minute" questions.

B. An **abbreviated physical exam** should be performed just prior to the procedure to confirm previous findings and assure no interval change.

1. An evaluation of the planned **access vessel** (e.g., femoral artery) is critical in the preprocedure holding area. The absence of or

diminution in this pulse should prompt reconsideration of the access site except in cases of access distal to known disease that is the target of intervention (e.g., femoral access distal to iliac disease that is target of intervention).

2. Distal pulses or Doppler signals should be confirmed prior to angiography and ankle-brachial indices (ABIs) recorded if lower extremity intervention is likely. **Comparison of the pulse examination before and after intervention** is essential care of the vascular patient. The absence of a pulse or Doppler signal after intervention implies embolization, vessel occlusion, or a poor technical result. ABIs are obtained in follow-up after lower extremity endovascular intervention and compared objectively with preprocedure values.

3. Newly recognized or poorly managed medical conditions such as severe hypertension, arrhythmia, diabetes mellitus, or acute worsening of renal insufficiency may require delaying the angiogram or cancelling it altogether.

4. Patients with foot ulcers or gangrene should have their wounds reassessed, as they may benefit from debridement prior to or just following the endovascular procedure in an appropriate operating room.

C. **Previous open surgical or endovascular procedures** are particularly relevant and should be reviewed as part of this preprocedure routine. Vessels that have been accessed multiple times in the past, or the presence of an extremity bypass, may affect the location and method of access for angiography. For example, previous aortobifemoral bypass will present challenges related to scar and the number of patent lumens at the femoral level (e.g., prosthetic bypass limb and the native femoral or external iliac lumen). An aortic bypass graft or stent-graft creates a narrow aortic bifurcation that generally prevents placement of a sheath "up and over" into the contralateral limb of the prosthetic graft. The locations of prior endovascular interventions, along with balloon and/or stent sizes, and complications from prior procedures should also be recorded, noting previous access problems.

D. **Allergy to iodinated contrast material** should be ascertained and can occur in 2% to 5% of patients. These reactions are usually mild, with itching and urticaria. Rarely, more severe anaphylactic reactions occur, manifested by wheezing, bradycardia, and hypotension. Patients with prior contrast reactions are at higher risk for recurrent allergic complications with angiography. In this high-risk group, it is generally recommend that a "prep" consisting of steroids and diphenhydramine (Benadryl, Johnson and Johnson, New Brunswick, NJ) be administered prior to the angiogram. One such regimen includes 50 mg of prednisone by mouth 13, 7, and then 1 hour prior to the procedure (Greenberger protocol). A single dose of 25 to 50 mg of diphenhydramine may also be given 1 hour prior to administration of contrast. When an urgent angiogram or CTA is needed, an urgent prep can be administered with intravenous doses of diphenhydramine (50 mg) and hydrocortisone (200 mg) but may be less effective. Frequently, patients scheduled to receive iodinated contrast are queried as to a history of seafood or topical iodine (e.g., Betadine®, Purdue Pharma LP, Stamford, CT) allergy. It is a myth that these particular allergies have any relationship to contrast allergy and patients do not require a special "prep" prior to contrast exposure. Contrast allergy is mediated by a separate, non-IgE pathway and is largely driven by the osmolality of contrast relative to blood.

E. The patient should be questioned as to his or her **current medications**.

1. Care should be exercised in the use of iodinated contrast in patients taking **metformin** or metformin-containing medications. This oral

agent is used to treat non–insulin-dependent diabetes mellitus and metabolized renally. Patients on metformin are at risk for a rare, but potentially lethal, lactic acidosis that can be precipitated by contrast agents. Patients with underlying renal insufficiency are at risk for worsening renal dysfunction after exposure to iodinated contrast (contrast nephropathy). In such cases, metformin cannot be excreted normally and can lead to increased lactate production by the intestines.

The Food and Drug Administration (FDA) required labeling changes that replace serum creatinine (SCr) with the measure referred to as estimated glomerular filtration rate (eGFR) as the best parameter used to determine appropriateness of treatment with metformin in patients with renal insufficiency. The calculation of eGFR takes into account age, race, and sex, as well as SCr, providing a more accurate assessment of kidney function. The eGFR should be calculated before patients begin treatment with metformin and annually thereafter. Regardless of the need for an iodinated contrast agent, metformin is now contraindicated in patients with an eGFR less than 30 mL/min/1.73 m^2, and starting the drug in patients with an eGFR between 30 and 45 mL/min/1.73 m^2 is not recommended. Metformin should not be administered for 48 hours after an iodinated contrast imaging procedure (e.g., angiogram or CTA) in patients with an eGFR less than 60 mL/min/1.73 m^2, and the eGFR should be reevaluated before the medication is restarted.

2. **Anticoagulants** such as warfarin or direct factor Xa inhibitors should be stopped before procedures that involve arterial access. This usually means stopping the medication for 2 to 4 days prior to the procedure to allow them to be cleared from the system. In the case of warfarin, most prefer the international normalized ratio (INR) to decrease below 1.5 prior to the performance of elective arteriography. The indications for anticoagulation must also be considered prior to stopping the blood thinner before an elective procedure. In some patients, such as those with mechanical heart valves or recent, serious thrombotic or embolic events, it may not be safe to discontinue anticoagulation and other strategies will need to be considered. For example, a heparin "window" can be used in patients at high risk for thrombosis or thromboembolism. In these cases, the patient is kept fully anticoagulated on intravenous unfractionated heparin (UFH) while the oral warfarin or factor Xa inhibitor is stopped. UFH has a short half-life (90 minutes) compared to warfarin (36 hours) and factor Xa inhibitors (9 to 14 hours), so that it can be stopped just hours prior to the angiogram and started soon after the procedure (i.e., creating a window of time during which the patient is not anticoagulated and the procedure can be performed). Low molecular weight heparin allows some patients at moderate risk for stopping anticoagulation to "bridge" at home with daily or twice daily subcutaneous injections instead of coming to the hospital for intravenous heparin.

3. **Antiplatelet agents** such as aspirin and/or clopidogrel (Plavix) are commonly taken by patients with peripheral vascular disease. In rare cases, these medications can be stopped prior to angiography, but in most instances, the interventionalist prefers the patient to continue the antiplatelet medications up to and immediately following the angiogram. Prior to certain endovascular interventions such as stenting procedures, many physicians ensure that antiplatelet agents are "on board" or even administer higher doses immediately before or

after the procedure. There is no consensus on the use of antiplatelet agents and angiography. At present, each case must be assessed, balancing the risk of bleeding with thrombosis. Patients with a personal or family history of **bleeding problems** should be carefully evaluated with a platelet count and coagulation studies (prothrombin time and partial prothrombin time). A hematology consultation should be sought if heritable bleeding disorder is suspected.

F. **Renal function** is grossly assessed by measuring SCr and blood urea nitrogen (BUN), although the more sensitive measure is calculation of eGFR. The National Kidney Foundation recommends using the CKD-EPI Creatinine Equation (2009) to estimate GFR, and this equation and GFR calculators can be easily accessed at various websites (e.g., https://www.kidney.org/professionals/KDOQI/gfr). Contrast material can be nephrotoxic, especially in the elderly, patients who are dehydrated, those with diabetes, and patients with renal insufficiency. In higher-risk patients, **adequate urine output** (0.5 mL/kg/h) should be established prior to contrast angiography, often by starting an IV and giving intravenous hydration with isotonic fluid such as 0.9% normal saline. Both oral acetylcysteine (Mucomyst, Bristol-Myers Squibb, New York, NY) and intravenous fluids containing sodium bicarbonate (to alkalinize the urine) are fairly innocuous treatments that have been studied and utilized extensively with the intention of reducing contrast nephropathy. However, recent randomized data from the PRESERVE trial have debunked the benefit of acetylcysteine and sodium bicarbonate over simple hydration with intravenous normal saline. Contrast nephropathy is defined as a 25% increase in SCr typically within 3 to 7 after contrast administration. Patients with baseline renal disease are at greatest risk for contrast nephropathy. The mechanism is believed related to vasoconstriction as well as direct toxicity to renal epithelial cells.

G. **Skin preparation** of the access or puncture site should include cleansing with an antiseptic soap such as chlorhexidine. In the case of femoral access, both groins should be prepped.

H. **Preprocedural antibiotics are not necessary** for routine angiography. However, antibiotics may be beneficial prior to implanting a permanent intravascular stent or if the access site includes puncturing a previously placed prosthetic graft.

III. **RISKS.** The main risks of angiography are hemorrhage from the access site; allergic reactions to the contrast material; thrombosis of the punctured vessel; and embolization of a thrombus, air, or atheromatous material from or around the catheter. In experienced hands, these complications occur in 1% of all cases. Mortality is less frequent (0.05%), but is a risk that the patient must understand.

IV. **SELECTION OF ACCESS VESSEL.** Every endovascular procedure begins with intravascular access. Although percutaneous access is usually straightforward, this basic technique can also be foreboding and should be accomplished with the aid of **ultrasound guidance.** The most frequent complications of angiography occur at the access site (2% to 4%) and include hematoma, pseudoaneurysm, and arteriovenous fistula. Careful selection of the access vessel is critical to the safety and success of the angiogram. The most commonly selected vessels for arteriography are the femoral and brachial arteries.

A. **The common femoral artery** is accessible and large enough to accommodate sizeable sheaths. The primary disadvantage of femoral access includes the risk of retroperitoneal hemorrhage, which can occur with an inadvertent high puncture and access into the external iliac artery under the inguinal ligament. In contrast, low puncture or access into the superficial femoral artery increases the risk of pseudoaneurysm, vessel dissection, and thrombosis.

The technique of femoral artery access requires careful attention to anatomic landmarks, including those on the patient's skin and those identified by fluoroscopy and on transcutaneous ultrasound. The optimal site for access into the common femoral artery is just below the inguinal ligament at the level of the femoral head. At this level, the **femoral artery courses over the medial one-third of the femoral head** (Fig. 9.1), and access at this location improves the effectiveness of "closure devices" or manual compression of the vessel when the access sheath is removed following the procedure. Fluoroscopic confirmation of this location is simple and important to avoid misadventures associated with punctures based solely on the inguinal skin crease, which is often misleading. A line between the anterior superior iliac spine and the pubic tubercle marks the inguinal ligament, and by using a hemostat placed at the planned puncture site and fluoroscopy, one can confirm that the access is over the femoral head. This technique is helpful in obese patients in whom the skin landmarks are distorted as well as in patients with diminished pulses.

Use of B-mode ultrasound is also important for arterial access, and at the femoral level demonstrates the firmer, pulsatile, and noncompressible common femoral artery lateral to the more compliant and compressible common femoral vein. B-mode ultrasound should also be used to show the origin of the deep femoral artery that is an important distal landmark

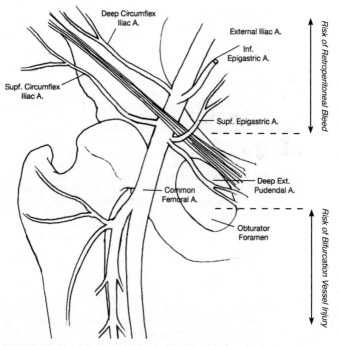

FIGURE 9.1 Bony landmarks are useful for identifying the level of the common femoral artery. The inguinal ligament runs between the pubic tubercle and the anterior superior iliac spine, marking the top of the common femoral artery. High puncture or laceration of the inferior epigastric artery can lead to serious retroperitoneal bleeding. Puncture at or below the femoral bifurcation is also to be avoided.

(i.e., the access point should be proximal to the deep femoral artery origin). In experienced hands, ultrasound-guided vascular access will also show direct entry of the echogenic needle into the pulsatile artery as well as passage of the small wire through the hollow-tip needle into the vessel.

B. Arterial access can be accomplished in a **retrograde** or **antegrade** manner, and consideration of these options should be made prior to attempting to enter the vessel. **Retrograde arterial puncture** refers to the needle being placed opposite the direction of blood flow. For lower extremity arterial disease, the femoral artery opposite the more symptomatic leg is often selected for retrograde puncture. This allows for performance of an aortogram and runoff or imaging of the most symptomatic lower extremity without interference from the femoral access sheath. Access via the contralateral femoral artery also offers working room, if needed, to treat the symptomatic leg by going "up and over" the aortic bifurcation. An **antegrade stick of the femoral artery** is placed in the direction of blood flow down the symptomatic lower extremity and allows for a focused unilateral arteriogram. The antegrade technique does not image the aortoiliac segments proximal to the femoral artery, which would generally be mapped out on either a prior CTA or diagnostic angiogram. The antegrade approach provides a shorter, more supportive platform when treating severe disease or total occlusions of the distal femoral, popliteal, and infrapopliteal arterial segments. Antegrade access generally requires more precision to allow access of the common femoral artery in a more proximal location away from the femoral bifurcation and profunda femoris artery. Even with accurate access, directing the wire into the superficial—not the deep—femoral artery can be challenging, because of limited working room between the entry site and the femoral bifurcation. Because of these technical challenges, antegrade femoral access has a slightly higher risk of access site complications compared with the more standard retrograde access. **Pedal access** (access via the dorsalis pedis or posterior tibial artery) has gained momentum in treatment of complex tibial disease, as small wires can more easily traverse vessel occlusions without diversion into collaterals that are frequently encountered from above.

C. **Brachial artery access** may be selected in patients with poor femoral pulses or with other compelling reasons to avoid access in the groin, such as the presence of a bypass graft. Additionally, downward sloping vessels such as the mesenteric arteries are often easier to enter with wires brought from a more cephalad position afforded by brachial access. The portion of the brachial artery just above the antecubital crease is superficial and suitable for access. We prefer **access through the left brachial artery over the right in order to** avoid traversing the origins of the common carotid arteries with wires and possibly sheaths. Right-sided brachial access requires crossing both common carotid artery origins with these devices and harbors a small risk of causing a stroke from embolization of atheromatous plaque or debris. The smaller size of the brachial artery makes access more challenging, and accurate entry into the brachial artery should be facilitated with ultrasound guidance. The brachial artery can rarely accommodate larger than a 6- or 7-Fr sheath, which may curtail procedures requiring larger devices unless an open exposure of the artery is performed to allow direct repair after removal of a larger sheath. Lower extremity interventions cannot usually be performed from a brachial approach due to the limited length of endovascular devices. The location of the brachial artery and its proximity to the median nerve in a small fixed space (i.e., the brachial sheath) in the arm necessitates good hemostasis following access sheath removal. In contrast to femoral access hematomas, which are most often managed without surgery, even a small hematoma over the brachial artery (i.e., brachial sheath hematoma) can result in median nerve compression requiring operative intervention. The interventionalist should have a high level of suspicion for brachial sheath hematoma in a patient complaining of persistent hand pain, paresthesias, or motor dysfunction, even with minimal bruising or swelling. Pulse examination will be normal. Without surgery, median nerve compression can lead to the **orator's hand posture**, with permanent inability to pinch together the thumb and index finger.

V. METHODS

A. **Pain or discomfort associated with angiography** is related to vessel puncture, sheath placement, and contrast injection and is usually minimal and transient. Occasionally, the use of balloon angioplasty and/or stents may result in visceral pain if the vessel wall is stretched significantly. Pain accompanying contrast injection is reduced with the use of **iso-osmolar or only slightly hyperosmolar contrast agents.** If an older hyperosmolar contrast agent is used, the patient may experience an intense hot or burning pain that lasts for several seconds. In most cases, the patient's pain and anxiety can be managed with the oral or IV administration of a short-acting benzodiazepine or use of an intravenous dose of a short-acting narcotic such as fentanyl. It is rare for an intravenous sedative such as propofol (Diprivan, AstraZeneca, Wilmington, DE) to be required. Local anesthetic is used around the puncture site, and in many cases, it is all that is required. Transient visceral pain with balloon angioplasty or stenting is mediated by adventitial receptors and indicates vessel stretch. Severe or persistent pain following angioplasty or stenting suggests rupture or impending perforation of the vessel requiring further monitoring and investigation.

B. A variety of available **nonionic contrast agents** are much improved over older ionic contrast agents. Many of the nonionic agents are iso-osmolar or only slightly hyperosmolar, which represents the greatest improvement over older agents, which were hyperosmolar and painful. Excreted by the kidneys, contrast agents can induce acute renal dysfunction in patients with or without preexisting renal insufficiency. Individuals with known renal failure, proteinuria, diabetes mellitus, and dehydration are at higher risk. Postangiographic renal dysfunction peaks at 48 hours and can be minimized by intravenous hydration and limited contrast loads. Contrast-induced nephropathy is usually transient and improves within a week's time. Alternatively, carbon dioxide gas can provide good images of the major abdominal and leg arteries with no risk of renal injury (i.e., CO_2 angiography). The gas is injected into the vessel and displaces the blood, rather than mixing with blood as standard contrast does. Special modifications are needed with digital subtraction angiography in order to create the best images, and the value of CO_2 angiography also depends on technician and operator experience.

C. **The modified Seldinger's technique** with ultrasound guidance is used to gain access to the vessel (Fig. 9.2) and entails puncture of the anterior wall of the vessel with a hollow, beveled needle. Once the echogenic needle is visualized entering the vessel with ultrasound and pulsatile flow from the hub of the needle is confirmed, a guidewire (e.g., floppy J-wire) is advanced through the needle into the vessel. Next, the needle is withdrawn over the stationary wire while manual pressure is held over the entry site to prevent bleeding. A sheath that contains a soft, tapered inner dilator is then placed over the stationary wire into the lumen and the inner dilator of the sheath removed. **The sheath acts as a working port within the vessel, through which catheter and wire exchanges can be made with minimal bleeding or trauma to the vessel wall.**

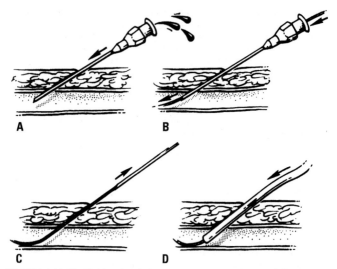

FIGURE 9.2 Modified Seldinger's technique for percutaneous angiography. **(A)** Introductory needle is passed into femoral or brachial artery. **(B)** Smaller flexible guidewire is passed through the introductory needle into the artery. **(C)** Introductory needle is withdrawn over the guidewire, which is left in the artery. **(D)** Larger flexible angiographic sheath or catheter is passed over the smaller guidewire into the artery.

The smallest sheath that can effectively accomplish the goals of the angiogram should be selected to minimize access site complications. If initial passage of the wire into of the artery is impeded, the needle may not be completely within the lumen, in a side branch of the artery, or up against a plaque. Advancing the wire under these circumstances can cause damage, and any resistance to wire advancement should lead to examination under fluoroscopy to avoid coiling of the wire, which can be seen with extraluminal placement or dissection. In these cases, the wire is removed and the arterial back-bleeding again confirmed. The endovascular specialist may try to angle the bevel of the needle in a different direction or withdraw the tip slightly, in an effort to enter the true lumen and then reinsert the wire under fluoroscopic or ultrasound guidance, aiming for resistance-free placement. In instances where blood flows freely from the needle but the wire will not pass, a small contrast injection under fluoroscopy may help identify the problem. Failure of these simple maneuvers should prompt withdrawal of the needle, manual pressure, and a new puncture.

The original Seldinger's technique is worth mentioning for historic purposes and involves not only puncture of the anterior vessel wall but also the back wall of the artery as well (**double-puncture technique**). With this technique, the needle is withdrawn until a flash of pulsatile blood confirms intraluminal placement. Deliberate use of the double-puncture technique is best avoided, as bleeding from the posterior wall puncture can be a problem.

Difficult arterial access may also be due to poor pulsation or large body habitus. In these situations, bony landmarks in relation to the chosen access location and ultrasound guidance are especially helpful. In more difficult cases, the endovascular specialist may wear a lead glove and attempt to access the artery under real-time fluoroscopy. Calcium deposits in the femoral and iliac arteries may actually form a cast of the vessel that can also be used as a guide to the vessel using fluoroscopy. The importance of establishing safe intravascular access cannot be underestimated, as complications from angiography arise from flawed access choices or technique.

D. Once access is established, an **aortogram with lower extremity runoff** is performed by positioning a flush catheter with multiple side holes in the aorta above the level of the renal arteries (radiographically above L2 level). A contrast bolus is rapidly injected through the catheter to define the anatomy of the aorta and iliac vessels. Subsequently, this catheter can be repositioned lower to the aortic bifurcation, and additional contrast boluses are timed to properly acquire radiographic "runs" of the lower extremities.

It may be necessary to use a curved catheter to get "up and over" the aortic bifurcation when additional imaging or intervention is planned on the contralateral leg. In general, catheter or sheath advancement should be done over a wire in order to avoid vessel injury from "snowplowing" or dislodging atheroembolic material upon advancement. A catheter can be placed closer to the vascular bed of interest. For example, having a catheter in the popliteal artery will provide excellent images of the tibial vessels that otherwise may "washout" with a more proximal catheter. The locations and degree of stenosis and/or occlusion in the arterial tree are noted. It is essential to identify precisely which arteries are spared of disease, particularly when revascularization to a target artery is planned. Different projections in the anterior-posterior and oblique planes may be necessary in order to clarify the anatomy. Lastly, the wire, catheter, and sheath are removed, and either manual pressure or a closure device is applied to the access site.

VI. VENOGRAPHY

A. Diagnostic venography of the extremities typically consists of two parts, **ascending and descending**, and may also be referred to as **phlebography**. This two-staged exam allows for study of venous anatomy and patency by injecting contrast from venous access distal in the extremity to proximal in the direction of venous flow (i.e., ascending). Typically, the descending venogram is performed from a remote venous access site to allow injection of contrast down the extremity against the flow of venous blood to assess competence of the venous valves. Traditionally, ascending and descending venography is performed on a tilt table to allow gravity-induced changes in venous flow during different stages of the exam. While duplex has nearly replaced venography in the diagnosis of deep vein thrombosis (DVT) and venous reflux, there has been a resurgence of venography performed in conjunction with catheter-directed thrombolytic treatment for acute venous thrombosis. Venography is also useful in complicated venous cases to define lower extremity anatomy for patients with venous obstruction or those needing deep venous reconstruction (Chapter 19).

B. **Patient Preparation and Risk.** Steps in preparation for and the risk of venography are nearly the same as those for arteriography and include recognition of contrast allergies, renal insufficiency, and need for a suitable puncture or access site. About 3% of venographic studies will be complicated by minor allergic reactions, **contrast-induced thrombophlebitis** or thrombosis, or contrast extravasation at the puncture site.

C. **Methods.** The quality and safety of leg venography can be optimized by paying attention to the previously mentioned aspects of the technique.

1. **Ascending venography** is performed by injecting contrast into a vein on the distal extremity in a direction away from the foot. The patient should be positioned at 30- to 45-degree reverse Trendelenburg on a tilt table, with no weight bearing on the affected limb. Weight bearing causes the gastrocnemius and soleus muscles to contract, preventing adequate filling of some deep veins. For general diagnostic purposes, a vein on the dorsum of the foot is punctured with a 21-gauge needle. Rarely, a cut down exposure of the great saphenous vein at the ankle is necessary. Diluted nonionic contrast in a volume of 60 to 90 mL per extremity is usually suitable and may reduce the risk of contrast-related phlebitis. Views of the superficial and deep veins can be obtained without a tourniquet unless leg swelling is severe and causes increased compartmental pressures. In this situation, an ankle tourniquet to occlude the superficial system is used to promote better filling of the deep veins. Images of the leg are made with external and internal rotation of the foot, and the same views are obtained over the knee and thigh. Finally, the pelvic film is exposed after the table is returned horizontal and the leg elevated. The venous system is flushed with 60 mL of normal saline at the completion.

    Ultrasound-guided popliteal vein access with the patient in the prone position is often chosen for catheter-directed thrombolytic treatment of acute DVT involving the proximal femoral and/or iliac veins. A form of ascending venography, this approach provides excellent support for crossing acute venous thrombus with wires, catheters, and mechanical thrombectomy devices and provides optimal imaging of the proximal femoral, iliac, and even caval circulation.

2. **The normal ascending venogram** is able to image the lower extremity up to and including the inferior vena cava. During normal ascending venography, the deep and superficial veins are opacified. Deep venous trunks in the calf are paired, the smallest being the anterior tibial veins. These deep leg veins have smooth, straight walls except where the valves are positioned and then a beadlike appearance of the vein can be appreciated. Venous sinuses within the muscle of the leg are large and fusiform in the young but appear smaller with advancing age. The popliteal and femoral veins are usually single but may be paired in some individuals. Normally, contrast should flow quickly up the deep system after leg elevation, allowing for visualization of the proximal femoral, iliac, and even caval circulations. For more complete opacification of these proximal venous segments, and depending upon the size and location of the distal access vein in the leg, it may be necessary to place a sheath to allow placement of a catheter near or into the proximal venous segment of interest. Injection of contrast into a catheter placed more proximally allows more full and complete filling and imaging of these venous segments. Alternatively, the proximal venous segments may be imaged as part of the descending venogram.

3. **Descending venography** of the lower extremity is performed by accessing the contralateral femoral vein and crossing over the bifurcation of the inferior vena cava with a wire and catheter. This allows placement of a catheter above the venous segment of interest for injection of contrast to assess for valvular reflux. Once the catheter is placed above the segment of interest, the patient is positioned in a steep reverse Trendelenburg position (i.e., head up), while diluted contrast boluses are injected through the catheter and images recorded. The patient may perform a **Valsalva maneuver**, which increases intra-abdominal pressure and transiently halts venous emptying

from the legs to increase the sensitivity of descending venography. In the setting of normal valvular function, the contrast will only descend as far as the next set of competent valves, which prevent flow down the venous segment. Conversely, in the setting of valvular incompetence, contrast will flow down the venous segment of the leg until a competent set of valves intervenes.

4. **Acute lower extremity deep venous thrombosis** is confirmed by filling defects in the deep veins on more than one view. The contrast column will end abruptly when the thrombosis obstructs the vein. Deep veins may also fail to opacify because of external compression from muscle swelling in the fascial compartments. Chronic changes from **postthrombotic syndrome** reveal well-developed venous collaterals and partial recanalization with intraluminal webs or synechiae. Chronic venous insufficiency as a result of primary valvular degeneration or postthrombotic syndrome is evident by the degree of contrast reflux visualized on descending venography.

5. **Upper extremity venography** can accurately diagnose and potentially treat central venous stenosis or thrombosis. Although duplex is the initial test of choice in these situations, the intrathoracic position of the central veins makes them difficult to examine directly with ultrasound. The use of chronic central venous catheters for parenteral nutrition, chemotherapy, and dialysis predisposes the subclavian and innominate veins to stenosis and/or thrombosis, which may require central venous angiography to diagnose. In such cases, an often distended superficial arm vein may serve as a site for access and injection of diluted contrast. **Ultrasound-guided basilic vein access** allows placement of a sheath, wire, and catheter into more proximal segments for imaging and potential treatment. The presence of a dialysis fistula or graft in the arm provides an obvious site for venous access and intervention in select cases. In the case of acute **axillo-subclavian venous thrombosis, also referred to as Paget-Schröetter syndrome,** distended antecubital veins may make venous access easier. Venography in this scenario is often combined with catheter-directed thrombolysis to treat the acute DVT, which often forms as a result of thoracic outlet syndrome. In the absence of acute axillo-subclavian venous thrombosis but suspected thoracic outlet syndrome, diagnostic venography should include provocative maneuvers (abduction and external rotation of the arm), which may provide the diagnosis.

Selected Readings

American College of Radiology Committee on Drugs and Contrast Media. *ACR Manual on Contrast Media, Version 10.3.* https://www.acr.org/Clinical-Resources/Contrast-Manual. Accessed January 2018.
Searchable, online 100-page guide addresses issues related to all contrast agents used in radiological procedures.

Barrett BJ, Parfrey PS. Preventing nephropathy induced by contrast medium. *N Engl J Med.* 2006;354:379-386.
Case vignette introduces a review of contrast nephropathy with emphasis on preventative measures.

Garrett PD, Eckart RE, Bauch TD, et al. Fluoroscopic localization of the femoral head as a landmark for common femoral artery cannulation. *Catheter Cardiovasc Interv.* 2005;65:205-207.
Femoral angiograms were reviewed in 126 patients to assess location of common femoral artery bifurcation relative to fluoroscopic landmarks.

Kalish J, Eslami M, Gillespie D, et al.; on behalf of the Vascular Study Group of New England. Routine use of ultrasound guidance in femoral arterial access for peripheral vascular intervention decreases groin hematoma rates. *J Vasc Surg.* 2015;61:1231-1238.

This large study using the Vascular Quality Initiative database lends support to routine use of ultrasound-guided femoral access.

Kennedy AM, Grocott M, Schwartz MS, et al. Median nerve injury: an underrecognised complication of brachial artery cardiac catheterisation? *J Neurol Neurosurg Psychiatry.* 1997;63:542-546.

Interesting small case series demonstrates the importance of recognizing small antecubital hematomas; the classic "orator pose" complication is shown in photograph.

Lasser EC, Berry CC, Talner LB, et al. Pre-treatment with corticosteroids to alleviate reactions to intravenous contrast material. *N Engl J Med.* 1987;317:845-849.

This original, randomized, placebo-controlled study examined the effectiveness of steroids for prevention of iodinated contrast allergy.

Pasternak JJ, Williamson EE. Clinical pharmacology, uses, and adverse reactions of iodinated contrast agents: a primer for the non-radiologist. *Mayo Clin Proc.* 2012;87:390-402.

Excellent primer on iodinated contrast, including prevention and treatment of contrast reactions.

Rupp SB, Vogelzang RL, Nemcek AA, et al. Relationship of the inguinal ligament to pelvic radiographic landmarks. *J Vasc Interv Radiol.* 1993;4:409-413.

Cadaveric study proving that puncture above the inguinal ligament can cause retroperitoneal bleeding.

Weisbord SD, Gallagher M, Jneid H, et al.; PRESERVE Trial Group. Outcomes after angiography with sodium bicarbonate and acetylcysteine. *N Engl J Med.* 2018; 378:603-614.

Randomized trial demonstrates no benefit for sodium bicarbonate or acetylcysteine over normal saline for prevention of contrast-related acute kidney injury.

Catheter-Based Technology and Postprocedure Care

To participate in a discussion of endovascular therapies or to take part in endovascular procedures, the vascular interventionalist or trainee must have a fundamental understanding of equipment and techniques. This chapter is designed to prepare the reader with that basic familiarity and understanding and includes sections on catheter-based technologies and thrombolytic therapy. Additionally, this chapter provides an overview of postangiogram care and complications specific to endovascular procedures. As a starter and because the use of catheters in these cases is ubiquitous, the term ***catheter-based*** should be considered synonymous with **endovascular** procedures.

I. **BASIC EQUIPMENT.** The increased use of endovascular procedures to treat vascular disease and certain patterns of vascular injury has driven the development of a large number and different types of catheter-based technologies. Competition to "build the better mousetrap" has led to an increased number of new endovascular tools, some of which are interchangeable or provide multiple options for a given diagnostic or therapeutic objective. The wide range of endovascular technologies can seem at first overwhelming. However, a basic understanding of few basic categories of endovascular tools is all that is necessary to establish a fundamental understanding of endovascular procedures, an understanding one can expand with more time and experience. The following section describes these core tools that are used as part of nearly all endovascular procedures: **sheaths, wires**, and **catheters** (Table 10.1). Categories of therapeutic technologies, including **balloons, stents, covered stents, or stent grafts**, and **intravascular ultrasound** are described followed by an introduction of the basic concepts related to **catheter-directed thrombolysis**.

The nuances of different device brands are not discussed here, as the purpose of this chapter is to provide an overview of each category of equipment. Where brand names are mentioned, these may imply a frequent practice of the authors but are not intended to promote superiority of a particular device. In many cases, the obvious utility of catheter-based interventions has led to usage prior to FDA approval for such indications. For example, bare metal stents were originally FDA approved only for use in the biliary tree and covered stents for the tracheobronchial tree. **The following discussion includes some off-label use of catheter-based technology, and the reader is advised to consult the individual manufacturer's guidelines and instructions for use (IFU) for each device prior to its use.**

A. **Sheaths.** The primary function of **sheaths** is to maintain hemostatic access to the inside of the vessel once entry has been accomplished by the modified **Seldinger's technique**. Sheaths act as ports through which wires, catheters, and other devices can be exchanged without causing trauma to the vessel or significant blood loss. The hemostatic valve at the end of the sheath through which these devices are passed from outside of the patient to inside the blood vessel is often referred to as the diaphragm. A side port

TABLE 10.1	Categories of Catheter-Based Tools

Access needles
  18 gauge
  21-gauge Micropuncture kit
Sheaths—4 Fr and greater
  Short straight (10–12 cm and 22–25 cm lengths)
  Long straight (90 cm)
  Preshaped crossover sheaths (45–60 cm)
Wires—0.014–0.035 inches diameter (regular and exchange length)
  Hydrophilic (e.g., glide wire)
  Nonhydrophilic (i.e., working wires)
  Starter (e.g., starter J-wire or Bentson wire)
  Stiff (e.g., Amplatz, Cook, Inc., Bloomington, IN)
Catheters
  Nonselective flush (e.g., straight, pigtail, Omni)
  Selective/end hole (e.g., angled glide, Bernstein, Cobra, Simmons)
  Infusion (e.g., multi-sidehole thrombolytic)
Guide catheters
Balloons
  Compliant
  Noncompliant
  Cutting
  Drug coated
Stents
  Balloon expandable
  Self-expanding
  Covered (i.e., stent grafts)
Intravascular ultrasound (IVUS)
Atherectomy devices
Mechanical thrombolysis (arterial or venous)
  AngioJet™ (Boston Scientific, Marlborough, MA)
  EkoSonic™ endovascular system (BTG Interventional Medicine, London, UK)
  Penumbra Indigo® (Penumbra, Inc., Alameda, California)
Access or puncture site closure devices

positioned toward the end of the sheath allows it to be flushed proximal to the diaphragm and allows one to transduce and measure the pressure within the vessel. **Sheaths are sized based on their inner diameter with 1 Fr unit equaling 0.33 mm.** This is important to keep in mind, understanding that a 5-Fr sheath has a 1.65 mm inner diameter but an outer diameter that creates a slightly larger opening in the vessel. The majority of diagnostic procedures are performed through 10- to 12-cm-long sheaths, with longer ones (e.g., 45 and 90 cm) available to provide a platform for more involved endovascular procedures at distances farther from the access site. Sheaths that are shaped with preformed curves are also available, such as the popular "crossover" sheath that has a wide U shape for optimal positioning over the aortic bifurcation into the contralateral iliac or femoral artery. Using this longer preformed sheath allows one to more easily access remote vascular beds to perform an angiogram and/or catheter-based interventions (e.g., the leg opposite the side of femoral artery access).

The smallest sheath suitable for the task at hand should be used in order to minimize the size of the hole in the vessel and decrease the risk of access site complications. The most common sheath sizes range from 4 to 10 Fr. Very large diameter sheaths up to 24 Fr are necessary to accommodate devices for endovascular aneurysm repair.

B. **Wires.** Endovascular interventions are initiated with placement of a wire maneuvered into a desired location using fluoroscopic guidance. Once the wire is in the desired location, the endovascular tool needed to accomplish the next step (e.g., catheter, balloon, or stent) may be placed over the stationary wire through the sheath, with the wire acting as a rail on which the device travels. Once a wire has been positioned to its desired location, it should not be advanced or withdrawn until the given intervention is complete (i.e., it should remain stationary). Meticulous **wire control** or **wire management** is important to avoid injury to vessels or structures beyond the desired location and is critical once placed beyond a stenosis targeted for therapy. Should the wire be inadvertently pulled back proximal to such a lesion, regaining wire access may be difficult; multiple wire passes can cause adverse events such as embolization or vessel dissection.

Wires are sized based on their diameters and lengths. The most common wire diameters are 0.035, 0.018, and 0.014 inches. Because they are the largest, 0.035-inch wires are most easily handled and can be used for the majority of basic diagnostic and large vessel interventions. Because of their small size, 0.014-inch wires are more difficult for the less experienced endovascular specialist to handle and maneuver. The 0.014-inch wires were originally designed for use in the coronary arteries and are therefore compatible with smaller profile balloons, stents, and other endovascular devices. A benefit unique to the 0.014-inch wire pertains to **monorail catheter technology**. The monorail mechanism allows the wire to exit from an opening of a device (e.g., catheter, balloon, or stent) much closer to the forward tip of the device instead of out the back or rear of the device (Fig. 10.1). This technique allows for more rapid exchanges over a shorter length of wire, reducing manipulation and making the exchange easier for one individual to accomplish. The 0.014-inch wire system is most often used in small vessels (e.g., carotids or tibials) or when wire movement must be kept to a minimum (e.g., renals). The "working wires" for the endovascular specialist include **standard** (145 to 180 cm), and longer lengths also referred to as **exchange lengths** (240 to 300 cm). Exchange length wires are necessary when performing over-the-wire interventions at a distance far enough from the sheath such that catheter or balloon exchanges can be made without losing wire access. **The length of wire needed for a given procedure can be estimated using the following formula: distance from the access site to the target lesion location + length of the catheter + 10 cm.**

Wire properties also vary with respect to their **steerability, trackability**, and **stiffness.** Starter wires are used at the onset of vascular access to facilitate sheath and initial catheter placement. A typical starter wire has a low degree of stiffness with a floppy, straight, angled, or J-shaped tip that makes initial intravascular passage atraumatic. Wires with an angled tip are more steerable in that the interventionalist can turn the tip in a desired direction as the wire is advanced, allowing it to navigate circuitous turns. Wires with a hydrophilic coating are useful for negotiating tortuous vessels and tight stenoses and for selecting or entering the orifice of target vessels. **Hydrophilic wires** are frictionless or slick when kept wet, which is a necessary step to maintain their handling and trackability. Because these wires are often too slick to manipulate with the user's fingers alone, tools referred to as **torque devices** may be used to grip and effectively steer or spin the tip of the hydrophilic wire. Care must be taken

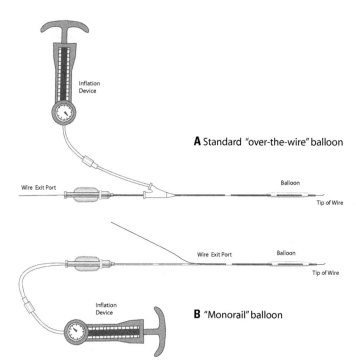

FIGURE 10.1 **(A)** "Over-the-wire" balloons typically go over a 0.035- or 0.018-inch wire, which exits at the end of the balloon. **(B)** Monorail technology utilizes a 0.014-inch wire that exits via a side port in the balloon.

with hydrophilic wires, as they are prone to enter the subintimal plane. This can be advantageous if a subintimal angioplasty is desired, but it can also create unwanted dissections or even vessel perforations. The stiffness of a wire's body depends on its diameter and composition, although the segment at the leading edge is almost always floppy.

Once the starter and hydrophilic wires have gained access to the desired intravascular location, an exchange to a more **stiff wire** is often performed to allow endovascular work over a rail with more substance. Specifically, stiff wires are often necessary to negotiate a sheath into position at a distance far from the access site without losing wire position. Stiff wires also tend to straighten tortuous vessels and provide appropriate support for the deployment of larger endovascular devices, such as endografts (i.e., for aortic aneurysm repair). Examples of more stiff wires in order of increasing rigidity include the **Rosen, Wholey, Meier, Amplatz,** and **Lunderquist** wires. Finally, specially designed **pressure wires** are available that can be placed to measure intravascular pressure waveforms at their distal segments or tips. These wires are useful to directly measure intravascular pressure and to determine the presence or absence of a pressure gradient across a narrowing or stenosis.

C. **Catheters and Guiding Catheters.** Catheters are long, flexible tubes with hollow lumens that are placed over and used to direct wires through vessels or across stenoses or occlusions. Once the wire has been removed from the catheter, contrast may be injected through the lumen for performance

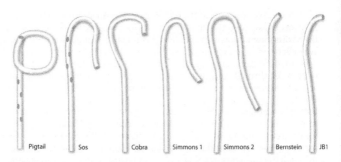

| Pigtail | Sos | Cobra | Simmons 1 | Simmons 2 | Bernstein | JB1 |

FIGURE 10.2 A sampling of commonly used catheter shapes. Catheters with a complex curve must be reformed to their preformed shape in vivo (e.g., Vitek, Simmons).

of angiography (Fig, 10.2). Catheters are sized based on their outer diameter and come in two general categories, **nonselective flush catheters** and **selective end-hole catheters**. Nonselective angiography is performed through flush catheters, which have multiple side holes near the tip and can accommodate high-pressure, high-flow injections without causing catheter motion (also referred to as catheter whip) within the vessel during injection. Flush catheters are designed to image larger, high-flow vessels such as the aorta and vena cava and come in various lengths and shapes, including the straight flush catheter, the pigtail flush catheter and the Omni SOS catheter (AngioDynamics, Latham, NY). A wide assortment of selective or end-hole catheters is available to permit the endovascular selection or cannulation of different types of vessels in various anatomic locations. The choice of a particular catheter depends on the diameter and tortuosity of the main access vessel and the angle of takeoff of the branch vessel targeted for cannulation. Most often, several different catheters may be suitable for engaging a given vessel, such that the interventionalist's preference and familiarity with the catheter is a major factor in its success. Once the catheter is engaged in the orifice of the desired vessel, the wire may be removed and a selective angiogram performed or advancement of the catheter over the wire can continue into a more distal position. Catheters with a single curve such as the **angled glide, visceral selective (VS)**, or **cobra catheters (C1-3)** are advanced by simply pushing them forward over the wire. Catheters with a complex curve must be reformed within the vessel once the wire is withdrawn. Paradoxically, some complex curve catheters must be withdrawn by the endovascular specialist in order to allow them to advance into the vessel. Examples of complex curve catheters are the **Simmons** and **Vitek catheters**.

Guiding catheters, sometimes simply called guides, are essentially larger and sometimes preshaped catheters through which other devices such as balloons and stents may be passed. **Like catheters (and unlike sheaths), guides are measured according to their outer diameter.** Therefore, an 8-Fr guide that has a 2.66 mm outer diameter will fit through an 8-Fr sheath that has the same inner diameter. The inner diameter of the guide is of course smaller and determines what size devices may pass through. Also, like catheters, guides come in a variety of preformed shapes, which facilitates placement in angled orifices such as the renal and mesenteric arteries. Although guides can be positioned directly over a wire into a vessel's orifice, unlike sheaths they typically do not come with a tapered inner dilator. Therefore, there is an increased risk of atheromatous embolization with this maneuver because of the step-off (i.e., size mismatch) between the wire and the opening at the end of the guide. An alternative technique involves telescoping the guide over a catheter and wire. The catheter is then withdrawn, leaving the guide in position to conduct interventions. A **Tuohy Borst** adapter may be placed over the wire and attached to the external end of the guide to prevent back-bleeding. This device allows injection of contrast through its side port into the guide to facilitate angiography while the wire remains in place, exiting out the back end of the Tuohy Borst.

D. **Unfractionated heparin** (UFH) is used during many peripheral interventions to prevent thrombus formation; however, consistent recommendations for its use and dosage are lacking. Higher doses of UFH (75 to 100 mg/kg) are often used for carotid interventions and femoral or tibial angioplasty in which the catheters or wires occlude or nearly occlude the target vessel or when prolonged interventions are anticipated. Lower doses (50 mg/kg) may be suitable for more straightforward cases such as limited iliac angioplasty. The authors also suggest low doses of systemic heparin when working through larger femoral sheaths (7 Fr or more) or when working through smaller brachial artery access. Heparin may be directly reversed with the use of **protamine** at the end of the procedure or simply allowed to wear off over a period of 1 to 2 hours prior to removal of the access sheath. Protamine binds to heparin at a ratio of 1 mg protamine to 100 U heparin and may induce histamine release leading to hypotension and (rarely) anaphylaxis. As such, 50 mg of protamine would neutralize 5,000 units of heparin; however, the time since the heparin dose should also be considered. The half-life of unfractionated heparin varies (30 minutes to 2 hours), depending on the dose.

E. **Vasodilators** can be used in select cases to alleviate distal vessel spasm related to catheter or wire manipulation. **Nitroglycerine** can be delivered through the sheath or catheter directly into the blood vessel in increments of 50 to 100 μg. The main side effect of nitroglycerin is headache related to vasodilation. When the hemodynamic significance of a mild or moderate stenosis visualized on arteriography is in question, pressures should be transduced proximal and distal to the stenosis. This can be accomplished by transducing the end of the catheter when it is beyond or distal to the stenosis and then slowly withdrawing the catheter more proximally across the stenosis. A pressure wire may also be used to measure the pressure proximal and distal to the identified stenosis. A **resting mean arterial pressure gradient** of greater than 5 mm Hg or **systolic pressure gradient** greater than 10 to 15 mm Hg across a stenosis is considered hemodynamically significant. If there is no resting gradient identified across a moderate stenosis, **intra-arterial papaverine** (10 to 30 mg) can be administered in attempt to unmask the gradient. Papaverine causes distal vasodilation, thereby increasing the velocity across any proximal stenosis mimicking the effects of walking or exertion. A mean arterial pressure gradient of greater than 10 mm Hg or more than 15% following administration of papaverine is considered significant.

II. **CATHETER-BASED THERAPEUTIC TECHNOLOGIES** can be used in cases of acute or chronic occlusive disease, aneurysms, and for select patterns of vascular injury. Once the endovascular specialist has decided to proceed with a catheter-based intervention, the tools for that intervention need to be selected. If a diagnostic angiogram or CTA has already been performed, the basic equipment for the case can be decided upon in advance and set aside. When the intervention is done at the same sitting as the diagnostic angiogram, the interventionalist should take a few minutes to mentally plan an approach to the lesion. The plan should then be discussed with personnel in the catheterization laboratory or operating room. The staff's understanding of the "game plan" encourages active involvement and anticipation of the methods and tools needed to accomplish the treatment goal.

A. **Indications for Angioplasty.** Angioplasty is used to dilate or recanalize arteries or grafts in nearly every anatomic region of the body. Catheter-based interventions generally have lower morbidity and mortality than open surgical approaches and in some cases are less expensive since the length of hospitalization is shorter. Patient recovery is usually excellent, with ambulation occurring on the same or the following day. However, endovascular therapies may be less durable than operative revascularization, depending on the vascular pathology and location being treated. The specific indications and options for intervention depend on the area being treated and are discussed in detail in the chapters on specific diseases. Guidelines such as the **Trans-Atlantic Inter-Society Consensus (TASC)** provide recommendations for catheter-based versus surgical treatment of lower extremity occlusive disease (see Chapter 13). For example, a short common iliac stenosis is best treated by endovascular revascularization, whereas open surgery (aortobifemoral bypass) may be more fitting for very diffuse aortoiliac and femoral occlusive disease. Nonetheless, the decision for or against a catheter-based intervention should be carefully considered in the context of the anatomy, patient comorbidities, and the skill set of the interventionalist. Finally, success of an intervention should be more than just radiographic and should include documentation of improved symptoms and clinically relevant hemodynamic measurements such as ankle-brachial indices, Doppler waveforms, pulse volume recordings, or transcutaneous oxygen measurements.

B. **Percutaneous transluminal angioplasty (PTA)** is the most fundamental and popular technique used for treating vascular occlusive disease and generally uses polyethylene catheters that have an inflatable balloon near the tip. Balloon angioplasty represents a variation of the original transluminal arterial dilatation described by **Dotter and Judkins.** The Dotter technique used a relatively large 12-Fr Teflon catheter introduced over an inner 8-Fr catheter and passed through the stenosis to dilate. No balloon was involved. **Gruntzig** popularized balloon catheters in the late 1970s, and their use now is common practice.

The first step in PTA is to cross the lesion with the wire as described in the previous section. An angled hydrophilic or glide wire is particularly effective in this maneuver and can be steered into and beyond the stenosis, often with the aid of a gripping or torque device. An angled catheter can also be used to direct or steer a straight hydrophilic wire to the appropriate position to navigate across the lesion. Alternatively, the endovascular specialist may enter a subintimal plane when crossing chronic total occlusions (CTO) (e.g., **subintimal angioplasty**) (Fig. 10.3). With this technique, the wire is directed into an eccentric plane at the start of the lesion forming a loop in the subintimal plane. A catheter can then be used to follow the wire until it reenters into the true lumen beyond the stenosis or occlusion. A characteristic "give-way" sensation followed by smooth passage of the wire and catheter signals the interventionalist that the true lumen has been reentered. Contrast should be injected into the catheter once the lesion has been crossed to confirm reentry or positioning into the true lumen of the vessel on the other side of the target lesion. Once the wire and catheter have crossed the lesion, a wire exchange can be performed through the catheter to allow placement of a more substantive working wire over which the balloon angioplasty catheter can be placed. Both transluminal and subintimal angioplasty are successful for treating aortoiliac and infrainguinal disease.

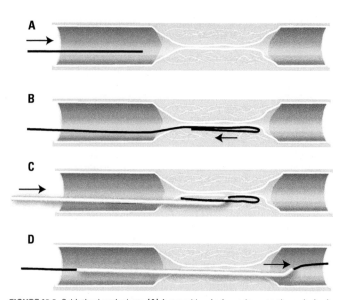

FIGURE 10.3 Subintimal angioplasty. **(A)** A steerable wire is used to enter the occlusion in an eccentric plane. **(B)** The wire begins to loop once in the subintimal plane. **(C)** A catheter is advanced over the wire into the subintimal plane. **(D)** After the wire is felt to reenter the lumen, contrast is injected into the catheter to confirm intraluminal placement. The wire is replaced, and the catheter is removed. The wire is maintained past the lesion for the duration of the intervention.

The mechanisms by which PTA dilates a stenotic vessel are complex. **First, balloon dilatation causes a focal dissection,** disrupting the plaque and the artery wall. With rupture of the plaque and partial separation from the media, there is stretching of the adventitia to increase the cross-sectional area of the lumen (Fig. 10.4). **Second, the intimal plaque protrudes into the lumen,** accounting for the angiographic appearance of local flaps and dissection channels visualized in some cases. **Third, remodeling occurs** by adherence of the intimal flaps with little change in plaque volume. Thus, long-term patency depends on sufficient stretching of the vessel and an adequately remodeled lumen. Restenosis may occur because of insufficient dilatation (compliance), from extension of dissection channels into nondilated segments and from **myointimal hyperplasia.** Essentially, myointimal hyperplasia is a vessel's complex response to injury (i.e., angioplasty or surgery) with smooth muscle proliferation and subsequent restenosis of the vessel. Excessive myointimal hyperplasia can lead to severe stenosis and failure of the intervention. In fact, early and midterm angioplasty or bypass failures are largely attributed to myointimal hyperplasia and have therefore been the target of drug-eluting technologies.

The selection of a balloon for angioplasty is based on the diameter of the vessel (oversized by 1.1 times) and length of the lesion. A variety of techniques can be used to measure or estimate the normal diameter of the target vessel so that the appropriate diameter balloon may be selected. These include marking tapes and catheters with radiopaque markers at known distances from one another and use of the known sheath tip size. Intravascular ultrasound (IVUS) is a technology that allows more

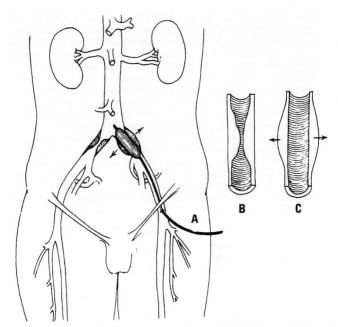

FIGURE 10.4 Percutaneous transluminal angioplasty (PTA). **(A)** By the Seldinger's technique, a catheter with an internal flexible guidewire is passed into and gently insinuated through the area of arterial stenosis. **(B, C)** The balloon is inflated to several atmospheres of pressure. When the PTA is complete, the arterial lumen is larger and the local artery is stretched.

accurate measurement of vessel diameter from within and can also be used to estimate balloon size. Balloon sizes commonly used for peripheral interventions range from 2.5 to 10 mm in diameter and 20 to 200 mm in length. Often, for peripheral interventions, a simple over-the-wire approach is taken with the balloon. When minimal wire movement is important, and for smaller vessels, the **monorail balloon catheter** compatible with a 0.014-inch wire may be chosen (Fig. 10.1). Just like the monorail catheters described previously, the monorail balloon devices have a side port for exit of the wire so that only the initial 20 to 30 cm of the catheter are involved with each exchange.

Once the balloon is positioned within the target lesion, an inflation device is used to expand it to a desired pressure. Every balloon has a **nominal pressure** at which its full or prescribed diameter is reached. The **rated burst pressure** is the pressure below which the balloon is guaranteed not to rupture with 95% confidence. Typical nominal and burst pressures are 6 to 8 and 12 to 16 atmospheres, respectively, and these numbers are affected by the balloon's compliance (change in volume/change in pressure) or degree of softness. **Highly compliant balloons** are softer and track easily due to their composition but will also expand beyond their designated diameter and length at higher pressures. For this reason, more compliant balloons are generally not effective for angioplasty of inflexible calcified stenoses. Large compliant balloons such as the Coda® (Cook Medical, Inc., Bloomington, IN) and Reliant™ (Medtronic, Inc., Minneapolis, MN) are useful for gently expanding stent grafts after endovascular aneurysm repair and can also be used to temporarily occlude the aorta or other bleeding or injured arteries. **Noncompliant balloons** are stiffer and are better and more effective for angioplasty of tight stenoses, as they expand to their predetermined diameter without elongating. Rigid or resistant stenoses can occur in some native arterial lesions as well as with in-stent or recurrent stenosis due to neointimal hyperplasia. These types of rigid or recalcitrant stenoses may be seen at the venous anastomosis of hemodialysis grafts and may have elastic recoil that does not respond to traditional angioplasty. Such lesions can be treated with ultra-high-pressure, noncompliant balloons with rated burst pressures from 20 to 30 mm Hg. Alternatively, **cutting balloons** have several microblades circumferentially positioned on a balloon, such that longitudinal incisions are made in the plaque with balloon inflation. This technology can also be helpful to overcome the rigidity of very fibrous lesions.

C. **Stents** are cylindrical tubes composed of a wire latticework that can be deployed within a vessel in order to overcome elastic recoil and expand the vessel's lumen. Stents are broadly categorized as either **balloon expandable** or **self-expanding** and either **covered** or **bare metal**. Most stents are composed of either stainless steel or the metal alloy referred to as nitinol. Placement of endovascular stents falls into one of two strategies: **selective stenting** or **primary stenting**. Selective stenting refers to the practice of stent placement only in response to an inadequate technical result seen on completion angiography following PTA. The usual criteria for selective stenting are a residual stenosis or dissection from the angioplasty that compromises 30% or more of the lumen. The presence of a residual pressure gradient also indicates an imperfect PTA result and may be an indication for stent placement. In some cases, the original intent is to **primarily stent** the target lesion. With improved stent technologies and the demonstrated effectiveness of primary stenting, this practice has become more common over time. In some cases, the target lesion may need to be **predilated** with an undersized balloon to create a small channel within the stenosis in order to position the stent. In these cases, the term primary stenting still applies.

Similar to balloons, stents are available in a variety of lengths and diameters. Typically, the stent is oversized slightly for the diameter of the vessel and should nearly match the length of the lesion so that normal segments of vessel are not stented unnecessarily. In cases of selective stenting, a device that has a 1 to 2 mm greater diameter than the angioplasty balloon is generally selected. It is important to recognize the different properties and applications of balloon-expandable and self-expanding stents (Table 10.2).

Balloon-expandable stent technology originated with the Palmaz design. Today, these devices are typically made of stainless steel and are premounted on a less compliant balloon that matches the diameter and length of the stent. When this balloon is inflated, the stent expands simultaneously and is deployed at the time of angioplasty. Balloon-expandable stents can be precisely positioned by the operator, which is critical in certain locations such as the renal and mesenteric arteries and aortic arch vessels. Traditionally, balloon-expandable stents are thought to have the advantage of more precise control and exact placement compared to their self-expanding counterparts. Balloon-expandable stents can also be expanded beyond their prescribed diameter (i.e., **overexpansion**) by inflating a balloon with a diameter 1 to 2 mm larger than the stent once it is initially deployed. Overexpansion will result in some **shortening** of the stent as the lattices withdraw from the ends as the diameter expands beyond

Bare Metal Stents Are Either Balloon Expandable or Self-expandable, and Different Properties Influence Their Selection for Use.

Property	Balloon Expandable	Self-expandable
Precision of deployment	Excellent	Fair
Radial force	Very strong	Moderately strong
Trackability in tortuous anatomy	Poor	Fair to good
Crushable with external compression	Significantly	Minimally
Continuous self-expanding properties	No	Yes
Can be enlarged beyond set diameter	Yes[a]	No
Conformability to the vessel	Absent	Excellent[a]
Flexibility	Poor	Fair to good

[a]Balloon-expandable stents can be further enlarged by using a larger balloon. Self-expanding stents will conform to a smaller portion of the vessel if a size discrepancy exists. However, an undersized self-expandable stent cannot be further expanded and is vulnerable to migration.

the designed measurement. These stents are vulnerable to deformation or compression from external forces, and placement of balloon-expandable devices in locations where they could be crushed or fractured, such as an extremity, should be avoided.

Self-expanding stent technology stemmed from the original **Wallstent** design, and most are made of nitinol, a metal that assumes its preformed shape when warmed to body temperature. Although the initial **radial force** or **hoop strength** of self-expanding stents is not as great as the balloon-expandable devices, the self-expanding component of the design works to assume the prescribed diameter and shape over time. In contrast, the balloon-expandable stents, which have greater initial radial force, do not increase in size after placement. Self-expanding stents are generally more flexible than balloon-expandable devices and therefore are better suited for tortuous anatomy. Common locations for self-expanding stents include the carotid arteries, arteries of the extremities, and iliac veins. Intuitively, certain anatomic areas contain flexion or compression points and may not be well suited for stenting. Examples of such locations are the thoracic outlet, common femoral artery, and popliteal artery. There are concerns for stent fracture and early stenosis that must be balanced with the risks of alternative treatment such as open reconstruction or bypass. Some interventions can be performed as **hybrid, open-endovascular procedures** in which one portion of the procedure is open surgical and the other endovascular. An example of this tactic is a retrograde iliac artery stent placement during the same procedure as an open femoral artery endarterectomy.

Covered stents are made of a wire exoskeleton covered by plastic (expanded polytetrafluoroethylene). Covered stents are often referred to as stent grafts and can be used to reline or to exclude a portion of an artery from the circulation. One such application is the treatment of a **pseudoaneurysm**. A pseudoaneurysm is a localized outpouching or area of bleeding from a disrupted artery or artery-graft anastomosis that is contained only by the adventitia or surrounding tissues. Traumatic pseudoaneurysms or arterial disruptions from penetrating or blunt trauma or from iatrogenic injury (postcatheterization) are often suitable for catheter-based treatment. In these cases, a covered stent can be deployed across the pseudoaneurysm to exclude it so that it thromboses, while maintaining axial flow through the main vessel lumen. Similarly, an **arteriovenous fistula** from penetrating injury can be treated by placement of a covered stent on the arterial side, effectively sealing the fistula. The choice of catheter-based versus open surgical therapy is often influenced by the location of the lesion. **Endovascular aneurysm repair** is based on the principle of aneurysm sac exclusion with modular stent graft components. Along the same lines, covered stents (Viabahn®, W.L. Gore and Associates, Flagstaff, AZ) have been used as an alternative to surgery in patients with popliteal artery aneurysms, with promising results. The use of covered stents has been extended to occlusive disease, specifically in the iliac and superficial femoral artery distributions. A theoretical disadvantage of covered stents in the treatment of occlusive disease is the coverage of potentially important collateral or side-branch vessels, although relining of the diseased segment is intuitively appealing. Prospective clinical studies have been performed demonstrating that primary stenting of iliac artery occlusive disease with covered stents is as viable and effective as bare metal stenting. Similarly, the practice of primary covered stenting of some superficial femoral stenoses or occlusions has been shown safe and effective in the short term.

D. **Miscellaneous. "Debulking" technologies** such as **laser therapy** and **atherectomy** that vaporize or excise atheromatous plaques are intuitively appealing. A prospective study of the excimer laser in the superficial femoral artery (SFA) failed to show superiority when compared with PTA with selective stenting, although the need for stenting in patients treated with the laser was reduced. Several atherectomy devices are available for use in the periphery. Additional studies comparing debulking therapies to PTA/stenting need to be performed before their widespread use can be advocated. Locations considered unfavorable for stenting, such as the popliteal or tibial vessels or bifurcation stenoses, may benefit from technologies that reduce the need for stent placement.

Some innovative strategies target myointimal hyperplasia, the principal cause of midterm angioplasty failures—a true Achilles' heel of vascular intervention. **Cryoplasty** is a technology that uses a combination of angioplasty with freezing in order to enact both a physical and a biological response (apoptosis) in attempt to decrease rates of intimal hyperplasia and restenosis. Clinical trials have not shown any clear advantage of cryoplasty over standard PTA with or without stenting. **Drug-eluting technologies** release antiproliferative agents (e.g., **sirolimus, paclitaxel**), and these stents have been shown to reduce the short-term risk of restenosis in the coronary arteries. Drug-eluting stents have also been applied in the superficial femoral artery with advantageous results over bare metal stents. The paclitaxel is released from the stent into the surrounding tissue and targets microtubules at a cellular level to inhibit proliferation. Based on similar science, **drug-coated balloons** have been developed with promising results in the femoral-popliteal arteries, while avoiding the need for permanent metal implantation.

Intravascular ultrasound or IVUS provides internal imaging and measurement of vessels and has the potential to be useful in a range of clinical applications. Because IVUS images are in cross section, they can provide additional information not seen on two-dimensional angiography. Technical results after angioplasty can be assessed using IVUS to determine if significant residual stenosis or dissection exists and stent apposition can be assessed for completeness. IVUS is useful for verifying measurements of length and diameter for stent graft repairs of aortic aneurysms. In these instances, the origin of the renal arteries can be identified and the exact neck diameter can be measured from inside the aorta and the presence of plaque or thrombus can also be identified. IVUS is also used following catheter-directed thrombolysis of deep vein thromboses (DVTs) to assess completeness of the therapy and identify external compression that may not be present on standard venography (e.g., May-Thurner syndrome).

III. **CATHETER-DIRECTED THROMBOLYTIC THERAPY.** Despite widespread interest in thrombolytic drugs, their role in peripheral arterial and venous disease is relatively selective. Currently, the most commonly used thrombolytic agents are urokinase and various forms or generations of **recombinant tissue plasminogen activator (r-tPA)**. The use of any of these agents must be undertaken with careful consideration of their pharmacokinetics, indications, and possible complications. The main complication of pharmacologic thrombolysis is bleeding. The administration of systemic intravenous doses of thrombolytics is not effective and not advised for peripheral vascular thrombosis. Rather, **catheter-directed thrombolysis** can be performed in either the arterial or venous system. Traditionally, this technique is performed by the infusion of thrombolytic drugs via a multi-sidehole catheter into the thrombosed vessel. Alternatively, mechanical thrombectomy devices may be used alone or in combination with thrombolytic agents and often decrease the need for thrombolytics and thus lower the risk of bleeding.

A. **Pharmacokinetics.** Thrombolytics are plasminogen activators that lead to clot lysis by enhancing the fibrinolytic system via conversion of plasminogen to its active form, plasmin. These agents not only act on plasminogen within a clot but also on plasminogen throughout the circulation, and systemic fibrinolysis may result. **Streptokinase** must first form an activated complex with plasminogen, which completes the conversion of excess plasminogen to plasmin. This agent was discovered in 1933 and was the original thrombolytic agent used for acute myocardial infarction. Streptokinase is no longer used in the United States, primarily because of high antigenicity and allergic response with repeated exposure and the availability of better drugs. **Urokinase** acts by directly cleaving plasminogen to plasmin, with higher affinity for fibrin-bound plasminogen than streptokinase.

Various forms or generations of **r-tPA** are most commonly used for catheter-directed thrombolysis. These forms of r-tPA are more specific for plasminogen bound to fibrin clot than the other lytic agents. As such, although some systemic fibrinolysis occurs with r-tPA analogs, it happens to a lesser degree than that observed with the other drugs; an advantage that reduces systemic bleeding complications.

The half-life for most thrombolytic drugs is short: streptokinase, 10 to 12 minutes; urokinase, 11 to 16 minutes; r-tPA analogs, 5 to 15 minutes. Consequently, the effect of the drugs dissipates rapidly, although depleted fibrinogen levels may take at least 24 hours to normalize. In the authors' experience, the need to use ε-**aminocaproic acid** (**Amicar**; Xanodyne Pharmaceuticals, Inc., Newport, KY) or fibrinogen concentrates to reverse the effects of thrombolysis is rare.

B. **Indications.** Selective use of catheter-directed thrombolysis in cases of severe proximal DVTs actively reduces if not eliminates thrombus burden, thereby preserving venous endothelial and valvular function. Although initial concerns regarding bleeding complications limited widespread use of thrombolysis, recent data suggest that serious bleeding mishaps are rare. Furthermore, the effective use of **mechanical thrombectomy devices** (Table 10.1) can reduce the amount and duration of catheter-directed thrombolysis, decreasing the risk of bleeding. This therapy is also effective in treating acute axillo-subclavian vein thrombosis associated with central venous catheters or effort thrombosis from thoracic outlet syndrome. In summary, catheter-directed thrombolysis for the treatment of acute DVT is considered in symptomatic patients with extensive iliofemoral DVT, not only for symptomatic relief but also to potentially reduce long-term morbidity associated with postthrombotic syndrome. Catheter-directed thrombolysis is also appropriate for some cases of massive or submassive pulmonary embolism.

Acute arterial ischemia is often the result of thrombosis of a diseased native vessel or embolic from another source. Catheter-directed thrombolysis is most effective for acute, not organized, thrombus and has good limb salvage rates compared to open surgical methods. Other uses of thrombolysis for acute arterial occlusion are situations for which surgery has traditionally poor results or for which high operative mortality makes a nonoperative approach attractive. Acutely thrombosed popliteal aneurysms with tibial artery thrombosis and thrombosis of bypass grafts or stents are examples of patients that can benefit from an endovascular approach.

C. **Methods.** In the setting of arterial or venous occlusion, catheter-directed thrombolysis occurs as the drugs are delivered via continuous infusion through a catheter with multiple sideholes directly into the thrombus (e.g., Craig-McNamara™ catheter, Medtronic, Minneapolis, MN). The infusion catheter is placed within the thrombus over a selecting wire via standard endovascular techniques and comes in variable infusion lengths (5 to 50 cm). Different catheter-directed thrombolytic regimens have been described—including those using mechanical adjuncts—and the options for any given patient will depend on the location, duration, and extent of thrombosis as well as the experience and capability of the endovascular specialist and his or her institution. One regimen administers a dose of 2 mg r-tPA in the first hour, followed by 1 mg/h for 8 to 12 hours, an approach which is aimed at minimizing the risk of bleeding complications. For the r-tPA analog reteplase, an initial catheter-directed dose of 5 units followed by 0.25 to 0.5 units/h for 8 to 12 hours has also been described. (**Note: rt-PA doses are in mg, and reteplase doses are in units.**) Lower doses are generally used for prolonged infusions, venous cases, and when drugs are combined with mechanical thrombectomy devices. Intra-arterial delivery of a small bolus of thrombolytic can also be used during an open revascularization operation to eliminate distal thrombus (e.g., after an open surgical thromboembolectomy).

Mechanical thrombectomy devices have evolved to become quite useful in the management of thrombotic conditions, either alone or in combination with thrombolytic drugs. These devices are especially useful in patients who have contraindications to thrombolytic medication, such as those with bleeding diathesis or a history of gastrointestinal bleeding, a recent stroke or recent surgery. When used as a mechanical adjunct, these devices hasten the process of clot lysis by debulking and directly removing thrombus from the vessel lumen. One such device works by instilling a high-velocity saline jet into the thrombus, resulting in a vacuum effect, such that the macerated clot can be aspirated into the catheter (e.g., AngioJet™ and AngioJet™ ZelanteDVT™ devices, Boston Scientific, Marlborough, MA). The EkoSonic™ endovascular system (BTG

Interventional Medicine, London, UK) uses targeted ultrasonic waves in combination with clot-dissolving drugs to better disseminate the drug into the clot. The Penumbra Indigo® (Penumbra, Alameda, California) uses an aspiration catheter and separator system connected to high level, continuous suction. There is a small risk of distal embolization (2% to 5%) during these procedures that may be reduced by a period of pharmacologic thrombolysis (i.e., use of an r-tPA analog). Technical success and limb salvage with mechanical thrombolysis is promising and comparable with pharmacologic thrombolysis alone.

Several laboratory tests, **hemoglobin, fibrinogen level, fibrin split products (also referred to as fibrin degradation products), and platelet count,** should be monitored during the performance of catheter-directed thrombolysis to assess for potentially dangerous systemic effects of the procedure. The fibrinogen level (normal 150 to 400 mg/dL) is important because a level less than 150 mg/dL and definitely less than 100 mg/dL is indicative of systemic, and potentially dangerous thrombolytic activity (i.e., risk of bleeding complication). A fibrin degradation level of greater than 10 mg/L and definitely greater than 40 mg/L is also indicative of an unwanted systemic effect of the thrombolytic therapy. In addition to laboratory measures of systemic thrombolysis and coagulopathy, attention should be paid to the total dose and total time of thrombolytic therapy. Clinical studies and experience have shown that the risk of bleeding complications from the puncture site and from spontaneous intracranial and retroperitoneal hemorrhage begins to increases significantly with a total thrombolytic dose of more than 30 to 40 mg of alteplase and 15 to 20 units of reteplase and treatment durations that extend beyond 24 to 36 hours.

When catheter-directed thrombolysis is initiated, heparin is commonly administered through the access sheath to prevent clotting in the sheath. This also requires close attention as too high of a dose will increase the risk of bleeding complications. One strategy is to begin a low-dose heparin infusion (300 to 500 units/h) through the access sheath to avoid **pericatheter thrombus formation** while following the PTT to ensure the heparin dose does not become supratherapeutic (i.e., maintain PTT around 50 seconds).

D. **Complications.** Catheter-directed or regional thrombolytic therapy may be complicated by bleeding, thrombosis, or embolism in 10% to 15% of patients. Access site bleeding is the most common problem. Distal emboli are often small and sometimes can be resolved with continued thrombolytic administration. Nonetheless, about 5% of patients will require some type of surgical intervention to manage these complications. The most devastating bleeding complications associated with catheter-directed thrombolysis are those related to **intracranial hemorrhage.** Although this complication is rare (0.5% to 1%), it can occur as a result of too high a dose of thrombolytic drug over too long a period of time and is prone to occur in the elderly and those with underlying hypertension or previous history of stroke. The rare occurrence of intracranial hemorrhage emphasizes the care that must be taken when evaluating patients for this therapy and the attention to detail that must occur among all medical providers on the team once therapy is initiated.

IV. **POSTANGIOGRAM CARE.** Any patient who has undergone angiography should be monitored hourly for at least 4 to 6 hours as most early complications become evident during this time period. Nursing personnel can perform most postprocedure checks, but a physician or physician assistant/nurse practitioner should also examine the patient during this immediate recuperative period, as they are likely to be the ones on-call for complications arising after patient discharge. The baseline postprocedure exam should include **(a) evaluation of the patient's general appearance and mental status (especially after cerebral studies), (b) heart rate, (c) blood pressure, (d) inspection of puncture or access sites, (e) palpation of extremity pulses (including Doppler signals), and (f) a check of the hematocrit if there are any signs of bleeding.**

In addition, adequate hydration should be maintained for 12 to 24 hours after the procedure, since contrast material causes a diuresis and can lead to dehydration. The combination of diuresis and the nephrotoxicity from the contrast material can damage renal function, especially in patients with diabetes mellitus or baseline chronic kidney disease. In higher-risk patients, the authors often maintain an intravenous infusion for 4 to 6 hours after the angiogram. Oral fluids are also encouraged for 24 hours after the procedure to maintain hydration.

Sheath removal and access site management. At the completion of a catheter-based procedure, the final step is **sheath removal.** If the procedure has been done in the lower pressure venous system (i.e., a venogram or intervention on the venous system), the access sheath can be removed and manual pressure held for hemostasis. For nearly all scenarios of venous access, including those with larger sheaths and even those in which anticoagulation has been used, removing the sheath and holding 5 to 10 minutes of manual pressure is sufficient to seal the access site.

In contrast, removing the access sheath following endovascular procedures performed in the higher-pressure arterial system (i.e., arteriography or arterial intervention) is more involved and includes several important considerations. To achieve an adequate and safe seal of the arterial entry site, one must consider the following factors: **size of access sheath, whether or not anticoagulation was used during the procedure (and when it was last administered), and if arterial access was achieved at a "virgin" site or at a site of previous interventions or operation (i.e., "redo" access site).** Larger sheaths have greater risk of bleeding once removed, a risk that is compounded when the patient received heparin or other anticoagulant during the procedure (especially when the heparin has not worn off or is being continued). It is also recognized that arterial access in a "redo" site or site where there exists a previous vascular reconstruction (i.e., prosthetic graft) is associated with higher rates of complications.

The development of different percutaneous closure devices and their improved reliability can facilitate management of the access site and allows the patient to ambulate sooner after the procedure. Nonetheless, such devices do not necessarily decrease access site complications, and it is still important for all members of the team to give careful consideration to the arterial sheath removal and care for the patient afterward.

Percutaneous vascular closure devices come in three categories: **(a) extravascular sealant or plug, (b) mechanical seal or clip, and (c) suture mediated.** Most of the commonly used devices are now sold as an advanced generation, and most have improved significantly over each iteration of their development. All the percutaneous closure devices have instructions for use (IFU) that should be read and include recommendations on the range of sheath size defects each can effectively close. Generally speaking, the extravascular sealant or plug devices are able to close arterial defects left by 5- to 7-Fr sheaths. Most of the mechanical seals or clip devices are able to close a defect left by sheaths in the 7 to 8 Fr range, and the suture-mediated products are able to close a defect left by a sheath as large as 10 Fr. By placing two suture-mediated devices in the arterial defect at the time of gaining initial access (i.e., the "preclose" approach), defects left by sheaths as large as 20 Fr can be safely closed after their removal.

If the procedure is a basic arteriogram performed through a 5-Fr sheath and no anticoagulation is used, the sheath can be pulled at the end of the case and manual pressure held for 20 to 25 minutes to achieve a safe arterial seal. In these cases because no closure device was used, we generally recommend the patient lay supine for 4 to 6 hours after pressure has been held. If an extravascular sealant or plug device is used in these cases, the patient can be mobilized sooner, usually after 2 to 4 hours of laying still. If an endovascular procedure has been performed through a 5- to 7-Fr sheath, including administration of heparin, one of the closure devices should be considered. Alternatively, one can wait until the heparin effect dissipates and then pull the sheath and hold manual pressure for 20 to 25 minutes followed by 6 hours of bed rest. Some type of closure device should be used if the arterial procedure required an 8-Fr or larger sheath. Although percutaneous closure devices reduce time to hemostasis and help with early mobilization of the patient, they add to the cost of the endovascular case. In addition, closure devices can be maldeployed resulting in arterial occlusion or hemorrhage and rarely may become infected. For these reasons, some endovascular specialists still prefer using the manual pressure technique for basic 5 to 6 Fr cases in which no heparin was used.

V. COMPLICATIONS

A. **Neurologic Deficits**. Aortic arch and selective cervical arteriography can result in transient or permanent central neurologic deficits that may occur immediately at the time of the angiogram or minutes to hours after the case. Neurologic deficits that happen during the study are most likely embolic from dislodged atheroma or catheter thrombus. Meticulous care must also be taken during arch and carotid angiography to assure that no air is injected through the imaging catheter, as air embolization can cause severe neurologic complication during such procedures. Delayed neurologic deficits may also be secondary to hypoperfusion or thrombosis associated with contrast-induced diuresis and dehydration.

Peripheral nerve symptoms can also result from vascular access in the brachial or femoral arteries. Transient neuropraxia can occur from irritation of adjacent nerves or one of their branches from the needle puncture itself or from blood extravasating out of the vessel puncture site. **After brachial puncture, any hematoma that compresses the median nerve causing persistent pain or other neurologic change should be decompressed in the operating room.**

B. **Hemorrhage**. Small hematomas and ecchymosis at the access site are not uncommon. However, an expanding hematoma indicates continued bleeding into the perivascular spaces and a more urgent situation. The first treatment for a hematoma should be the reapplication of manual pressure for 20 to 30 minutes. Significant hypertension or coagulopathy should be corrected, as these contribute to bleeding from the puncture site. Expanding or pulsatile hematomas should be evaluated immediately by ultrasound. Often, a pseudoaneurysm can be closed by ultrasound-guided compression with the ultrasound probe or using ultrasound-guided thrombin injection into the pseudoaneurysm. In some patients, an acute arteriovenous fistula may also resolve with ultrasound-guided compression. Significant retroperitoneal hemorrhage can also occur after angiography, particularly after accessing the femoral or external iliac artery in a too proximal location (i.e., a "high stick"). Early indications of bleeding may be persistent back pain, tachycardia, hypotension, and anemia. Flank ecchymosis is a delayed finding. CTA will demonstrate a retroperitoneal, periaortic, or psoas muscle hematoma and initial supportive treatment consists of correction of any coagulopathy, transfusion of blood products as needed, and bed rest. Most episodes of minor retroperitoneal bleeding resolve by the time they are discovered. Ongoing bleeding or hemodynamic instability indicates a significant femoral or iliac injury and requires immediate angiography or open operation. Repeat arteriography in this situation would be aimed at identifying and sealing the bleeding site with a covered stent.

C. Diminished or absent pulses (compared with baseline) following the angiogram suggests partial or complete arterial occlusion. Although spasm may occur, it is rarely the cause of diminished pulses persisting beyond 30 to 60 minutes after the arteriogram. **The most common causes of compromised extremity blood flow after angiography are (a) arterial injury (intimal flap); (b) thrombus adherent to, or as a result of, the sheath or catheter; (c) arterial occlusion associated with a misplaced percutaneous closure device; and (d) hematoma compression of the arterial wall.** Stent thrombosis can occur in the early postintervention period and is usually secondary to a technical defect, poor inflow or runoff, or failure to administer adequate anticoagulation or antiplatelet therapy. Antiplatelet therapy with at least aspirin is recommended after angioplasty and/or stent placement to reduce the thrombotic risk. **Clopidogrel** (Plavix) is often prescribed in addition to aspirin after catheter-based interventions at a dose of 75 mg daily. A loading dose of 300 mg may be administered in some cases, when the patient is not already on steady-state dose. The added benefit of clopidogrel in preventing thrombosis after intervention is not necessarily proven, but it makes empiric sense and thus is often used.

If there are questions about extremity perfusion following an endovascular procedure, the physician or other members of the care team should make good use of the continuous wave Doppler device. Ankle-brachial indices can be rapidly performed for an objective measure of perfusion (i.e., provides a number or ratio) and can often be compared with a similar measurement taken prior to the endovascular procedure. An acutely ischemic limb (painful, pallid, pulseless) following endovascular intervention necessitates urgent reintervention, either with repeat arteriography or surgery.

D. A pulsatile mass at the access site represents either a hematoma transmitting a pulse from the artery underneath or a **false aneurysm** (pseudoaneurysm). This is a difficult distinction to make in the early postprocedural period, and a duplex ultrasound is a favorite diagnostic modality. In some situations, small (<3 to 4 cm) acute hematomas can be eliminated by **ultrasound-guided compression** using the ultrasound probe. Although this process may take more than an hour and can be uncomfortable for the patient, the success rate is greater than 90%. Small pseudoaneurysms (<2 cm) frequently resolve with time and should be reimaged with ultrasound within weeks of the procedure. Pseudoaneurysms that are initially missed and then noted at a later examination should be repaired about 6 to 8 weeks after the arteriogram. By this time, local inflammation generally has resolved and dissection and repair may be easier. Chronic pseudoaneurysms have a developed capsule that is not likely to resolve with ultrasound-guided compression. If the pseudoaneurysm has a narrow neck, **ultrasound-guided injection of thrombin** (0.1 cc at a time of diluted 5,000 IU in 5 cc) is a very effective means of treatment, as flow in the pseudoaneurysm will cease with administration of a small amount of thrombin. Any postarteriogram hematoma that suddenly causes pain and local subcutaneous hemorrhage is a ruptured pseudoaneurysm and usually requires urgent surgical evacuation and repair of the artery. Pseudoaneurysm rupture is most likely to occur within 7 to 10 days of the initial angiogram. For this reason, it is the authors' suggestion that all patients with a significant hematoma receive close follow-up in the days and week after the procedure.

E. **Infection.** If appropriate sterile technique at the time of the endovascular procedure is used, local access site infection is very unusual. Sterile technique and preparation includes (a) cleansing the site with a surgical scrub soap before the study, (b) standard sterile preparation with a chlorhexidine-based prep at the time of the study, and (c) standard surgical attire for members of the endovascular team. In uncommon cases in which there is cellulitis around the desired vascular access site, the procedure should be delayed if elective, or if urgent, a different access site chosen. **If an endovascular procedure is being performed through a previously placed prosthetic graft (i.e., a synthetic graft or patch in the femoral position), the patient should receive a dose of prophylactic antibiotics prior to the beginning of the case.**

Selected Readings

Babapulle MN, Eisenberg MJ. Coated stents for the prevention of restenosis: part I. *Circulation.* 2002;106:2734-2740.
Brief basic science and histological description of myointimal hyperplasia.

Comerota AJ, Gravett MH. Do randomized trials of thrombolysis versus open revascularization still apply to current management: what has changed? *Semin Vasc Surg.* 2009;22(1):41-46.
Critical synopsis of older clinical trials on thrombolysis for arterial limb ischemia that incorporates discussion of modern techniques.

Curi MA, Geraghty PJ, Merino OA, et al. Mid-term outcomes of endovascular popliteal artery aneurysm repair. *J Vasc Surg.* 2007;45:505-510.
Feasibility and outcomes after repairing popliteal aneurysms with covered stent-grafts.

Dake MD, Ansel GM, Jaff MR, et al.; Zilver PTX Investigators. Paclitaxel-eluting stents show superiority to balloon angioplasty and bare metal stents in femoropopliteal disease: twelve-month Zilver PTX randomized study results. *Circ Cardiovasc Interv.* 2011;4:495-504.
Randomized trial showed one-year patency of drug-eluting stents in superficial femoral artery is 83% compared to 65% in optimal PTA group.

Koreny M, Riedmuller E, Nikfardjam M, et al. Arterial puncture closing devices compared with manual standard compression after cardiac catheterization: systemic review and meta-analysis. *JAMA.* 2004;291:350-357.
Meta-analysis of 4000 patients comparing "closure devices" with manual compression after femoral access.

Lakhter V, Aggarwal V. Current status and outcomes of iliac artery endovascular intervention. *Interv Cardiol Clin.* 2017;6:167-180.
Discussion of endovascular management of iliac disease with technical emphasis.

McCaslin JE, Andras A, Stansby G. Cryoplasty for peripheral arterial disease. *Cochrane Database Syst Rev.* 2013;11(8):CD005507.
Summary of seven randomized trials could not demonstrate superiority of cryoplasty over standard angioplasty.

Nadal LL, Cynamon J, Lipsitz, et al. Subintimal angioplasty for chronic total occlusions. *Tech Vasc Interv Radiol.* 2004;7:16-22.
Early experience with subintimal angioplasty with description of basic technique.

Ouriel K, Veith FJ, Sasahara AA; for the Thrombolysis or Peripheral Arterial Surgery (TOPAS) Investigators. A comparison of recombinant urokinase with vascular surgery as initial treatment for acute arterial occlusion of the legs. *N Engl J Med.* 1998;338:1105-1111.
Multicenter, randomized TOPAS trial examined the safety and efficacy of catheter-directed thrombolysis for acute arterial occlusions with duration of less than 14 days, finding no significant difference in amputation-free survival between thrombolysis and surgery.

Schillinger M, Minar E. Percutaneous treatment of peripheral artery disease: novel techniques. *Circulation.* 2012;126:2433-2440.
Modern review of data regarding endovascular technology, including stents, drug-coated technology, and atherectomy.

Scott EC, Biuckians A, Light RE, et al. Subintimal angioplasty for the treatment of claudication and critical limb ischemia: 3-year results. *J Vasc Surg.* 2007;46:959-964.

Experience with an "endovascular-first" approach to lower extremity arterial occlusive disease using subintimal angioplasty technique.

Sohail MR, Khan AH, Holmes DR, et al. Infectious complications of percutaneous vascular closure devices. *Mayo Clin Proc.* 2005;80:1011-1015.

A cautionary appraisal of the incidence and natural history of "closure device" infections.

The STILE Investigators. Results of a prospective randomized trial evaluating surgery versus thrombolysis for ischemia of the lower extremity: the STILE trial. *Ann Surg.* 1994;220:251-268.

Along with the TOPAS trial, one of the original trials that examined safety and efficacy of catheter-directed thrombolysis for arterial ischemia.

Tonnessen BH. Iatrogenic injury from vascular access and endovascular procedures. *Perspect Vasc Surg Endovasc Ther.* 2011;23:128-135.

Incidence and management of common iatrogenic injuries that the vascular specialist will encounter.

Vedantham S, Goldhaber SZ, Julian JA, et al.; ATTRACT Trial Investigators. Pharmacomechanical catheter-directed thrombolysis for deep-vein thrombosis. *N Engl J Med.* 2017;377:2240-2252.

Contemporary, randomized trial with 2-year outcomes for DVT treatment using either catheter-based thrombolysis or anticoagulation.

Basic Fluoroscopic Concepts and Applied Radiation Safety

Most patients who require an intervention for severe or refractory vascular disease will eventually undergo some type of angiographic procedure in the endovascular suite or operating room. **Fluoroscopy refers to the digital or photographic formation of images using electromagnetic radiation and is the main principle behind angiography, which pertains specifically to imaging of the blood vessels.** With the aid of devices and contrast material within the vessel lumen (i.e., endovascular), fluoroscopy becomes angiography and allows the physician to see the contour of the vasculature to diagnose, quantify, and even treat disease. While angiography has led to remarkable advances in the treatment of vascular disease, its expanded use must be viewed in balance and with recognition of the potentially harmful effects of radiation to both the patient and the interventional team.

This point is relevant given that much of the recent enthusiasm for angiographic procedures has outpaced awareness of basic radiation terminology and radiation safety. In contrast to even a decade ago, when most angiographers had formal instruction in radiology and were dedicated to interventional fluoroscopic procedures, today's endovascular specialist has a more diverse training and practice background. Although well versed in the natural history of vascular disease and the range of management options, the endovascular specialist may not have had dedicated schooling in radiation science. In lieu of such formal training, basic concepts are often passed down to trainees by mentors who may not stress a basic understanding of a few key radiologic principles. While practical, this method may not be ideal in a time when the number and complexity of endovascular procedures is increasing along with the diversity of physicians enlisting to perform them.

The intent of this chapter is to recognize this important aspect of vascular care and to present basic radiation terms and concepts including the effects of radiation on patients and the interventional team. Basic steps toward radiation safety are presented, including steps to minimize radiation risk. To cover the entire field of interventional fluoroscopy is beyond the scope of this chapter, and therefore the reader is encouraged to use this as a primer to familiarize and to stimulate additional reading.

I. BASIC RADIATION CONCEPTS

A. X-rays are a form of electromagnetic radiation.
The main characteristics of x-rays are similar to those of visible light, and radiation is frequently quantified in a unit called a photon. **A single photon is a quantum of electromagnetic radiation containing a defined amount of energy, in this instance defined in terms of electron volts (eVs)** (Table 11.1). The stronger the radiation source, the more the photons per second can be produced. It takes thousands of x-ray photons per square millimeter to form a single fluoroscopic frame that is thousands of times greater than the energy contained in a photon of visible light. X-ray photons used for imaging have energies that range from 10,000 to 150,000 eVs. The source of radiation or x-ray tube converts electrical energy into electromagnetic quanta, and heat

T A B L E 11.1	Basic Radiation Terminology	
Term	**Definition**	**Unit of Measure**
Electromagnetic radiation	A form of energy emitted from a source	Photons or electron volts
Exposure	A measure of the quantity of radiation present at a particular location and formally determined by air ionization	KERMA (joules/kg of air)
Absorbed dose	Amount of energy absorbed from the radiation source at a point divided by the mass of the tissue at that point	Gray
Dose equivalent	A quantity defined for radiation protection purposes that expresses on a common scale for all types of radiation the irradiation incurred by exposed persons	Sievert or rem

KERMA, kinetic energy released per unit mass of air.

is generated as a side product. Radiation is the transport of this energy away from the x-ray tube by these electromagnetic quanta. **The intensity of an x-ray beam decreases inversely as the square of the distance between the source and the measuring point (e.g., the greater the distance, the less the beam intensity).**

B. **Radiation units and nomenclature are found in the International System (SI) of Units (e.g., gray, sieverts) or conventional system (e.g., rad, rem)** (Table 11.1). The term **exposure** refers to the concentration of radiation field delivered to a given point, such as the surface of a human body. Most measurements of exposure are actually measurements of air dose that has very similar absorption properties to human tissue. Therefore, our standard measures of exposure are actually measures of the x-ray beam's ability to ionize air caused by the small amount of absorbed energy. The working unit of exposure is the **kinetic energy released per unit mass of air** acronym (KERMA), which is a measure of the energy in joules (J) deposited in a unit mass (kg) of air.

Radiation **absorbed dose** is the amount of energy absorbed from the radiation source at a point divided by the mass of tissue at that point. Surprisingly, a very small amount of energy is actually absorbed by or deposited into tissue during medical procedures. As mentioned, the amount of energy absorbed by tissue is similar to the amount of radiation energy absorbed by the surrounding air. **1 gray (Gy) = 1 joule of energy absorbed per kilogram of material.** A gray is a large unit of radiation. For perspective, *therapeutic radiation* for treatment of certain malignancies is delivered in 1 to 2 gray range fractions (e.g., total 50 Gy over weeks), meaning that 1 to 2 joules of energy are delivered per session per kilogram of radiated tissue. In contrast, a standard chest x-ray delivers a dose of approximately 100 µGy.

Taking into account all forms of radiation, including natural, industrial, nuclear, and others, different types of radiation produce vastly different biologic effects for the same number of Gy or dose. So the **dose equivalent (H)** was developed to account for this biologic impact for radiation protection purposes and is expressed in units called **sieverts (Sv)**. The dose equivalent expresses on a common scale for all forms of radiation the amount of irradiation incurred by exposed persons and was established by means of an experimentally defined quality factor. While quality factors for some forms of radiation such as alpha particles are as high as 20, conveniently the quality factor for medical x-ray energies is 1: 1 Sv = 1 Gy × quality factor. The equivalent dose is often presented on radiation safety reports to workers on a monthly or quarterly basis in Sv or rem (roentgen equivalent in man) with 1 Sv = 100 rem.

C. **Radiation measuring device.** A radiation measuring device called a **dosimeter is necessary to determine the dose of radiation emitted by any given source at a particular location.** Dosimeters come in different forms, depending upon the type and amount of radiation that will be monitored or measured. Some basic instruments directly measure the ionization produced in a defined volume of air (i.e., KERMA) within a cylindrical instrument called an ionization chamber. The Geiger counter is another type of radiation detection device, which uses a Geiger tube and associated electrical display components. While these devices provide an accurate representation of soft tissue dose, they are not designed to monitor lesser amounts of exposure to patients or providers on a routine basis.

The more familiar and clinically practical dosimeters are available on clips to be worn by the interventional team and sometimes patients in the endovascular suite or operating room. Thermoluminescent dosimeters determine the amount of radiation exposure to that point on the dosimeter by the degree of color change in the device (i.e., the greater the radiation exposure, the greater the change in color). These dosimeters, sometimes referred to as radiation badges, are used to sample radiation levels at various locations on the body and should be recorded or logged each month. Typically, these dosimeters are worn in three locations to assess exposure and to assure effectiveness of the lead shielding. Specifically, they should be worn on the collar outside of the thyroid shield of the neck, at the waist outside of the lead apron, and at the waist underneath the lead apron. These dosimeters report their dose in sieverts, and most have a minimal detectible level of 0.01 millisievert (mSv). The safety dose limits for occupational exposure with respect to different body areas (e.g., neck, body, and hands) recommended by the United States Nuclear Regulatory Committee and the International Commission on Radiation Protection are provided in Table 11.2 and are defined using mSv per year.

TABLE 11.2	Maximum Permissible Doses

Occupational Exposures

Whole body exposures: *effective* dose limits	20–50 mSv/y[a]
Partial body exposure: *equivalent* dose annual limits for tissues and organs	
Lens of the eye	150 mSv/y
Hands	500 mSv/y

Units shown in mSv, millisievert, or 1/1,000th of 1 sievert.
Adapted from the United States Nuclear Regulatory Commission Title 10 Part 20 and the International Commission on Radiation Protection.
[a]In conventional measuring system, 50 mSv = 5,000 mrem.

D. Components of basic imaging and the fluoroscopic device. It is important for the interventional team to have an understanding of the components of a fluoroscopic system in order to be effective in the operating room or endovascular suite while minimizing radiation exposure to all in the room. **The basic setup of a fluoroscopic system is diagrammed in Figure 11.1 and includes a generator and controls, an x-ray tube, a collimator, and an image receptor or image intensifier.** The purpose of the generator and its controls are to convert available electrical power into the exact form needed to operate the x-ray tube, which is typically underneath the patient (Fig. 11.1).

The **x-ray tube is a lead-shielded device with an exit port positioned toward the patient that converts the electrical energy from the generator into x-rays.** This process is very inefficient, with less than 1% of the applied electrical energy converted to x-rays and the remaining 99% converted into heat. Although x-ray tubes are designed to handle this heat byproduct, they can "overheat," especially during longer endovascular procedures, which may result in an aggravating system shutdown. Several maneuvers can be implemented by the endovascular specialist to minimize heat production. **These same maneuvers reduce the amount of radiation exposure** during a given case. **Specifically, use of the "pulse" mode instead of the continuous mode of imaging, and reducing the frames per second, reduces the amount of heat produced by the x-ray tube and exposure to the patient.** High level or boost fluoroscopy uses an even higher intensity of energy to generate more detail and should be used very rarely and only when such degree of image detail is necessary. Similarly, doses from **digital subtraction** "runs" may be up to five times higher than standard fluoroscopy and should be reserved for when this high level of resolution is required.

The **image intensifier** often called the "II" is an electro-optical device that captures and converts an x-ray image into a visible form. The size of the image intensifier has steadily increased with technology, which permits clearer and more comprehensive imaging of the abdominal, thoracic,

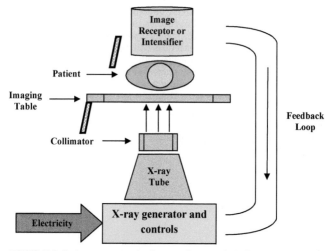

FIGURE 11.1 Basic components of a fluoroscopic system including x-ray generator and controls, x-ray tube, and image intensifier. The dark hatched objects represent lead shields or drapes that accompany most imaging units and tables. The x-ray tube is typically located underneath the bed unless rotated.

and peripheral vessels. However, with such large image intensifiers—most are now at least 15 to 17 inches in width—use of collimators becomes even more important in order to focus the radiation field to clinically relevant areas. **Moving the patient toward the image intensifier will broaden the image field and reduce intensity of the radiation beam and the amount of scatter, while improving its clarity.**

Therefore, optimal positioning of a patient for standard posteroanterior imaging is with the table raised away from the x-ray tube ("table up") and the II positioned close to the patient ("close the gap").

The x-ray beam collimators (i.e., filters) control and minimize the size of the x-ray beam and, when used effectively, will decrease radiation dose and scatter during an endovascular procedure. These tools are important because x-rays are emitted uniformly from the generator and are designed to radiate the entirety of the image intensifier, sometimes irradiating a field larger than the image receptor. Focusing or collimating down to only the area of clinical interest reduces the radiation field and scatter, while subject contrast is improved and the image quality is enhanced. **Radiation scatter is the secondary radiation that arises after the x-ray beam contacts the patient.** These photons of electromagnetic radiation are less intense than the primary x-ray beam but still constitute a radiation risk. Scatter is always more intense on the side where the x-ray beam contacts the patient. This side of the imaging setup is referred to as the *zone of high-intensity scatter,* which is often underneath the imaging table (Fig. 11.2). The area between the patient and the image intensifier (the "II")

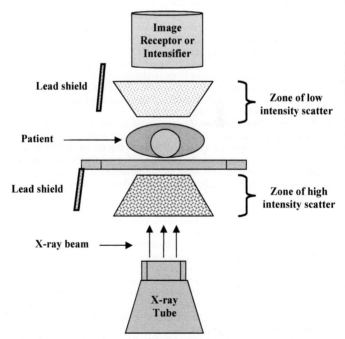

FIGURE 11.2 Zones of high- and low-intensity radiation scatter in relation to the x-ray beam and patient position. Note the zone of high-intensity scatter is on the side where the radiation strikes the patient, which is under the imaging table in this figure.

constitutes the *zone of low-intensity scatter*. During lateral projections (e.g., mesenteric stenting), the operator should be on the opposite side from the x-ray tube (same side as the II) to minimize his or her scatter exposure. Understanding these zones will help the interventionalist and assistants effectively position and shield themselves to minimize exposure. Lead shields and drapes should be placed between the operator and the patient to reduce scatter.

The endovascular specialist should develop a checklist in his or her mind pertaining to these simple components of the fluoroscopic system for optimization of images and reduction of radiation exposure. A review of the following points prior to any imaging series will serve the interventionalist, the patient, and others in the room well during endovascular procedures:

1. Collimator position
2. X-ray beam setting (i.e., standard pulse mode emits less radiation)
3. Frames per second (i.e., lower FPS for less radiation production and exposure)
4. Position of the patient in relation to the image intensifier
5. Use of appropriate lead shielding, garments, and eyewear
6. Magnification (magnification can increase penetration and dose)
7. Angle of beam (steeper angle travels through more tissue at higher dose)

II. **RADIATION BIOLOGY, INCLUDING GENETIC AND CARCINOGENIC EFFECTS OF RADIATION**

A. **Radiation effects on human tissue are referred to as either deterministic or stochastic.** Deterministic effects have a *radiation threshold* below which there is no probability of harmful effect. However, once the threshold has been reached, there is a direct relationship between further radiation dose and the adverse biologic effect. The most common deterministic effect of radiation is skin erythema (at risk with >2 Gy) or burns that can progress to dermal necrosis with higher levels of exposure. In contrast, the stochastic effect is related more to chance than to a known effect of an increased dose up to and beyond a threshold. An example of this is a mutation occurring from a single or random dose of radiation that results in a mutation leading to malignancy.

B. **Direct and indirect ionization.** Absorption of radiation by living cells can result in an interaction with an important target molecule in one of two ways, direct or indirect. **Direct ionization means that the energy from the x-ray is directly absorbed by the target molecule. Indirect ionization refers to x-ray absorption and damage to the water around the molecule.** The indirect radiation and breakdown of water within living cells and tissue is called radiolysis, which results in the formation of damaging ions called free radicals. Studies have shown that radiation damage to living tissue occurs mostly (about 80%) from indirect radiation, while the minority (about 20%) occurs as a result of direct radiation effects.

C. **A variety of molecules or cellular structures can be affected by radiation, although DNA appears to be the main target.** DNA, which exists in the form of a double helix within the nucleus of the cell, contains the operation plans for cellular life as well as the genetic code for reproduction. Direct or indirect radiation damage can break the structure of DNA so it is unable to program these activities. While most cells can repair minor or single-strand breaks in the DNA, more significant injury to both strands of the double helix often results in permanent damage.

The effect of radiation on cells is influenced by how rapidly they are proliferating and the sensitivity of specific cell types to radiation. In general, rapidly dividing cell types such as skin cells are more sensitive to radiation than cell types that are less active. Other organ types that are known to be sensitive to radiation exposure are the thyroid, the breast, the lens of the eye, the lung, and the bone marrow. **Two modes of cellular death can occur after exposure to radiation: reproductive death and apoptosis.** Reproductive death refers to proliferative cells that have sustained various levels of DNA injury—some of which may be repaired initially—that ultimately results in failure to proliferate and cell death. Apoptosis is programmed cell death, which is a more uniform and active process in which organized cellular events take the cell down a definite path of demise.

D. **Radiation biology is the study of how living cells and organisms react to radiation.** At the cellular level, one can conceptualize one of four outcomes that can occur following radiation exposure or damage.

1. If the damage is to **critical cellular components,** or is too great, the cell can no longer function and dies.
2. Some radiation damage may be repaired fully by the cell with **no identifiable adverse effects.**
3. The damage may be repaired and the cell survives, but with **decreased function or capacity.**
4. Damage may be partially or incorrectly repaired resulting in a **mutation.** In this last group of radiation-induced cellular injury, a malignancy or cancer can develop years later. **Genetic mutations can occur in cells that are damaged by radiation but do not die or repair themselves correctly following exposure.** A mutation from radiation occurs due to a nonlethal, nonrepaired flaw in the DNA, which results in a failure to produce a protein that is necessary to support or control cell proliferation. In instances where the mutation results in failure to control or shut off a cell line, these cells will proliferate unchecked, resulting in malignancy or cancer. Although the understanding of the link between radiation exposure and cancer is relatively limited, there are specific types of cancers known to be related to radiation exposure.

   It is important for the vascular physician to realize that the levels of radiation exposure associated with cancer are generally much higher than those encountered during medical fluoroscopy. However, they are worth noting if for no other reason than to underscore the seriousness of radiation exposure and the importance of protective measures. The thyroid gland may be the most radiation-sensitive tissue and is known to be associated with radiation-induced malignancy. The first human cancer to be linked to radiation exposure was skin cancer, which continues to receive considerable attention given its prevalence and relation to sun exposure. Other forms of cancer that have a recognized association with radiation exposure include bone cancer, lung cancer, and leukemia (i.e., bone marrow).

E. **Radiation injury with the use of medical fluoroscopy** occurs most commonly in the skin and the lens of the eye. This is because radiation exposure to providers and patients occurs at the surface where radiation first makes contact. Skin injury from radiation is particularly prone to occur in those with underlying collagen vascular diseases such as lupus erythematosus and scleroderma and those with diabetes mellitus. Skin injury can range from mild erythema and hair loss, which result from as little as 2 to 3 Gy, to dermal atrophy, induration, and even necrosis, which can occur with doses in the 10 to 15 Gy range.

   Cells that make up the lens of the eye are also prone to radiation injury, which causes them to lose their clarity or lucency. **Because these cells are continually produced and form layers on the lens over time, if a**

significant number of cells are adversely affected, an opacity, or cataract, can form. A cataract may or may not impair vision and generally requires radiation doses in excess of 1 Gy delivered at one time in an otherwise healthy lens. The threshold for induction of cataracts is greater when the radiation exposure is in lower doses over extended periods. The time between radiation exposure and diagnosis is delayed, often more than 5 and 10 years for cataracts caused by lesser doses received over extended periods.

III. **PRACTICAL RADIATION SAFETY.** With the above concepts of imaging systems and radiation biology in mind, the goal in the interventional suite or fluoroscopy-equipped operating room is to facilitate patient care while minimizing the risk of radiation exposure. The risks associated with radiation exposure underscore points made throughout this handbook that indications for angiographic procedures must be sound and that noninvasive, nonradiographic alternatives should be used to their fullest extent. Patients with vascular disease often undergo multiple angiographic interventions as well as CT and x-ray imaging that increases overall radiation exposure. Assuming that the endovascular procedure is indicated or must be performed to provide optimal care, **interventionalists should expect or be willing to accept a risk of radiation exposure that is as low as reasonably achievable (ALARA).**

Regulatory authorities define a maximum permissible dose of radiation per year (Table 11.2). These levels are an *absolute maximum*, which no individual radiation worker should come close to on an annual basis. Establishing the lowest level (i.e., ALARA) is somewhat arbitrary but should be a number that careful practitioners know and strive for in their practice. For example, in well-designed endovascular rooms, interventionalists usually have total body doses of 0.5 to 15 mSv per year (50 to 1,500 mrem). Consistently meeting an established ALARA goal requires some amount of discipline and good endovascular habits, some of which have been mentioned briefly in previous sections. The five main operational factors to reduce radiation dose that each team member should consider prior to any endovascular procedure are **distance, time, shielding, beam management, and situational awareness** (Table 11.3).

A. **Beam management by the primary operator includes stepping on the pedal and producing x-rays only when necessary.** The temptation to "stay on" the pedal or to inadvertently step on the pedal when no one is looking at the image screen should be eliminated. This often requires a team effort and a willingness to remind the primary operator to get "off the pedal" when this occurs. Collimating the x-ray beam to tightly image only the necessary anatomy reduces the intensity of stray radiation and increases image quality. Use of low-dose or pulsed imaging is also a useful beam management tool that reduces radiation dose during the initial or final parts of some procedures.

T A B L E 11.3	Elements of Practical Radiation Safety

Beam management
Situational awareness
Distance
Time
Shielding (structural and wearable)

B. **Situational awareness includes physicians and supporting staff knowing when the fluoroscopic unit is active.** This is typically keyed by a light and a characteristic noise, but the primary operator should also state that he or she is ready to begin the imaging so everyone in the room is aware. Typically, there is a light on the outside of the endovascular room to alert those who may consider coming into the room that imaging is taking place. The operator needs to be aware of the position of his or her technicians and other assistants in the room so that imaging does not occur while a nurse is tending to the patient in direct line or in close proximity of the x-ray beam.

C. **Distance from the radiation source should be maximized understanding that doubling the distance from the source of radiation decreases the intensity fourfold.** For example, increasing one's distance from the emitting beam from 1 to 2 m decreases the intensity from 100 mGy/h to 25 mGy/h. Patient proximity to the image receiver or imaging intensifier is also important. An increase in the distance between the patient and the image intensifier increases the required x-ray beam output and scatter. Positioning the patient close to the image intensifier (Fig. 11.1) is an easy way to reduce radiation requirements and exposure risk. Whenever possible, the interventionalist and team members should step away from the beam source to reduce their exposure as per the inverse-square law.

D. **Time of radiation use is also a key component to operational safety and is closely related to beam management.** Time in this context relates both to the operator's initiation of the x-ray beam and time that assisting staff are in areas of higher radiation risk. Familiarity with the system is important in order to maximize tools such as last image hold, replay, and adjuncts that can accentuate certain aspects of the previously taken and stored image. Use of these adjuncts maximizes clinical decision-making with the fewest number of fluoroscopic images and radiation time. Finally, the alarm that sounds with each 5-minute interval of time should serve as a reminder for the primary operator that judicious use of fluoroscopic time is an important part of operational safety.

E. **Shielding comes in all shapes and sizes,** including fixed shields that come from above (i.e., ceiling mounted) to rest between the primary operator and the patient and those that originate from the imaging table itself (Fig. 11.1). Movable shields should also be available for staff members to stand behind during the imaging. Ideally, most team members should be able to provide their assistance (e.g., record the case log) outside of the imaging room. These individuals can enter the room to provide supplies or patient adjustments when the beam is off.

The lead apron, the mainstay of wearable shielding, is at least 0.5 mm thick and provides a barrier between the radiation source and the interventionalist. This form of shielding should be updated occasionally and is ideally fitted to the individual. Shielding can be compromised if the apron is ill-fitted or outdated, as the lead shielding elements can fracture which creates gaps in the barrier. Most current two-piece aprons are lighter than older models, offering more comfortable shielding with less associated musculoskeletal aches and pains. An extension of the lead apron is the thyroid shield, which should also be at least 0.5 mm thick and worn consistently during fluoroscopic procedures. Lead garments should be imaged annually to look for cracks or defects in the shielding, and defective garments replaced. Leaded eyeglasses should complete the shielding assembly. Although their effectiveness in preventing radiation-induced cataracts is debated, some form of protective eyewear is required for compliance with universal precautions and leaded glasses should be the component of choice.

Selected Readings

Pei H, Cheng SWK, Wu PM, et al. Ionizing radiation absorption of vascular surgeons during endovascular procedures. *J Vasc Surg.* 2007;46:455-459.

Study examined radiation exposure for different endovascular procedures in a group of four different vascular surgeons.

Sigterman TA, Bolt LJ, Snoejs MG, et al. Radiation exposure during percutaneous angioplasty for symptomatic peripheral arterial disease. *Ann Vasc Surg.* 2016;33:167-172.

Study shows range of radiation exposure to patients with various peripheral procedures.

Sprawls P. *The Physical Principles of Medical Imaging.* 2nd ed. 1995. Retrieved from http://www.sprawls.org/resources. Accessed March 2018.

Excellent resource for the student of basic radiation and imaging, available online courtesy of the Sprawls Educational Foundation.

Reed AB, Killewich LA, Brown KR. Radiation safety in vascular surgery. *J Vasc Surg.* 2011;53(suppl):1S-46S.

In 2011 the Society for Vascular Surgery Women's Leadership Committee published a 46 page educational supplement on radiation – an excellent primer or refresher for the vascular interventionalist. Sample topics are highlighted:

Tonnessen BH, Pounds L. Radiation physics. *J Vasc Surg.* 2011;53:6S-8S.

Basic electromagnetic radiation concepts.

Mitchell E, Furey P. Prevention of radiation injury from medical imaging. *J Vasc Surg.* 2011;53:9S-14S.

Tips for reducing exposure and proper fluoroscopic management during angiography; graphic shows best practice for patient positioning relative to C-arm.

Shaw P, Duncan A, Vouyouka A, Ozvath K. Radiation exposure and pregnancy. *J Vasc Surg.* 2011;53:28S-34S.

Well-researched resource for pregnant workers and patients.

12 Great Vessel and Carotid Occlusive Disease

Today, the incorporation of medical management and that of open and endovascular therapies for cerebrovascular disease makes the vascular specialist an integral member of the health care team treating these patients. The necessity of this involvement has been proven by the success of carotid, aortic arch branch, and vertebral artery revascularizations for the relief of symptomatic, stenotic, or ulcerated arterial lesions, aneurysms, and vascular tumors located in these vessels. The vascular and endovascular surgeon may also be consulted to evaluate patients with asymptomatic cerebrovascular disease, to provide a risk assessment, as well as to help determine the appropriateness of intervention for stroke-risk reduction. Currently, evaluation and analysis of the selection and performance of carotid angioplasty and stenting (CAS) versus carotid endarterectomy (CEA) and medical management continues to alter the landscape in which extracranial cerebrovascular disease is treated.

In this chapter, common clinical presentations that suggest extracranial brachiocephalic, carotid, or vertebral artery disease are discussed. Certain principles of current care that facilitate an appropriate, smooth, and safe procedure for the patient are highlighted. Finally, the management of the most common early and late complications of carotid interventions is summarized.

I. COMMON CLINICAL SCENARIOS

A. **Symptomatic carotid disease.** Symptomatic carotid occlusive disease consists of **transient ischemic attacks (TIA)** and **stroke, or cerebrovascular accident (CVA).** The socioeconomic, health care administrative, and individual health care importance of stroke is clear. In the United States, over 790,000 CVAs occur annually and result in 140,000 deaths. In the United States, there are roughly 7 million stroke survivors with varying degrees of disability and the yearly economic burden of stroke is approximately 45 million dollars. Worldwide stroke is the second leading cause of death, estimated to occur in just over 17 million people per year, leading to death in over 6 million. Approximately 80% of CVAs are due to ischemic stroke, or thromboembolic events, and extracranial atherosclerosis is a major contributor. Most strokes, 75%, occur in those who have had no prior neurologic symptoms. The anatomic distribution of cerebrovascular atherosclerosis has been studied, and the breakdown by location in those with disease is as follows: carotid bifurcation 38%, intracranial 33%, arch branch based 9%, and proximal vertebral 20%.

1. **Symptom classification.** Classically, a **TIA** is defined as acute neurologic symptoms lasting less than 24 hours that completely resolve. However, the duration usually is measured in minutes, not hours. The term reversible ischemic neurologic deficit **(RIND)** has been used to describe neurologic symptoms that last longer than 24 hours but then rapidly resolve. **CVA** is defined as neurologic symptoms lasting longer than 24 hours with evident structural infarction. The term **crescendo TIA**, or stuttering TIA, is used when TIAs occur more frequently (progressive over 24 to 48 hours), yet there remains complete reversal of neurologic symptoms in between. **Stroke-in-evolution** is when there is no resolution of symptoms, but rather they wax and wane indicating ongoing neuron ischemia and neural tissue at risk of infarction. These are highly unstable situations. Symptoms reflective of thromboembolic events due to disease in the carotid artery or anterior circulation include hemiparesis, hemiparesthesias, transient monocular blindness **(amaurosis fugax [AF])**, or difficulties with speech **(aphasia)**.

2. **Outcomes of TIA.** Approximately 75% to 80% of patients who suffer a stroke have had no type of preceding transient neurologic symptoms. However, the corollary is that if a patient experiences a TIA, the risk of stroke is significant. Studies have delineated a 30% to 50% 5-year risk of stroke once TIA occurs. In fact, recent evidence suggests that a significant proportion of this risk occurs within the first several weeks after TIA with, perhaps, a **10% to 25% risk of CVA within 1 month of the event**. Some have even suggested that 5% to 10% of this risk is within hours of the event. It is, thus, critical to identify and evaluate these patients. Unfortunately, TIAs are not specific for the presence of significant carotid artery stenosis or ulcerated plaques. Only about 50% of patients with TIAs will have a tight, or hemodynamically significant, carotid stenosis (<2 mm; ≥50%), occlusion, or ulcerated plaques. The remaining 50% of patients have thromboembolism from other sources such as the heart, aortic arch, intracranial vascular disease, or no evident etiology. TIAs from alternate site thromboembolism or hypercoagulability also commonly lead to stroke. However, patients with no evident etiology for their TIAs and relatively normal carotid arteries on evaluation usually follow a more benign course; they seldom suffer a stroke.

   TIAs may be either hemispheric or retinal in nature. In up to 25% of patients presenting with symptomatic carotid bifurcation atheroma, visual disturbances are the presenting symptom. **AF** is the most common of these ocular manifestations. Transient hemianopsias and other subtle visual field defects occur less frequently. Classic amaurosis is described as a "shade coming down over the eye" for a few seconds to minutes at a time and is due to embolism to the ophthalmic artery. While the natural history of AF is somewhat more benign than hemispheric TIAs, it is still significant. The stroke risk once AF arises is roughly 6% to 8% per year, or roughly half that in those with cerebral TIAs. And, in those experiencing visual symptoms due to cerebrovascular disease, a significant group (25%) will ultimately suffer permanent visual loss.

3. **Stroke recurrence.** The importance of identifying those with CVA and cerebrovascular atherosclerosis, particularly within the extracranial arteries, is due to the significance of stroke recurrence. Without treatment, those with CVA will have another stroke at a

rate of between 10% and 20% per year, thus the 5-year gross risk is somewhere between 50% and 100%. The mortality associated with this second CVA is a staggering 35%, and events beyond the second are more than 60%. Hence, the institution of therapy is imperative.

4. **Unusual presentations and symptoms of cerebrovascular disease.** Rarely, deterioration in visual acuity may be due to chronic ocular ischemia (COI). Severe bilateral occlusive disease leads to a supply/demand mismatch in the retina with an increase in metabolic demand. COI is the name of the constellation of signs and symptoms related to this. Findings may include eye pain, venous stasis retinopathy, central or branch retinal artery occlusions from stagnant flow, ischemic optic neuropathy, narrowed retinal arteries, retinal microaneurysms, retinal hemorrhages, iris neovascularization (**rubeosis iridis**) with neovascular acute angle glaucoma, iris atrophy, corneal edema, and cataracts. This syndrome only occurs in 3% to 4% of those with cerebrovascular disease. Without treatment, permanent blindness occurs uniformly. Another rare ocular symptom that may occur is **"bright light AF."** This occurs because of the poor retinal blood flow causing complete white out blindness when the retina is stressed, such as going outside into the sunlight. Frequently, the vascular specialist may be asked to comment on the presence of **Hollenhorst plaques** and retinal artery occlusions seen on fundus examination without evidence of COI. Less than 10% of these patients will have significant carotid stenosis ipsilateral to these findings.

There are a few other uncommon symptoms of cerebrovascular disease that may be attributed to significant carotid occlusive disease. One is jaw claudication with eating due to poor external carotid artery (ECA) flow to the masseter muscle. Focal seizure activity has been noted due to atheroembolism from carotid artery disease. Presyncope or syncope, sometimes called drop attacks and cognitive impairments, may rarely occur secondary to poor perfusion from significant bilateral cerebrovascular disease.

B. **Asymptomatic carotid disease**. Extracranial cerebrovascular disease may also be identified in those who have no symptoms directly attributable to their arterial stenoses. Overall, only 1% of the population over the age of 65 harbors carotid occlusive disease. Yet, when focusing upon those with cardiovascular risk factors such as hypertension, hyperlipidemia, and cardiac disease, this figure rises substantially to nearly 20%. This is the reasoning behind cerebrovascular screening programs, which allow recognition of those at highest risk of stroke, followed by the initiation of therapy for stroke-risk reduction. The most common initiating event for those undergoing evaluation for asymptomatic carotid stenosis is bruit on physical examination. **Carotid bruits** are present in approximately 5% of the general population over 50 years of age. However, only 23% of bruits are found to be associated with a hemodynamically significant stenosis (≥50%), and less than half of significant stenoses occur in the presence of a bruit. There is no correlation between the loudness of a bruit and the degree of narrowing. Thus, a bruit is neither sensitive nor specific for significant carotid stenosis; still, with the ease of noninvasive imaging, the status of the carotid artery when a bruit is detected is relatively simple. A neck bruit may originate from the carotid arteries or be transmitted from the aortic arch or heart, such as with transmitted murmurs (Fig. 12.1).

Also, not infrequently, vascular specialists are asked to consult on patients with atypical symptoms, and noninvasive imaging is performed to establish the status of the carotid arteries. Usually, the symptoms are found to be unrelated to the carotid arteries, yet a stenosis is identified.

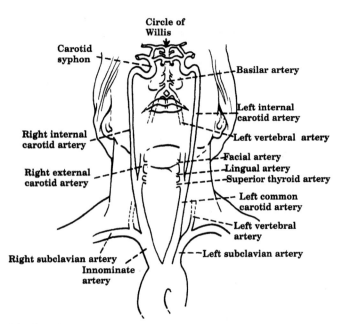

FIGURE 12.1 Anatomy of the aortic arch and extracranial cervical arteries. The internal carotid artery has no branches in the neck.

When asymptomatic carotid stenoses are identified, some 10% to 15% will progress to a severe category. Therefore, the management of those with asymptomatic carotid artery stenosis has become a very germane issue.

II. IMAGING OF CEREBROVASCULAR DISEASE

A. Duplex ultrasound. With the advent of noninvasive vascular laboratories and the establishment of duplex ultrasonography, this is the initial imaging modality of choice for most patients in which a diagnosis of carotid artery disease is entertained (see Chapter 5). Duplex ultrasound combines brightness-mode (B-mode) ultrasound with pulsed wave Doppler to produce a real-time gray scale image of the arteries, as well as spectral analysis of flow. Many criteria have been espoused that attempt to identify and quantify the degree of carotid stenosis using duplex ultrasound. This is an ongoing process and requires regular correlation with other imaging modalities in order to solidify each noninvasive laboratory's exactness. When performed by skilled vascular technologists, this imaging approach is quick, sensitive, specific, and highly accurate, and carries little risk. Indirect evidence of arch-based and intracranial stenosis may be present but no direct imaging in these areas is possible. Transcranial Doppler may be performed in conjunction to further ascertain intracranial disease, but it cannot delineate lesion anatomy or true disease burden. Two commonly used criteria include the modified University of Washington criteria, and the Society of Radiologists in Ultrasound (SRU) criteria (Table 12.1). A greater understanding and study of duplex ultrasound in carotid occlusive disease, as well as its ease, has led to sensible surveillance regimens in those with cerebrovascular disease. This is now standard practice both in those found with moderate carotid stenosis and after carotid surgery (Table 12.2).

TABLE 12.1 Modified Washington Duplex Criteria

Stenosis	PSV	EDV	Spectrum
Normal	<125 cm/s		Normal with no plaque
1%–15% (B)	<125 cm/s		Normal with plaque
16%–49% (C)	<125 cm/s		Broadening
50%–79% (D)	>125 cm/s	<140 cm/s	Broadening
80%–99% (D+)	>125 cm/s	>140 cm/s	Broadening
Occluded (E)	No flow	No flow	No flow

Society of Radiologists in Ultrasound Consensus Criteria

| Degree of Stenosis (%) | Primary Parameters | | Additional Parameters | |
	ICA PSV (cm/s)	Plaque Estimate (%)[a]	ICA/CCA PSV Ratio	ICA EDV (cm/s)
Normal	<125	None	<2.0	<40
<50	<125	<50	<2.0	<40
50–69	125–230	≥50	2.0–4.0	40–100
≥70 but less than near occlusion	>230	≥50	>4.0	>100
Near occlusion	High, low, or undetectable	Visible	Variable	Variable
Total occlusion	Undetectable	Visible, no detectable lumen	Not applicable	Not applicable

PSV, peak systolic velocity; EDV, end diastolic velocity; cm/s, centimeters per second; CCA, common carotid artery; ICA, internal carotid artery; ECA, external carotid artery.
EDV: 80 cm/s ~ 60%; 100 cm/s ~ 70%.
ICA:CCA PSV ratio: 3.2 ~60%; 4.0 ~70%.
[a]Plaque estimate (diameter reduction) with gray scale and color Doppler US.

TABLE 12.2 Standard Carotid Surveillance Protocol

Clinical Group	Frequency of Surveillance Duplex
B lesion and C lesion	Every 1–2 y
D lesion without CEA	Every 6 mo
Post CEA	Every 6 mo for 2 y, then yearly or based on contralateral stenosis
Contralateral carotid occlusion	Every 6 mo
Post CAS	Every 6 mo

CEA, carotid endarterectomy; CAS, carotid angioplasty and stenting.

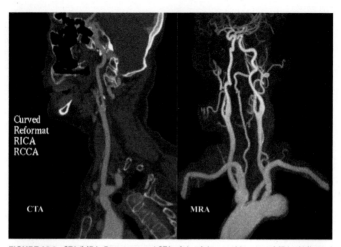

FIGURE 12.2 CTA/MRA: Reconstructed CTA of the right carotid system. MRA of bilateral carotid bifurcations, aortic arch, and brachiocephalic vessels. CTA, computed tomography; MRA, magnetic resonance arteriography.

B. **Computed tomography (CT/CTA) and magnetic resonance arteriography (MRI/MRA).** Anatomic definition and direct imaging of the brain, intracranial vasculature, arch branches, and aortic arch are valuable benefits of CTA and MRA (Fig. 12.2). Up to 10% of the time, arch branch–based disease is found to be present. In 2% to 5% of carotid bifurcation stenoses, either a tandem intracranial stenosis or intracranial aneurysm exists distal to the carotid lesion. Further, the status of the brain and recent or past CVA can be identified, which is particularly important in symptomatic cerebrovascular disease. With CTA, infarction cannot always be identified immediately as it often takes 24 to 48 hours for evidence of stroke to be present using this imaging modality. A benefit of CTA is the imaging of intracranial bleeding. Atherosclerotic calcification can limit CTA's ability to characterize stenoses. MRA, on the other hand, using diffusion-weighted technology, can illustrate and describe infarction immediately. A drawback to MRA is its notorious overrepresentation of stenoses. This is due to the fact that magnetic resonance (MR) technology depends on electron polar changes with magnetic field pulses. In standard magnetic resonance, blood flow is thus represented as signal dropout or a black appearance, since electrons do not stay in one place in the blood. If not timed appropriately, flow attributes may not be portrayed correctly, so this technology is highly institution and personnel dependent.

C. **Arteriography.** The stroke risk associated with cerebrovascular arteriography is 1% to 2%. Access site and other complications can occur in up to 3%, which led to the development of other less invasive methods of imaging. Yet, there remain several situations where arteriography is helpful and finalizes cerebrovascular imaging. These include discordant or unreliable noninvasive studies, a high carotid bifurcation, no clear lesion end point seen, concern for either intracranial or arch-based/great vessel disease, the possibility of nonatherosclerotic etiologies of disease, suspected posterior circulation disease as the symptom cause, and recurrent stenosis. As CTA/MRA has improved, these former reasons become increasingly infrequent. The usual indication today for arteriography is potential for endovascular treatment such as CAS or vertebral origin stenting.

III. TREATMENT OF CAROTID OCCLUSIVE DISEASE

A. **Medical therapy.** Risk factor modification is clearly indicated in patients with cerebrovascular disease (see Chapter 6). Many already have risk reduction therapies in place for hypertension, hyperlipidemia, and coronary artery disease at the time of diagnosis of carotid, great vessel, and vertebral artery disease due to the association with other cardiovascular processes. Statin therapy has been shown to be beneficial in carotid occlusive disease both in primary and postprocedural roles. Antiplatelet drugs such as aspirin and clopidogrel retard platelet aggregation and may prevent microemboli that cause TIAs and strokes. This has made these agents critical components of maintenance therapy after neurologic events and diagnosis of asymptomatic stenosis. Aspirin reduces the risk of continuing TIAs, stroke, and death by approximately 20%, compared to controls. In a randomized, blinded trial of clopidogrel (Plavix, Sanofi Pharmaceuticals, Inc., New York, NY, USA) versus aspirin in patients at risk of ischemic events (CAPRIE), clopidogrel (75 mg daily) reduced the relative risk for ischemic stroke, myocardial infarction, and vascular death by 24%. After CEA, antiplatelet therapy reduces risk of stroke and to a lesser degree restenosis. It appears likely that antiplatelet therapies modestly reduce the risk of stroke in both symptomatic and asymptomatic individuals with cerebrovascular disease, and are indicated with minimal bleeding risk.

Heparin or warfarin sodium (Coumadin, DuPont Pharmaceuticals Company, Wilmington, DE, USA) can also control TIAs in at least 90% of patients with recent onset. Warfarin also has proved effective in reducing serious cerebral infarct from 45% in untreated patients to 24% in treated individuals over 5 years. Of course, the main disadvantage of long-term Coumadin therapy is compliance and bleeding complications in about 15% of patients. Indeed, current recommendations from the multispecialty guidelines council have recommended heparin not be used in initial acute stroke management due to the hemorrhagic risk. Further, long-term medical therapy for secondary stroke prevention in carotid disease does not involve anticoagulation. It is based on antiplatelets, statin, and behavior modification.

B. **Surgical therapy.** Perhaps nothing in vascular disease has been scrutinized more closely than CEA. During CEA, the carotid artery is clamped and opened, and the atherosclerotic plaque is removed. Large, multicenter prospective, randomized trials comparing this operation plus antiplatelet therapy to antiplatelet therapy alone have provided many insights into this surgical option. In patients with a hemodynamically significant carotid stenosis, who have had a TIA or a stabilized, nondisabling stroke and are candidates for operation, CEA reduces the risk of recurrent stroke. This was clarified in both the **North American Symptomatic Carotid Endarterectomy Trial (NASCET)** and the **European Carotid Surgery trial (ECST)**. The **Veterans Affairs Trial 309 (VA 309)** also found a trend favoring surgery, but was halted when the initial results of NASCET and ECST were reported. NASCET's evaluation of those with high-grade ($\geq 70\%$) stenosis was stopped early as the risk of stroke at 2 years was 26% versus 9% ($p < 0.001$), and mortality 12% versus 5% ($p < 0.01$), in the medical and surgical arms, respectively. Stroke-risk reduction increased as the degree of stenosis became greater. Thus, those with the most significant degree of stenosis gleaned the highest degree of absolute benefit. For those with carotid stenosis of 50% to 69%, NASCET revealed a significant reduction in ipsilateral stroke (15.7% vs 22.2%; $p = 0.045$) and any stroke or death (33.3% vs 43.3%; $p = 0.005$) with CEA at 5 years. Although still statistically noteworthy, the absolute risk reduction was less than in those with higher-grade stenoses and was not as evident until the later points of follow-up.

In ECST and the VA 309, similar outcomes were found. Data generated from the pooling of these three trials have confirmed the stepwise augmentation in stroke-risk reduction with CEA by increasing stenosis degree. Carotid stenosis of 50% was confirmed to be the point at which CEA yields significant absolute 5-year stroke-risk reduction compared with medical therapy. Above 60% to 70% was the degree to which significant 3-year absolute stroke-risk reduction occurred. Benefits of CEA in the symptomatic prospective, randomized trials appear to be greatest in men, those with recent stroke, and hemispheric symptoms.

When symptomatic patients are encountered, several questions can lead to sensible management.

1. **Is there a significant carotid stenosis?** The imaging modalities discussed earlier are used. Duplex ultrasound is the first-line modality, which helps to delineate degrees of carotid stenosis and important plaque characteristics such as ulceration, as well as indirectly attempting to find evidence of proximal arch-based disease and poor vertebrobasilar flow. Additionally, the anatomic location of the carotid bifurcation and the presence of an identifiable lesion end point with normal appearing distal internal carotid artery (ICA) are important features. The spectral analysis of flow may reveal a resistive pattern suggesting distal intracranial disease. In many patients, particularly those with TIA, carotid duplex scanning may provide enough anatomic and functional information to proceed with CEA without alternative imaging.

   If any feature of the cerebrovascular circulation is not well appreciated, or there is concern for recent stroke, alternative noninvasive imaging is indicated. This consists of an MRA and/or a CTA. MR is used for acute stroke brain imaging and CTA for carotid artery anatomic detail. Findings that may necessitate carotid arteriography after duplex and/or CTA/MRA are as follows: discordant or unreliable noninvasive studies (i.e., the studies conflict one another), a high carotid bifurcation precluding complete duplex imaging, absence of a visible lesion distal end point on duplex or CTA/MRA, concern for tandem disease in the intracranial or intrathoracic carotid segments, suspicion of posterior circulation disease, and/or the presence of recurrent stenosis following CEA. In one or more of these instances, arteriography will finalize imaging and evaluation of the degree of stenosis and lesion morphology. Today, CTA and MRA have improved to the point most anatomic detail is understood well with these modalities. However, occasionally, arteriography may still be necessary, and may lead to endovascular therapies such as transfemoral or transcervical CAS.

2. **Are the symptoms actually consistent with TIA or CVA, or some other neurologic or psychosomatic complaint? Are they attributable to events ipsilateral to the carotid stenosis?** These questions are not always easy to answer. As noted, carotid distribution symptoms classically include unilateral hemiparesis, hemiparesthesias, speech disturbance, or AF. The symptoms that present confusion in determining whether a true TIA, or potential CVA, is being experienced are atypical complaints, especially dizziness, lightheadedness, presyncope, and unsteady gait. These posterior circulation type symptoms are rather common in elderly patients who may experience postural hypotension when arising quickly from a lying, sitting, or stooping position and other etiologies that produce these sensations. If a psychosomatic problem is suspected, a careful inquiry about family or work situations may disclose emotional stress that initiates the symptoms. If the patient is unsure of the symptoms, a family member who may have observed an attack can be very helpful.

3. **Are the neurologic symptoms chronic and stable or repetitive and progressive, and has the patient had a stroke?** If they represent TIA and are not suggestive of CVA and are not progressive, a more elective/urgent outpatient evaluation is appropriate. Remember, however, the newer, more worrying upfront risks of TIA. If the symptoms are concerning for a new or recent stroke or are progressive and repetitive, suggesting either crescendo TIA or stroke-in-evolution, immediate or urgent assessment is indicated. Thorough evaluation for TIAs may also require electrocardiographic monitoring (Holter monitor) to detect arrhythmias or echocardiography to rule out diseased heart valves or mural thrombus. Transesophageal echocardiography may also reveal ulcerative atherosclerosis of the aortic arch as a source of thromboemboli in some patients. Moreover, electroencephalography (EEG) is appropriate if a seizure disorder is suspected. Consultation with a neurologist or ophthalmologist may be helpful in evaluating patients if atypical neurologic or retinal symptoms are present. In those with atypical symptoms, or concern for stroke, computed tomography (CT/CTA) or MRI/MRA of the brain is useful to not only better clarify the extent of cerebrovascular disease but also to identify stroke and check for hemorrhage. MRI with diffusion weighting is particularly useful for this. It can identify stroke immediately while CT takes several days for the stroke to be evident.

If the patient has had a stroke, particular aspects are relevant to possible intervention and surgical therapy. First, it is important to understand how significant and debilitating the CVA has been and if there is still brain tissue at risk for infarction. In those with dense, complete deficits such as hemiplegia and/or loss of speech, it makes little sense to put the patient at risk for an operation if there is little hemispheric function left to lose. Indeed, the prospective, randomized trials studying CEA for symptomatic patients only included those with TIAs and "nondisabling" stroke. Poor outcomes due to hemorrhagic conversion in those with stroke and immediate surgical intervention were encountered before CT and MR technology were developed. Since that time, there has been much controversy with regard to radiographic features of CVA and the timing of CEA. No clear consensus has been reached with regard to the timing of CEA following hemispheric stroke. What is clear is that the larger the CVA, the more likely the patient is to have a permanent deficit. If there is any evidence of parenchymal hemorrhage associated with the stroke, or it is larger than 2 to 3 cm in size, it is probably wise to wait 4 weeks before CEA. If the stroke is small without hemorrhage, an earlier operation (within 14 days) can be performed.

Fortunately, scenarios where more emergent intervention is necessary are rare. Those with **crescendo TIA** should be immediately hospitalized for anticoagulation with heparin (loading dose of 5,000 to 10,000 units, with a continuous hourly infusion of 750 to 1,000 units) to achieve an aPTT of 60 to 90 seconds or an antifactor Xa level of 0.4 to 0.7 IU/mL. If the patient's condition is stable, an urgent MRA or CTA in conjunction with a duplex ultrasound usually is performed within 24 hours after admission. Arteriography is indicated if previously discussed features are present. Operative candidates with severe (>70%) carotid stenosis or shaggy, mobile, irregular ulcerative plaques undergo CEA when the surgical and anesthesia teams are optimized.

Management is more difficult if the neurologic symptoms are progressing, or waxing and waning, without complete resolution. These patients should be considered to have a **stroke-in-evolution**. Anticoagulation and emergent duplex ultrasound followed by immediate carotid surgery for severe carotid lesions and those with ominous plaque features may reduce the stroke severity and mortality in this group. However, the differentiation between a **stroke-in-evolution** and **completed stroke** is not always clear. This aggressive surgical strategy for crescendo TIA and stroke-in-evolution is related to a poor stroke and mortality rate with medical therapy alone in these patients. The reported mortality with these events is 50% to 80%, with up to 75% of survivors having a moderate to severe permanent neurologic deficit. Less than 5% to 10% will completely recover. With the institution of the treatment paradigm described, perioperative stroke and death rates of approximately 10% to 20% can be anticipated. While this is a considerable event rate after CEA, it may be the patient's best alternative. Also, **treatment of acute ischemic stroke with intravenous thrombolytic therapy (tissue-type plasminogen activator) is approved for selected patients with no evidence of intracranial hemorrhage or other contraindications when started within 3 hours of onset of symptoms.**

4. **What is the patient's operative risk?** Combined 30-day mortality and stroke in NASCET and ECST was 5.6% and 7.0%, respectively. In general, stroke/death rates for CEA in symptomatic patients should be 5% to 6% or less in order for the operation to make stroke-risk reduction sense. If the patient is a poor surgical risk from a comorbidity standpoint, CAS can be entertained. Antiplatelet and/or Coumadin therapy are medical alternatives that may be considered in this difficult scenario. Surgery or intervention should be reconsidered if antithrombotic/anticoagulant therapy fails to control the TIAs.

Based upon obtained imaging and surgical candidates with classic anterior circulation, carotid territory TIAs, or nondisabling stroke, we recommend CEA along with antiplatelet therapy for surgical correction of a stenotic plaque with ≥70% diameter reduction that correlates with the exhibited symptoms. In those with 50% to 69% diameter reduction, a more circumspect approach is used owing to the more modest risk reduction at later time points. If the patient clearly is healthy and has significant longevity, whereby they will glean the benefits that an operation can provide, CEA is undertaken. Other considerations causing us to lean toward surgical therapy include plaque morphology, such as ulceration or shaggy thrombus, contralateral ICA occlusion, and male gender, all of which may portend an increase in stroke risk for symptomatic patients. In those with less than 50% stenosis in the carotid artery, operation is not indicated except in very rare instances of ominous plaque morphology.

C. **Surgical therapy in asymptomatic patients.** The rationale for prophylactic CEA for high-grade asymptomatic carotid stenosis began with the classic observations of Dr. Jesse Thompson of Dallas, Texas. In his nonoperated group, 26.8% eventually had TIAs, 15.2% experienced a nonfatal stroke, and 2.2% had a fatal stroke. On the other hand, 90% of operated patients remained asymptomatic. Only 4.5% of the operated patients developed TIAs and 2.3% experienced a nonfatal stroke.

Subsequently, Strandness and colleagues at the University of Washington used duplex prospectively to study the natural history of carotid arterial disease in asymptomatic patients with carotid bruits. The presence of or progression to a greater than 80% internal carotid stenosis was highly correlated with development of TIA, stroke, and asymptomatic internal carotid occlusion in 46% of patients compared to those lesions of 0% to 79% stenosis (1.5%). The majority of adverse events occurred within 6 months of the findings of an 80% to 99% stenosis.

Trials comparing surgical and medical therapy for carotid stenoses in those without symptoms have also been accomplished. The risk of stroke with both medical therapy and operation is less in patients who are asymptomatic. Overall, the **Asymptomatic Carotid Atherosclerosis Study (ACAS), The Veteran's Affairs Asymptomatic Carotid Stenosis study, and the Asymptomatic Carotid Surgery Trial (ACST)** have indicated that in those with ≥60% asymptomatic stenosis, the risk of CVA at 5 years with antiplatelet therapy alone is 9% to 12%, or roughly 1.5% to 2% per year. With CEA added to antiplatelet therapy, this risk is reduced by half to 1% per year or 4% to 6% at 5 years. In ACAS, all in the surgical arm were required to undergo arteriography, yet some did not. In those who did, the risk of stroke with cerebral arteriography was 1.2%. The 30-day risk of stroke and death in the CEA group was 2.3%, and this was estimated to be 2.7% if all had an arteriogram. Thus, arteriography accounted for about half of asymptomatic perioperative events. In the ACST, enrollment was based upon duplex ultrasound. Arteriography was not required but some did undergo arteriography prior to CEA. The 30-day stroke and death rate was 2.8% in the surgical arm and 3.1% in all CEA procedures. As with the symptomatic trials, benefit with operation was not suggested in women.

Several points should be highlighted. First, duplex ultrasonography is an important diagnostic tool in asymptomatic patients, particularly when able to be used as a single modality prior to carotid surgery or to select those in whom the risk of arteriography is acceptable. It is worth noting that duplex criteria suggesting a stenosis of ≥80% correlated with an arteriographic lesion of 60% in ACAS. Second, the yearly risk of stroke in those with no symptoms is small. While the relative-risk reduction obtained with CEA is on the order of 50%, absolute stroke-risk reduction is only 1% to 2% per year. Therefore, to gain advantage from operation, patients must be selected well. They must be otherwise healthy and have a life expectancy of at least 5 years. Lastly, women must be looked at with some skepticism when evaluating them for prophylactic CEA and compelling reasons must be present. We believe that CEA in asymptomatic individuals with a carotid stenosis of over 60% is an essential component of therapy, particularly in men and those without considerable cardiac, pulmonary, renal, or other comorbidity, and the duplex ultrasound suggests the lesion to be 80%. This remains true only when the perioperative stroke and death rate can be 3% or less. Some physicians may be hesitant to recommend CEA for asymptomatic patients, but the natural history of this group does not appear to support this approach in otherwise healthy adults with good life expectancy. A major criticism of the asymptomatic trials today is that they were performed before the era of routine statin therapy and newer antiplatelet therapies. Medical therapy proponents suggest that the overall risk of stroke with medical therapy today is less than that simply with aspirin as in the trials. However, newer data also exist indicating that, even on medical therapy, both progression of the degree of stenosis as well as symptomatic conversion of severe stenosis warrants intervention.

D. Controversies in carotid occlusive disease

1. **Asymptomatic ulcerated plaque.** The natural history of asymptomatic ulcerated carotid lesions is not easy to define. Carotid ulceration is

difficult to detect or define well with duplex ultrasound and is usually large when seen with this modality. This imaging technique can define plaque morphology (homogeneous vs heterogeneous), but these characteristics do not always correlate with surface ulceration. Despite these limitations, some reports suggest that echolucent plaque, detectable by duplex ultrasound, increases the likelihood of future symptoms. Recent technologic advances have improved duplex resolution, but it remains overall a somewhat insensitive method to characterize ulceration. Arteriography also is not particularly accurate in defining ulceration, which may vary from a slight nonstenotic irregularity to a complicated ulcerated stenosis. CTA is best at defining overall characteristics associated with ulceration.

While carotid atherosclerotic ulceration has been shown to correlate independently with neurologic symptoms, the risk associated with lesions found in those who are asymptomatic remains somewhat controversial. Dr. Wesley Moore and colleagues classified asymptomatic ulcers without associated hemodynamically significant stenoses by their two-dimensional area on lateral arteriography: A, less than 10 mm^2; B, 10 to 40 mm^2; and C, more than 40 mm^2. They found that the yearly risk of stroke was less than 0.5% for A ulcers, 4.5% for B ulcers, and 7.5% for C ulcers. CEA was recommended for C lesions, and for B lesions if the patient was a reasonable operative candidate with good life expectancy. In general, ulceration may predict increased risk of neurologic events and should be considered in the treatment plan for those with carotid occlusive disease.

2. **Is a patient with cerebrovascular disease scheduled for other major surgery?** Controversy continues over whether patients with asymptomatic carotid stenoses are at increased risk for perioperative stroke at the time of other major surgery, especially any operation in which prolonged hypotension may occur. The major surgery of most concern has been cardiac and aortic operations. Many perioperative strokes occur in patients who were not suspected of having carotid disease prior to surgery. These strokes also are more commonly diffuse, or watershed than focal. Less than 2% of patients with no prior stroke or TIA undergoing major general or cardiovascular surgery suffer a perioperative stroke. With a history of prior neurologic event, this rate may increase to 4% to 6%. In those with a known hemodynamically significant carotid stenosis, the stroke risk for major surgery is 3%. With bilateral ≥50% carotid stenosis, this risk may increase to 4% to 5%. This risk can be as high as 7% to 9% in those undergoing coronary artery bypass grafting (CABG) with either carotid occlusion or prior stroke.

How then to proceed in patients undergoing major surgery with carotid occlusive disease? First, noninvasive carotid testing is performed to determine the hemodynamic significance of the carotid stenosis if this is not known. It is well established that there is little stroke risk in those undergoing general surgery if the patient is asymptomatic, and they should proceed to the intended operation. A caveat may be poorly compensated lesions, such as asymptomatic, severe bilateral disease, particularly in those in which the general surgery caries no immediacy. These should be surgically corrected before elective vascular surgery is attempted. The authors' stance has been to entertain carotid revascularization on at least one side prior to major general surgery. It seems logical to carry out CEA prior to any other surgery in those who are CEA candidates and would otherwise undergo CEA as this may, perhaps, negate any possible risk. This approach is unproven.

The issues surrounding those with cerebrovascular disease requiring heart operations, such as coronary artery bypass or valve replacement, deserve special mention. Roughly, half of strokes during CABG in those with a significant carotid stenosis are ipsilateral to narrowing and can be attributed to its presence. This special situation is confounded by the ability to perform these procedures in a combined fashion. In centers that carry out many combined CEAs with cardiac surgical procedures, the results are acceptable and can be quite good. However, this is not generalizable, and most evaluations suggest that the stroke/MI and death rate with staged procedures are likely superior to combining them. The first principle dictates to treat the symptomatic vascular territory first. Combined procedures are reserved for patients symptomatic in both territories, or those with severe bilateral asymptomatic carotid disease or contralateral ICA occlusion. Most surgeons agree that patients with symptomatic carotid disease should have CEA before other elective surgery is performed.

3. **Asymptomatic contralateral carotid artery stenosis.** Another controversial area in carotid surgery is the management of patients with asymptomatic contralateral carotid artery stenosis following a CEA. These patients may be at increased risk of TIAs and stroke. The outcome of such lesions again may depend on the hemodynamic significance of the asymptomatic lesion. Conservative management of nonoperated vessels opposite an endarterectomy appears appropriate until symptoms develop or a lesion greater than 80% is detected. We generally repair a hemodynamically significant contralateral carotid stenosis as a staged procedure. The endarterectomies are performed at least 5 to 7 days apart, although most patients require a longer recovery period between operations. If the contralateral stenosis is not hemodynamically significant, if the patient is not a good surgical risk, or if the first endarterectomy was complicated by cranial nerve injury, we follow the patient until symptoms occur or noninvasive studies document progression of the stenosis.

Study of duplex after CEA has informed us of several things. Progression of carotid stenoses is not uncommon and mandates surveillance in order to identify those who do progress. Further, flow velocity characteristics of the carotid artery contralateral to a severe carotid stenosis or occlusion may be artificially elevated due to increased blood flow demand on the "more open" side. The degree of stenosis by flow criteria may actually be lessened after CEA of the severe, contralateral side.

4. **Acute ICA occlusion.** It is uncertain whether thromboendarterectomy of an occluded ICA is advisable. Certainly, surgical repair of a thrombosed ICA in the setting of a completed stroke may be associated with intracranial hemorrhage and a high mortality risk. The natural history of untreated carotid occlusion is still debated. Approximately 25% of patients have TIAs, and 10% to 20% have a stroke with the occlusion event. Many patients, however, remain asymptomatic. Anticoagulation for 3 to 6 months followed by antiplatelet therapy remains the mainstay of the treatment paradigm.

A few reports indicate that thromboendarterectomy of a totally occluded ICA can be achieved with a reasonable morbidity and mortality rate and a 65% to 70% overall patency in severely symptomatic patients. Some have suggested that although the morbidity and mortality of operation in this setting is higher than without occlusion, these outcomes are better than without surgery. Retrograde filling of the ipsilateral intracranial ICA to its petrous or cavernous segment appears to be a good sign of operability. Timing of such surgery seems critical. Operation within 4 hours of acute symptoms has been recommended if this course of action is entertained. Not everyone agrees with this, and some have argued that after occlusion, the risk or recurrent ipsilateral events is relatively low.

An uncommon approach to management of the persistently symptomatic patient with an occluded ICA is ECA endarterectomy. ECA revascularization may relieve symptoms by increasing both the total and regional cerebral blood flow. The best results of external CEA are achieved when it is performed in the setting of an ipsilateral ICA occlusion and external carotid artery stenosis with demonstrated "internalization" of the ECA on duplex spectral flow analysis and identification of intracranial collateralization of the ECA on arteriography. In this setting, this procedure is usually performed to relieve retinal symptoms such as retinal TIA, bright light amaurosis, rubeosis iridis, or neovascular glaucoma. The ECA-ICA collaterals develop in the periorbital area to the ophthalmic artery, temporal area via leptomeningeal branches, and the dural vessels.

Finally, symptomatic patients with total internal carotid occlusion also may be relieved by extracranial to intracranial (EC-IC) anastomosis of the temporal artery to the middle cerebral artery. EC-IC bypasses generally are performed by a neurosurgeon experienced in microsurgical technique. We continue to see gratifying results in rare, select patients. However, the international randomized EC-IC bypass study failed to confirm that EC-IC anastomosis is effective in preventing ischemic stroke in patients with atherosclerotic disease in the carotid and middle cerebral arteries. Consequently, EC-IC bypass is rarely performed anymore. More recent randomized trials have also failed to show much stroke-risk reduction benefit. Thus, its use is on a select basis only. However, it remains a possibility in the rare, surgical treatment of progressively symptomatic ICA dissection when extracranial reconstruction becomes prohibitive.

E. **CAS.** Although the medical and surgical treatment of carotid occlusive disease has been well studied and effective treatment paradigms developed, the last two decades have seen the emergence of endovascular therapies as an alternative for treatment of cerebrovascular diseases. CEA removes the embolic source and relies on appropriate and "normal" healing of the endarterectomy, and CAS pushes, opens, and constrains the embolic source against the diseased arterial wall. **CAS** has been promoted as the preferred option in those who are "high risk" for CEA. There has been much debate as to what constitutes high-risk individuals in this relatively low-risk operation, and ongoing deliberations focus on what clinical factors may produce a scenario when CAS may be favored over other modalities of treatment.

To this end, many investigations have focused on noninferiority of CAS versus CEA in certain patient subgroups. Most early CAS investigations were industry sponsored and are specific to stent and embolic protection devices, in addition to combining end points and patient presentations. The most stirring industry-sponsored study to date is the stenting and angioplasty with protection in patients at high risk for endarterectomy **(SAPPHIRE)** trial. This study was supported by Cordis endovascular (a branch of Johnson & Johnson), and Cordis stents and embolic protection devices were used. It pitted CEA against CAS with embolic protection in those who were symptomatic with a ≥50% stenosis or asymptomatic with a ≥80% and had features that would place them at high risk for CEA. The main outcomes of stroke and death were not statistically different at 30 days and 1 year, thus CAS was not found to be inferior to CEA. However, when this end point was combined further to include MI, there was a trend favoring CAS in the perioperative 30-day period, and the incidence of stroke or death in 1 year was reported to favor CAS (12% vs 20%; p = 0.05). The occurrence of cranial nerve palsies was significantly less with CAS, and the need for revascularization of the carotid artery within 1 year of the treatment was statistically higher in those receiving CEA (4.6% vs 0.7%; p = 0.04). At 3 years, there was no difference between CAS and CEA groups in occurrence of death or stroke (p = 0.27).

This seemingly indicated that CAS is competitive with CEA in the early and midterm treatment of carotid stenosis (Fig. 12.3). Against the background of this literature, the U.S. Food and Drug Administration used this report to usher in the era of approval of CAS devices. Larger randomized trials of CAS versus CEA were born. The NIH sponsored carotid revascularization endarterectomy versus stenting trial (CREST) in the United States enrolled both symptomatic and asymptomatic patients, and in the European Union, the International Carotid Stenting Study (ICSS) was performed with symptomatic patients. The Asymptomatic Carotid Trial (ACT-1) looking specifically into treatment of asymptomatic patients was also performed in the U.S. ICSS suggested that occurrence of the composite of death, stroke, or myocardial infarction within 120 days of CAS was more frequent than with CEA (8.5% vs 5.2%, p = 0.006) largely due to stroke. ACT-1 reported 30-day composite outcomes of 3.3% for CAS and 2.6% with CEA (p = 0.60) with equal and low risk of stroke (2.8% vs 1.4%) or MI (0.5% vs 0.9%). CREST showed that the combined end point of death, stroke, or MI was statistically equal between treatment modalities (5.2% CAS vs 4.5% CEA, p = 0.38). However, CAS again led to more periprocedural stroke (4.1% vs 2.3%, p = 0.01), while CEA led to more cardiac events (2.3% vs 1.1%, p = 0.03). In CREST, postoperative MI with CAS or CEA was not influenced by symptomatic status. Neither was there a significant difference in 30-day stroke with asymptomatic patients (2.5% CAS vs 1.4% CEA, p = 0.15) in concordance with ACT-1. On the other hand, similar to ICSS, stroke occurred more frequently with CAS in symptomatic patients (5.5% CAS vs 3.2% CEA, p = 0.04). Late outcomes of all three trials indicate relative similarity between CEA and CAS in longer-term stroke-risk reduction and occurrence of restenosis. Suffice to say that proper selection for both CAS and CEA is important to good outcomes.

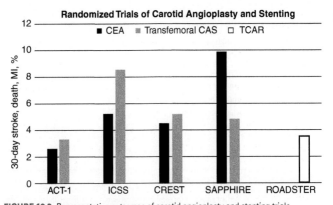

FIGURE 12.3 Representative outcomes of carotid angioplasty and stenting trials.

Stroke after transfemoral CAS occurs more often in the contralateral hemisphere compared to CEA, which is likely due to arch manipulation. Embolic protection devices do make a difference in the embolic rate during CAS. These include filters, occlusion/aspiration devices, and reversal of flow tools. **Current indications for CAS** continue to be better defined (Table 12.3). Anatomic factors in the carotid artery, aortic arch, descending aorta, and iliofemoral systems are very germane and may alter, or support, one treatment plan over another. Other issues, such as prior neck pathology requiring radiation or tracheostomy, or known contralateral laryngeal nerve palsy are more easily dealt with using CAS. Those with poor cardiopulmonary reserve may be better served with CAS. If the procedure seems anatomically feasible with minimal structural prohibitions, certain indications have become defined. Restenosis, prior radical neck surgery, an adverse neck due to tracheostomy and/or radiation, high carotid lesions at the C1-2 level making surgical exposure difficult, and significant cardiopulmonary comorbidities are reasons to proceed with CAS. It also appears that those patients who are 80 years of age or older do worse with transfemoral CAS. This may be due to more atherosclerotic disease and arch angulation in older people.

Over the last 15 years, use of transcervical CAS has been developed adding to treatment options for carotid disease. This is used in conjunction with reversal of flow, and is now commercially available in the United States and is commonly called TCAR (transcervical carotid revascularization). A small incision exposes the common carotid artery at the base of the neck between the heads of the sternocleidomastoid muscle. 5 cm of disease-free CCA is classically necessary for access. A short sheath is placed in the common carotid artery, and a sheath is placed in a common femoral vein. These are connected by flow tubing with a small filter to capture debris. Flow is controlled through the system by a small aperture which modifies tubing size. When the CCA is clamped below the sheath and flow is augmented in the system, blood flows in total reverse fashion from the distal carotid system through a filter and into the femoral vein. The carotid stent can then be delivered via the arterial sheath at the neck. Arteriography is possible through the neck with simple suspension of

TABLE 12.3	Current Recommendations and Potential Preferences for CAS vs CEA		
CEA Strongly Recommended	CEA Preferred	CAS Preferred	CAS Strongly Recommended
Age > 80 y	Inability to use EPD	High carotid bifurcation	Prior neck radiation
	Difficult aortic arch or carotid anatomy	Recurrent stenosis	Prior radical neck surgery
	Difficult vascular access	Neck immobility Significant cardiac or pulmonary disease	Tracheostomy stoma

Contralateral recurrent laryngeal nerve dysfunction.
CEA, carotid endarterectomy; CAS, carotid angioplasty and stenting; EPD, embolic protection device.
From Narins CR, Illig KA. Patient selection for carotid stenting versus endarterectomy: a systematic review. *J Vasc Surg.* 2006;44:661-672.

flow reversal in the system. The procedure can be done under local anesthesia with mild sedation. The CCA is then simply repaired with sheath removal. Using this technique, results from the ROADSTER trial in the United States reported 30-day stroke of 1.4%, stroke and death of 2.8%, and stroke, death, and MI of 3.5%. These are the best procedural results with any trial of carotid stenting to date regarding neurologic outcome. 1-year ROADSTER results show a very low risk of ipsilateral stroke. Like transfemoral CAS, further analysis of TCAR is ongoing.

IV. **VERTEBROBASILAR INSUFFICIENCY (VBI)**. Symptoms of **VBI** are characterized by ischemic events in the midbrain and cerebellum. These include ataxia, dysarthria, diplopia, dysphagia, vertigo, dizziness, drop attacks and gray outs with head rotation, instability of the patient in the upright position, visual changes, and bilateral paresthesias with occasional paresis. These may result from emboli (vertebrobasilar TIAs, or thromboembolic VBI) or hypoperfusion of the basilar artery and its branches (hemodynamic VBI). Overall, it appears that hemodynamic VBI is more common. Stroke in the posterior circulation accounts for 25% of CVAs, and the risks of stroke and related mortality after vertebrobasilar TIA appear similar to that of the carotid territory. However, vertebrobasilar stenosis and its treatment are much less well studied in contrast to the anterior circulation and carotid occlusive disease.

Subclavian stenosis proximal to the vertebral artery or stenosis of the origin of either vertebral artery may decrease vertebrobasilar flow. Additionally, only half of individuals have a "normal" circle of Willis, and collateral intracranial circulation between the anterior and posterior supplies may be compromised. Thus, hemodynamic VBI is especially likely to occur when carotid occlusive disease along with either vertebrobasilar or subclavian stenosis is present and collateral flow via the circle of Willis is inadequate.

In such cases, we generally repair the carotid lesions first, in the hope that increased collateral flow will alleviate the VBI. However, if both carotid and vertebral artery disease is present, consideration can be given to concomitant correction of both. Without significant carotid occlusive disease, or if the circle of Willis is not intact and appears to provide no considerable collateral flow, direct extracranial vertebral artery reconstruction should be considered. Proximal subclavian stenosis is usually corrected by carotid-subclavian bypass, subclavian-subclavian bypass, axillary-axillary bypass, or subclavian to carotid transposition. Stenosis at the origin of either vertebral artery may be managed by endarterectomy or reimplantation of the vertebral artery into the side of the common carotid artery (vertebral transposition). Anterior to posterior bypass grafts may be performed at either the low vertebral level, or at the skull base. Transposition of external carotid artery branches to the vertebral artery at the skull base have also been described. EC-IC anastomosis also may improve the posterior cerebral circulation. Finally, percutaneous balloon angioplasty and stenting of focal subclavian stenosis and vertebral artery lesions can be successful. Their utilization is well described but not well studied.

V. **GREAT VESSEL DISEASE AND SUBCLAVIAN STEAL SYNDROME**. Stenoses in the arch-based brachiocephalic vessels can lead to stroke, anterior or posterior circulation TIA, "watershed" ischemia of the brain noted during times of relative lowering of blood pressure, subclavian steal, and thromboembolic events or claudication in the arms. Indications for treatment of these lesions are based primarily in the symptomatic in order to prevent recurrent TIA, stroke, and upper extremity tissue loss. Similar to the treatment of lower extremity claudication, arch-based disease therapy may improve quality of life.

Left subclavian stenosis or occlusion is a common atherosclerotic lesion. Generally, it is asymptomatic and is discovered because the left arm blood pressure is lower than the right. Left arm claudication seldom is a significant problem, since the collateral flow to the left arm usually is well developed. However, for a few patients, proximal left subclavian occlusion may cause subclavian steal syndrome. Its clinical features are those of VBI such as dizziness, syncope, visual blurring, or ataxia, classically associated with vigorous left arm exercise. The mechanism of the syndrome relates to retrograde flow from the left posterior cerebral circulation down the left vertebral artery to the distal subclavian artery and arm. This "stealing" of blood from the brain to the left arm causes intermittent posterior cerebral ischemia. Another common scenario today is due to the standard use of the left internal thoracic artery for CABG. When a significant left subclavian artery stenosis develops proximal to such a LIMA graft, vigorous left arm use may lead to angina pectoris or "subclavian-coronary" steal. Should the stenosis become severe enough, unstable or early angina may develop regardless of arm use. This is clearly a more pressing issue in order to prevent acute myocardial infarction.

In our experience, classic subclavian steal syndrome is uncommon. Although many patients with subclavian occlusive disease have retrograde left vertebral flow on duplex, few have cerebral symptoms with arm claudication owing to the vast collateral flow in both the brain and the arm. If they do have cerebral ischemic symptoms, we perform a standard duplex carotid examination and either an MRA or CTA in order to further interrogate the arch and brachiocephalic vessels in addition to both the carotid and vertebrobasilar systems. Arteriography is utilized for evaluation when either the disease anatomy remains unclear or an endovascular option is entertained. Subclavian steal syndrome sometimes is relieved simply by correcting a severe left carotid stenosis, which improves collateral flow via the circle of Willis to the posterior brain. Significant arm claudication may be relieved by carotid-subclavian bypass, subclavian-subclavian bypass, axillary-axillary bypass, subclavian-to-carotid transposition, transluminal angioplasty and stenting, or direct anatomic reconstruction.

Overall, the treatment of arch-based disease has evolved as endovascular therapy has progressed. Anatomic surgical revascularization for arch-based symptomatic atherosclerotic lesions requires a median sternotomy and bypass grafting from the ascending aorta to each of the vessels beyond the blockages. Thus, it is imperative to have a CT of the aorta to confirm the ability to use proper side-biting cross-clamps for the proximal anastomosis. If lesions are focal in nature, classically the innominate artery, endarterectomy may be used. Arch-based grafting can be performed in conjunction with standard carotid bifurcation endarterectomy. Dacron and expanded polytetrafluoroethylene (ePTFE) prosthetic grafts are used.

Extra-anatomic open revascularizations such as the ones mentioned here for subclavian steal may also be used and are lower-risk procedures. Additionally, carotid-carotid bypass can be done. Should autogenous conduit for any of these open revascularizations be required, superficial femoral vein or paneled greater saphenous vein is an option if available. Patients undergoing operative revascularizations, particularly those based on the ascending aorta, must be evaluated for significant cardiopulmonary disease and risk stratified accordingly (see Chapter 7).

Endovascular methods, particularly balloon angioplasty and stenting, have been shown to achieve excellent immediate and midterm results. Due to this, operative anatomic reconstruction has been reserved for significant multivessel brachiocephalic disease. Creative techniques such as CEA with retrograde common carotid artery angioplasty and stenting are performed more and more commonly. The success of the neck-based extra-anatomic reconstructions and endovascular methods are particularly useful to avoid an increased morbidity and mortality with redo median sternotomy.

VI. OTHER CEREBROVASCULAR PATHOLOGIES

A. **Pulsatile masses.** Pulsatile masses near the carotid artery usually represent one of the following: true arterial aneurysms, carotid body tumors, local lymphadenopathy, or a prominent, tortuous carotid artery. After CEA, this may represent a patch pseudoaneurysm. Sonography, CT scanning, or MRI can generally differentiate between these etiologies. Carotid aneurysms are rare but dangerous since they may lead to rupture, cerebral embolization, thrombosis, and local pressure symptoms. The best surgical approach is resection and arterial restoration by direct end-to-end anastomosis or an interposition graft with either autogenous vein or ePTFE.

B. **Carotid body tumors (CBT)** are uncommon neoplasms of the neuroectoderm paraganglion cells, which make up the carotid body and are also referred to as paragangliomas. These tumors arise from the afferent ganglion of the glossopharyngeal nerve and are slowly progressive. CBTs are rarely malignant neoplasms. This occurs some 5% to 10% of the time, and in 8% of cases, they are bilateral. They can be associated with multiple endocrine neoplasia syndromes I and II, and, thus, familial tumors. Familial tumors have a higher incidence of being bilateral. Periadventitial resection sometimes requiring carotid artery replacement is recommended for all CBTs. The blood supply to these vascular tumors is from the external carotid artery, and preoperative embolization may be helpful when the tumor is over 5 cm in size. Radiation therapy appears to be of little value in their management, and observation is appropriate only for asymptomatic elderly patients who are poor surgical risks. The risk of stroke with CBT surgery is 5%, and the risk of cranial nerve injury is significant with some suggesting up to 40%.

C. **Carotid fibromuscular dysplasia (FMD)** is a relatively benign, often incidental, finding that rarely causes symptoms. Although carotid FMD may be associated with TIAs, the incidence of subsequent stroke is less than that seen with atherosclerotic carotid occlusive disease. Patients with FMD are more prone to ICA dissection. When neurologic or visual symptoms can be attributed to carotid FMD, they generally resolve without operation and recurrence is uncommon. We place these patients on antiplatelet therapy even when asymptomatic FMD is found. High-grade symptomatic FMD stenoses can be treated by operative probe dilation or internal carotid balloon angioplasty.

D. **Carotid dissection** may occur spontaneously or as a result of trauma with neck hyperextension. When spontaneous, it may be associated with hypertensive scenarios, inciting causes such as wretching or coughing, and connective tissue diseases. Most often, however, the causative piece remains unclear. Symptoms suggestive of dissection include headache, neck pain, and Horner's syndrome. Cranial nerve palsies and tinnitus, usually pulsatile, can also occur. Neurologic events arise due to either thromboembolic events or hypoperfusion. Initial treatment is anticoagulation as these are challenging to repair surgically. Serial duplex surveillance is suggested. With continued symptoms, either open repair, EC-IC bypass, or carotid stenting is indicated.

E. **Carotid kinks and coils.** Coils in the carotid artery arise from improper sequencing of cardiac descent and carotid uncoiling during embryologic development. Kinks are normally secondary to atherosclerotic plaque and arterial wall weakening with the degenerative process. Indications for surgical correction are the development of symptoms, significant stenosis falling within indications for CEA, or thrombus formation. Several repair techniques have been described, but all include the component of resection and reconstruction. Should endarterectomy be necessary, eversion endarterectomy with ICA resection and straightening is an excellent option.

VII. TECHNICAL ASPECTS OF CAROTID INTERVENTIONS

A. **CEA** is the most common open operation for extracranial cerebrovascular disease, and so we focus on principles of operative care for carotid reconstructions. These same principles also apply to other types of vertebral and subclavian revascularization.

1. **Preoperative preparation.** For elective cases, anticoagulants are discontinued 4 to 5 days prior to operation. Depending on the indication for Coumadin, either a heparin or Lovenox window can be used. Aspirin is continued throughout the course of operation. Clopidogrel (Plavix) is usually discontinued at least 5 days before surgery and aspirin instituted prior to discontinuation. The main exception is a patient with multiple recent TIAs or a severe carotid stenosis (<2 mm), who usually remains on heparin or clopidogrel accepting a slightly higher hematoma rate for a presumed decrease in neurologic events. There is mounting evidence that, if the patient is not already on statin medications, these should be instituted.

   Although neck infection is rare, several preventive measures are taken. The chin, neck, and anterior chest are shaved on the side of endarterectomy. This area is washed with a surgical scrub solution within 6 to 12 hours of operation. Preoperative parenteral antibiotics are started when the patient goes to the operating room; the antibiotic of choice usually is a cephalosporin or semisynthetic penicillin to cover skin flora.

   The patient is given non per os (nothing by mouth; NPO) status after midnight prior to operation. Stable or asymptomatic patients are admitted on the morning of operation. Some symptomatic patients will already be hospitalized for heparin anticoagulation. An intravenous infusion of balanced salt solution (e.g., 5% dextrose in Ringer's solution at 100 to 125 mL/h) is begun to maintain hydration. General narcotic premedications that may cause hypotension are avoided.

   On the day of surgery, a responsible member of the operating team is present in the operating room from the time the patient enters the room until the patient is transported to the recovery area. When the operation is complete, the surgical scrub remains sterile and the team maintains room preparation until the patient is awake enough for simple neurologic examination. An arterial line is generally inserted in the operating room. Occasionally, selected patients with severe cardiac disease (see Chapters 6 and 7) may also receive a Swan-Ganz catheter. A Foley bladder catheter is optional but may assist with blood pressure control since bladder distention may exacerbate hypertension in a labile patient.

2. **Operative principles**

   a. **General endotracheal anesthesia** is our preference, since it both provides the best control of the airway and best facilitates management of cardiorespiratory function. Other experienced surgeons prefer regional cervical block and local anesthesia. They believe that this provides a better hemodynamic course and direct neurologic monitoring.

b. **Carotid exposure** must be gentle and meticulous to avoid venous or nerve injury and dislodgement of atheromatous material from a plaque. Figure 12.4 demonstrates the relative positions of the major nerves of the neck that surround the carotid artery.

1. Branches of the **ansa cervicalis** (ansa meaning loop) provide innervation to the strap muscles and may be divided for better exposure, without a resulting neurologic deficit.

2. The **hypoglossal nerve** usually crosses the carotid artery cephalad to or near the carotid bifurcation. Most hypoglossal injuries are caused by retraction of the nerve. Clamp injuries may occur if the hypoglossal nerve is not dissected free from the common facial vein before this venous structure is divided. Hypoglossal injury results in weakness of the tongue on the operated side, with tongue deviation toward the side of the injury. This deficit may cause biting of the tongue while chewing, and the patient may have some difficulty swallowing or speaking. Bilateral hypoglossal nerve injury may be life threatening, since the tongue may prolapse posteriorly and obstruct the airway when the patient is supine.

3. The **vagus nerve** usually runs in the posterior carotid sheath behind the carotid artery. In 3% to 5% of cases, it swings anteriorly along the anterolateral surface of the carotid artery (anterior vagus nerve). The nerve must be dissected free from the carotid artery, especially at the proximal and distal extent of carotid dissection, where clamps may accidentally injure it.

4. Vagal injury is most commonly manifested by hoarseness, as the **recurrent laryngeal nerve** normally originates from the vagus in the chest and runs back to the vocal cord in the

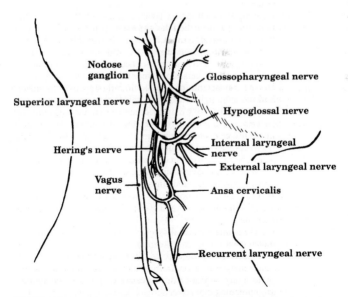

FIGURE 12.4 Nerves that may be encountered or injured during carotid endarterectomy and their typical relationship to the carotid arterial system.

tracheoesophageal groove. This cranial nerve injury is touted as the most common during CEA. The recurrent laryngeal nerve loops around the subclavian artery on the right side and the ligamentum arteriosum on the left. In roughly 1% or fewer cases, the laryngeal nerve is nonrecurrent and originates from the vagus nerve in the neck and passes posterior to the carotid artery.

5. The **external branch of the superior laryngeal nerve** travels behind the carotid bifurcation to the true vocal cord. This nerve innervates the cricothyroid muscle, which maintains the tone of the vocal cord. Injury may be avoided by careful dissection around the external carotid and superior thyroid arteries. Injury results in voice tone fatigue, especially after prolonged speaking or singing.

6. The **greater auricular nerve** is a sensory nerve to the skin overlying the mastoid process, the concha of auricle, and the earlobe. It lies on the anterior surface of the sternocleidomastoid muscle and may be injured when the neck incision is carried toward the mastoid process. Injury results in skin numbness around the lower ear and earlobe. This is the most common nerve injury during CEA.

7. The **mandibular branch** of the facial nerve runs forward from the angle of the mandible and parallel to the mandible. Injury results in weakness of the perioral musculature on the injured side. The patient may have a facial droop and drool from the corner of the mouth.

8. With very high internal carotid exposures, the **glossopharyngeal nerve** is at risk for injury. Injury to this nerve is rare but devastating and results in difficulty swallowing, which may preclude oral feeding and necessitate placement of a gastrostomy feeding tube. The glossopharyngeal nerve also provides a branch to the carotid sinus called **Hering's nerve**, which usually traverses posterior or deep to the ICA (Fig. 12.4). Use of local anesthetic to temporarily denervate the carotid bodies can help with blood pressure and heart rate control during CEA if dissection around the bulb causes bradycardia and hypotension.

9. During retraction of the cephalad sternocleidomastoid and internal jugular vein, the **spinal accessory** nerve may be encountered. In 20% of individuals, this courses over the jugular vein and is more superficial than the usual course underneath the vein, **posterior** to the ICA. Traction injury has rarely been reported and is usually manifest as shoulder pain and/or weakness or a sensation of neck or ear discomfort.

c. **Prevention of thromboemboli** obviously is essential if neurologic deficits are to be avoided. Thromboembolism is the most common etiology of postoperative stroke with CEA. The following measures should be taken to avoid thrombus accumulation and embolism.

1. During gentle carotid dissection, **suction** is used rather than blotting with sponges to keep the operative field dry. Vigorous manipulation of the carotid bifurcation may dislodge loose atheromatous material from an ulcerated plaque. We therefore prefer sharp dissection during carotid exposures and minimize any spreading maneuvers.

2. Before carotid clamping, **heparin** is administered intravenously and allowed to circulate for at least 3 minutes. Our usual dose

is a 5,000-unit bolus. Others use 100 units per kilogram for dosing.

3. The inside of the carotid artery is **irrigated** with heparinized saline to wash out any loose atheroma or clot both before a shunt is inserted and before the ICA is reopened.

4. Bleeding of the internal and external carotid arteries (back-bleeding) and forward bleeding of the common carotid artery flushes out any thrombus or atheroma that may accumulate behind vascular clamps. Carotid blood flow also is reinstated up the external carotid artery for a few cardiac cycles before opening the ICA. This sequence of reopening the carotid branches should allow any thromboemboli to go out through the external carotid artery and not directly to the brain.

d. **Cerebral protection** from clamp ischemia probably is best achieved by two methods: careful blood pressure control and cerebral monitoring of some type in conjunction with either selective or compulsory shunting. Clamp ischemia is based upon the limits of cerebral perfusion and is a lesser cause of stroke with CEA. Infarction of brain tissue occurs when the flow rate is reduced to 10 cc/100 g tissue/min for several minutes. Electrical quiescence takes place at 15 cc/100 g tissue/min.

1. Cerebral perfusion is directly related to **mean arterial blood pressure**, which was discussed in Chapter 8. Therefore, prior to carotid clamping, we remind the anesthesiologist to maintain the blood pressure in a normotensive to mildly hypertensive range (140 to 150 mm Hg systolic; mean arterial pressure of at least 80 mm Hg). If continuous EEG monitoring is used, a diffuse slowing pattern often can be eliminated by simply raising the patient's mean arterial pressure.

2. **Shunting** during CEA remains controversial. Experienced surgeons have demonstrated that with or without shunting, CEA can be performed with a low incidence of permanent postoperative neurologic deficit (1% to 3%). The key question is how to identify the few patients who will not tolerate carotid clamping long enough for the surgeon to complete endarterectomy without a shunt and, thus, allow for selective shunting. There are risks associated with shunting, which include thrombus formation with potential embolism and dissection. Under general anesthesia, the two most common methods to assess adequate cerebral perfusion during carotid clamping are carotid stump pressures and EEG monitoring. Our experience suggests that carotid stump pressures may not correlate with adequate cerebral perfusion as indicated by EEG monitoring. Consequently, we insert a shunt after carotid clamping if focal EEG changes occur and are not corrected by manipulation of anesthetic agents or blood pressure. If EEG monitoring is not available, a mean carotid stump pressure below 50 mm Hg may indicate inadequate cerebral collateral flow during carotid clamping.

Even without EEG changes, we often insert a shunt to allow for an unhurried endarterectomy and to provide an intraluminal stent, which, in our experience, facilitates a better closure of the ICA. For these reasons, in a teaching situation, we are more likely to use shunting. We also believe that routine shunting is advisable when the contralateral ICA is occluded and when the patient has had a recent stroke. Finally, in patients in whom the internal carotid plaque extends high into the carotid artery, an intraluminal shunt may make endarterectomy excessively difficult. In such cases, the endarterectomy of the distal plaque probably should be performed without a shunt in place. A shunt may subsequently be inserted to complete the operation.

Other techniques described for cerebral monitoring during CEA include the use of spectral analysis monitors, evoked potential monitoring, and cervical block, awake anesthesia. Spectral analysis quantifies bilateral hemispheric EEG tracings. Ischemia is manifest as lower number on the affected hemisphere. Evoked potentials may be motor (cortical) or sensory (peripheral) and search for latency and reduced strength or amplitude in peripheral nerve conduction. Monitoring and stump pressures all lead to a shunting rate above what is necessary clinically. One very successful strategy to maintain adequate cerebral perfusion during CEA that minimizes excess shunt use while avoiding hypoperfusion is use of regional cervical anesthesia in an awake patient. Problems are patient tolerance and the amount of dissection required to achieve a safe and complete operation.

8. **The endarterectomy technique** should achieve the two main goals of carotid artery reconstruction (Fig. 12.5). The first goal is adequate removal of the stenotic or ulcerated plaques. The carotid arteries are clamped sequentially, starting with the ICA to avoid embolism during further manipulation, and a longitudinal

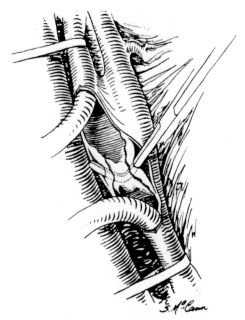

FIGURE 12.5 Standard longitudinal CEA with shunt. CEA, carotid endarterectomy.

arteriotomy is made from the distal common carotid past the stenosis to normal ICA. Since atherosclerotic lesions involve the intima and media, we generally remove the plaques down to the external elastic lamina. In our experience, such a deep endarterectomy plane has resulted in the removal of retained media fibers, which may cause recurrent myointimal restenosis, but it has not been associated with late aneurysm formation. In those with rough, irregular residual carotid artery walls, **dextran-40** is instituted for antiplatelet purposes during the procedure at a rate of 25 to 50 mL/h. This is continued as the patient's only IV fluid for 24 hours postoperatively. Its use must be selective for several reasons. It is highly hyperosmolar, and fluid overload and cardiac failure have been described. Prior to administration, a test dose must be given as anaphylaxis is also a known entity secondary to dextran.

The second goal is closure of the arteriotomy so that stenosis or thrombosis does not occur. A primary closure of the arteriotomy is usually adequate for very large (>6 mm) internal carotid arteries. Patches are used when primary closure would cause stenosis or in cases of redo endarterectomy. Patch angioplasty may protect against early thrombosis, and there has been a substantial trend toward more patching by all surgeons in the recent years. Clinical trials indicate that patching is extremely beneficial in the following situations:

1. Small internal carotid artery (<3.5 mm)
2. Long internal carotid arteriotomy (>3 cm)
3. Women who tend to have small arteries
4. Reoperative endarterectomies

Further trials have now clearly noted that recurrent stenosis is reduced with the use of patch angioplasty.

An alternative technique is **eversion CEA** (Fig. 12.6). In this procedure, the origin of the ICA as obliquely amputated at the carotid bulb. A circumferential endarterectomy is started in a similar plane and extended beyond the stenosis with the elevator. The ICA is then everted upon itself beyond the stenosis where an end point is identified and the plaque gently amputated or removed. It generally gives way quite nicely at the proper end point. The ECA and CCA may then undergo endarterectomy and the ICA is reverted, drawn to length and sewn directly back to the origin. Potential advantages of this technique include no need for prosthetic and the ability to resect redundant, kinked, or coiled portions of the ICA and essentially straighten it. Proponents believe it to have less restenosis than traditional, longitudinal CEA, and perhaps less stroke risk, but studies have generally shown equivalency. Disadvantages include a more challenging shunting technique and complete bulb dissection with more lability in blood pressure and heart rate afterward.

In our opinion, low-power magnifying glasses (magnification of 2 to 4) help us perform a more meticulous endarterectomy and arterial closure. Flow through the internal and external carotid arteries is assessed by a sterile continuous wave Doppler probe. Absence of flow or an obstructed, monophasic signal indicates thrombosis or stenosis, which requires immediate thrombectomy and a patch. Other methods of intraoperative assessment include arteriography or duplex ultrasound. Completion duplex ultrasound has become standard in many institutions and is an excellent, noninvasive way to further investigate the CEA site.

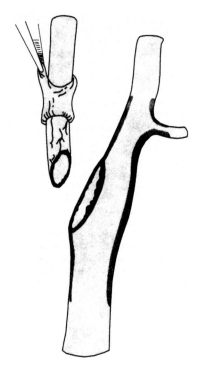

FIGURE 12.6 Eversion CEA. CEA, carotid endarterectomy.

f. **Recognition of postoperative neurologic deficit** ideally is made in the operating room if the anesthesiologist can awaken and extubate the patient early. This is the reason that the surgical technician and the back table as well as those in the operating room should maintain strict sterile methods until the patient appears neurologically intact. Otherwise, the patient is moved to the recovery area, and a neurologic examination of general motor function is made as soon as the patient is responsive. In our experience, the earliest signs of a neurologic deficit may be severe hypertension, difficulty in being awakened from anesthesia, or clumsiness of fine hand movement. This can be a tricky evaluation in those with recent stroke as it is not uncommon for them to awake with an exacerbation of their stroke symptoms. This is due to the ischemic penumbra of neurons surrounding the area of infarction whose metabolic function is affected by the decreased blood flow experienced, yet they are viable. This typically resolves in the first several hours to days after the operation.

The proper management of an **immediate postoperative neurologic deficit** must be individualized; however, the general tenet when this occurs is return directly to the operating room.

1. First, the patient's general **cardiorespiratory status** must be stabilized expeditiously. This includes stabilization of heart rate, blood pressure, pulmonary ventilation, and blood oxygenation.

2. Treatment then depends on the **location** of the neurologic deficit.

a. If the deficit is a **contralateral hemiparesis**, a technical problem at the endarterectomy site may exist. We generally have returned these patients immediately to the operating room to examine the endarterectomy site. Two tests may help determine whether the arteriotomy should be reopened. First, duplex ultrasound is a sensitive method to ascertain carotid thrombosis or a major filling defect due to thrombus or a technical problem (e.g., residual plaque). Second, an intraoperative carotid arteriogram may also be done if ultrasound is not available or equivocal. If these tests are not satisfactory, reexploration of the artery remains the only way to rule out technical error.

b. If the neurologic deficit is diffuse, the patient may have suffered an **internal capsule stroke**, usually caused by a hypotensive episode. Patency of the carotid arteries should then be assessed with duplex ultrasound. If the operated side is occluded, then reoperation is appropriate. If both carotid arteries appear widely patent, the patient should receive supportive care. CT/CTA of the brain should be performed once the patient is initially stabilized to search for hemorrhage and distal intracranial arterial patency, and again in approximately 12 to 24 hours to localize the cerebral infarct area and assess the amount of cerebral edema or hemorrhage.

Delayed deficits after CEA are typically defined as occurring 12 to 24 hours postoperatively. Duplex should be performed. If this appears to be fine, then CTA should be accomplished to evaluate the CEA site and the brain for hemorrhage and CVA. Any question of the CEA site should instigate arteriography. If this evaluation path reveals nothing, or CVA is seen on CT without concern for the CEA site, transthoracic and transesophageal echocardiography are done to assess for a cardiac source. Should no sources be identified, augmentation in antiplatelet therapy or anticoagulation can be instituted. Faults in the CEA site should lead to surgical correction and intracardiac thrombus treated with anticoagulation.

3. **Postoperative care**
   a. **Day of surgery.** All patients spend the first 12 to 24 hours after cerebrovascular surgery in an intensive recovery area, where vital signs and neurologic status can be continuously monitored. The head of the bed is elevated 30 to 45 degrees to diminish edema and facilitate deep breathing. Antiplatelet therapy is continued without interruption, and we generally try to keep the patient's systolic blood pressure below 150 mm Hg and above 100 mm Hg. This may require vasoactive intravenous medications the first 24 hours after CEA. The patient is kept NPO until the first postoperative morning since reexploration is occasionally necessary. While the patient is NPO, a maintenance intravenous infusion of 5% dextrose in water and one-half normal saline is run at 1 mL/kg/h. Antibiotics are continued for 24 hours postoperatively. Patients who have undergone staged bilateral carotid endarterectomies may be insensitive to hypoxia as a result of carotid baroreceptor trauma. Therefore, they must be observed for bradycardia, hypotension, and respiratory distress.
   b. **Postoperative day 1.** If a wound drain has been used, it is removed on the first postoperative day. Patients who are doing

satisfactorily resume a normal diet and all preoperative medications. Clopidogrel can be safely started 24 hours after CEA if there are no concerns for neck hematoma. If patients have resumed normal activities without complications or hemodynamic instability, they are discharged later the first postoperative day. Older patients with labile blood pressure or other medical comorbidities may stay an additional night.

c. **Discharge instructions.** Most patients are discharged within 24 to 48 hours after operation. Because the patient's full physical strength may not recover for 2 to 4 weeks, we generally advise patients to convalesce for that period of time before resuming normal working activities. This is particularly true for activities that require active neck motion, such as driving. All patients are rechecked as outpatients 3 to 6 weeks after surgery. They return to their local referring physician for long-term management of any medical problems and review and changes in antihypertensive medicines.

4. **Complications**
   a. **Early postoperative problems** are usually apparent on the day of surgery and require prompt recognition and treatment.
      1. **Immediate and delayed postoperative neurologic deficits** are discussed in the section on operative management (**p. 26**).
      2. **Hypertension** is a common postoperative problem that occurs in approximately 20% of patients who have CEA. Patients who were hypertensive before operation, especially if poorly controlled, are more likely to have severe postoperative hypertension. The incidence of neurologic deficit and death is significantly higher in these hypertensive patients. Therefore, we strive to maintain postoperative systolic blood pressure in a range mentioned earlier from the minimal normal preoperative recording to a maximum of 150 mm Hg. Alterations in blood pressure due to carotid sinus dissection may require antihypertensive medication manipulation.
      3. **Neck hematomas** may compromise breathing and swallowing. Patients with large neck hematomas should be returned to the operating room for evacuation. If a patient's respiratory status and hematoma are stable, no attempt at intubation should be made until the surgical team is ready to operate. In cases where respiration is desperately compromised or bleeding is profuse, nasotracheal intubation and control of bleeding in the recovery room may be necessary to save the patient and may require opening the neck. Smaller neck hematomas may be left alone and usually resolve in 7 to 14 days. They seldom are complicated by infection. If a pulsatile mass persists after the major portion of the hematoma resolves, a pseudoaneurysm should be suspected and evaluated by ultrasonography.
      4. **Local nerve injuries** following carotid operations probably are more common than generally recognized or reported. Some degree of cranial nerve dysfunction affects 5% to 20% of patients. The mechanism of injury usually is nerve retraction or clamping and not transection. Most cranial nerve injuries manifest as deficits in the recurrent laryngeal and the hypoglossal nerves. The injuries often are mild or asymptomatic and will not be detected unless one specifically examines for them. For example, one-third of recurrent laryngeal nerve injuries will go unrecognized unless direct laryngoscopy is

performed. **Therefore, all patients who undergo staged, bilateral CEA should be tested by direct laryngoscopy before the second operation.** Should dysfunction of the swallowing mechanism be suspected, formal swallowing study evaluation is indicated. Fortunately, most cranial nerve injuries resulting from retraction trauma will resolve in 2 to 6 months. Time and reassurance are all the treatment most patients require.

b. **Hyperperfusion syndrome** is a rare occurrence after CEA. It happens in 1% to 2% of cases and usually is seen 3 to 7 days after CEA. The complete syndrome occurs as a classic triad of headache, seizures, and intracranial hemorrhage. Hypertension usually accompanies the process. It is thought to be due to poor intracranial arterial autoregulation secondary to a significant period of time with reduced extracranial flow. Those at highest risk appear to be those with very high-grade carotid stenosis, severe bilateral carotid disease, and poorly controlled hypertension. Treatment is supportive and consists of blood pressure and seizure control, as well as evaluation for intracranial hemorrhage and significant cerebral edema by CT. Rarely, this may require neurosurgery.

b. **Late complications** of carotid artery reconstructions are uncommon or at least seldom cause symptoms.

1. **Recurrent carotid stenosis** that is symptomatic is rare, affecting only 1% to 3% of patients after CEA, and overall, the need for either operative or interventional therapy after CEA is 4% to 5%. Asymptomatic restenosis is detectable in 10% to 20% of patients followed by noninvasive carotid testing and is more common in women and active smokers. High-grade (≥80%) restenosis is also rare. The risk of a future stroke in this asymptomatic group appears to be low. Recurrent lesions have a striking predilection for the ICA near its origin and within the confines of the original endarterectomy site. Early recurrent lesions (<36 months) are predominantly a combination of intimal hyperplasia and surface thrombus. Features of recurrent atherosclerosis (abundant collagen, calcium deposits, and foam cells) are more pronounced in late recurrences.

An important feature that differentiates primary and recurrent atherosclerotic carotid lesions is the presence of surface and intraplaque thrombus in 90% of recurrent stenoses. Recurrent symptoms after CEA generally require repeat evaluation and arteriography. Recurrent stenosis is operatively repaired by repeat endarterectomy and patch angioplasty, or by patch angioplasty alone if an endarterectomy plane is not achievable. Segmental carotid resection and an interposition vein or ePTFE graft may also be performed. The rates of stroke and cranial nerve injury are slightly higher with reoperation. Alternatively, CAS can be utilized.

The need for long-term ultrasound surveillance of CEA sites is debatable. Since early restenosis is often a relatively benign process, asymptomatic restenosis does not mandate reoperation. However, contralateral atherosclerotic asymptomatic 50% to 79% stenoses have a significant risk of becoming symptomatic, especially if they progress. Consequently, we recheck carotid duplex scans on CEA patients every 6 months for 2 years and then yearly, and caution patients to report any ipsilateral, or contralateral neurologic or ocular symptoms.

Those undergoing carotid stenting should also be followed regularly (e.g., every 6 months).

2. **Carotid pseudoaneurysm** may occur after primary arterial closure or patch angioplasty. In general, such pseudoaneurysms should be repaired since mural thrombus may accumulate and cause cerebral thromboembolism. Large pseudoaneurysms also may cause local pressure symptoms. These require interposition grafting.

c. **Transfemoral carotid angioplasty and stenting (CAS)**

1. It is imperative that the patient be fully awake with little sedation. Generally, only local groin anesthetic is used at the arterial access site. Yet, these procedures should be done with an anesthetist comfortable with cardiovascular anesthesia. A full array of antihypertensive medications, pressors, heparin, and atropine and glycopyrrolate should be quickly available. Specifically, these are necessary to counteract the reflex bradycardia associated with carotid bulb angioplasty. In the past, transvenous pacemakers were placed prior to CAS; however, this is no longer advocated in the majority of cases.

2. This procedure begins with safe and adequate aortic arch and selective carotid and intracranial arteriography. Several technically challenging aspects of CAS have been categorized (Table 12.4). Each of these plays a role in successful performance of CAS, and one or several may preclude CAS. The use of embolic protection devices such as filters, occlusion-based technology, and reversal of flow devices is now considered standard, and a stenosis that is not amenable to their use should be questioned (Fig. 12.7). Unprotected predilation with a small balloon may facilitate proper positioning of the stent in certain cases of very severe stenosis. Arch anatomy may be especially challenging and has been graded based on degree of arch angle (Fig. 12.8). Specifically, the distance between the uppermost aspect of the aortic arch and the origin of the innominate and left common carotid arteries is one reliable predictor of difficulty in positioning of the necessary sheath proximal to the carotid stenosis. The greater this distance, the more acute the angle of the aortic arch and the more difficult

TABLE 12.4	CAS Technical Challenges
Technical Challenge	**Category**
High-grade stenosis precluding initial EPD	1
Complex arch anatomy	2
Compromised femoral access	3
Tandem stenoses	4
Circumferential calcification	5
Internal carotid tortuosity	6

CAS, carotid angioplasty and stenting; EPD, embolic protection device.
Adapted from Choi HM, Hobson RW, Goldstein J, et al. Technical challenges in a program of carotid artery stenting. *J Vasc Surg.* 2004;40:746-751.

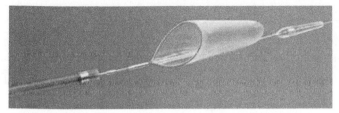

FIGURE 12.7 Example of a filter antiembolic device. (FilterWire EZ, Boston Scientific, Natick, MA, USA.)

the arch will be to maneuver. Type C arches represent the most difficult in this respect. Additionally, MRI/MRA data have shown that thromboembolic events leading to stroke during carotid stenting occur almost equally between hemispheres, which suggest that arch calcification and atheroma are important causes to consider. Novel carotid artery stenting with arm access sites is described. As noted above, with the increase in use of TCAR, many anatomic limitations can be overcome for CAS should CCA and bifurcation anatomy be amenable to this modality. Long, tandem stenoses generally fare worse using CAS. ICA tortuosity may make the stent placement difficult if not impossible, to achieve appropriate wall apposition. Creation of an area of malapposition may become a nidus for thrombus development and thromboembolic complications. Circumferential calcium is an anatomic scenario that may limit stent expansion and is at higher risk of rupture with balloon angioplasty, and should give pause to the consideration of CAS.

Platforms for CAS are based upon 6 Fr guiding sheaths and monorail systems (see Chapter 10). Brachiocephalic or common carotid artery access, trackability, and purchase may require 7 to 8 Fr sheaths. Systemic, intravenous heparin is given prior to selective catheterization of the brachiocephalic vessels. Activated clotting times can be monitored to keep this value above 250 seconds, and further boluses may be necessary. Some use GIIb/IIIa inhibitors, yet these are associated with increased hemorrhagic complications. Clopidogrel is

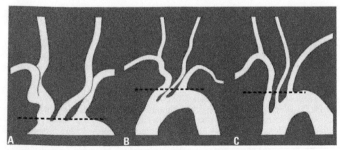

FIGURE 12.8 Arch anatomic classification: **(A)** brachiocephalic vessels originate at level of superior arch; **(B)** more acute arch angulation and innominate and left carotid originate below superior arch level; **(C)** severe arch angulation with all brachiocephalic vessels originating below level of superior arch.

continued through the procedure. If the patient is not on this, they are loaded with 300 mg by mouth the day prior to CAS. Self-expanding stents are used during carotid artery stenting and may have either an open or closed cell configuration. Open cell configurations tend to be more flexible; however, closed cells provide somewhat more radial strength and are better at "jailing" atherosclerotic plaque against the vessel wall and potentially reducing emboli. Filter distal embolic protection devices allow antegrade flow during the procedure, whereas occlusion-based distal embolic protection devices act like a clamp and cease antegrade flow in the ICA during the procedure. Reversal systems lead to retrograde ICA flow. Usually, stenoses require placing the stent across the origin of the external carotid artery. Tapered stents are now available designed for this purpose. We have avoided this if the ICA is straight enough and the lesion is higher in the ICA such as with restenosis.

3. **Unique complications** associated with transfemoral CAS compared to CEA include the potential for bilateral hemispheric events as mentioned previously due to aortic arch catheterization and manipulation and complications associated with the access site. These may comprise bleeding with hematoma, pseudoaneurysm, and arteriovenous fistula formation. These events occur in less than 4% of cases. If at all possible, one single stent should be used as multiple stents may increase the risk of thromboembolic complications. However, arterial dissection and stent misplacement may require further stent placement. Soft balloon angioplasty is critical as profound bradycardia and hypotension can occur. A unique advantage of CAS is the ability to accomplish intracranial arteriography before and after the procedure. This is, in our opinion, mandatory to document the state of the cerebral vessels and aid in the identification of distal emboli. Should "neuro rescue" be needed with distal thromboembolization, useful tools may include catheter-directed thrombolytic therapy, remote catheter mechanical thrombectomy, and intracranial angioplasty and stenting. Proper antiplatelet therapy and anticoagulation cannot be stressed enough for CAS.

Selected Readings

Bonati LH, Dobson J, Featherstone RL, et al. Long-term outcomes after stenting versus endarterectomy for treatment of symptomatic carotid stenosis: the ICSS randomized trial. *Lancet.* 2015;385:529-538.

Brott TG, Halperin JL, Abbara S, et al. 2011 ASA/ACCF/AHA/AANN/AANS/ACR/ASNR/CNS/SAIP/SCAI/SIR/SNIS/SVM/SVS Guideline on the management of patients with extracranial carotid and vertebral artery disease: executive summary. *J Am Coll Cardiol.* 2011;57:1002-1044.

Brott TG, Hobson RW, Howard G, et al. Stenting versus endarterectomy for treatment of carotid-artery stenosis. *N Engl J Med.* 2010;363:11-23.

Brott TG, Howard G, Roubin GS, et al. Long-term results of stenting versus endarterectomy for carotid-artery stenosis. *N Engl J Med.* 2016;374:1021-1031.

Blacker DJ, Flemming KD, Link MJ. The preoperative cerebrovascular consultation: common cerebrovascular questions before general and cardiac surgery. *Mayo Clin Proc.* 2004;79:223-229.

Capoccia L, Sbarigia E, Speziale F, et al. The need for emergency surgical treatment in carotid-related stroke-in-evolution and crescendo transient ischemic attack. *J Vasc Surg.* 2012;55:1611-1617.

Executive Committee for the Asymptomatic Carotid Atherosclerosis Study. Endarterectomy for asymptomatic carotid artery stenosis. *JAMA*. 1995;273: 1421-1428.

Hans SS, Jareunpoon O. Prospective evaluation of electroencephalography, carotid artery stump pressure, and neurologic changes during 314 consecutive carotid endarterectomy performed in awake patients. *J Vasc Surg*. 2007;45:511-515.

ICSS Investigators. Carotid artery stenting compared with endarterectomy in patients with symptomatic carotid stenosis (ICSS): an interim analysis of a randomized controlled trial. *Lancet*. 2010;375:985-997.

Karkos CD, McMahon G, McCarthy MJ, et al. The value of urgent carotid endarterectomy for crescendo transient ischemic attacks. *J Vasc Surg*. 2007;45:1148-1154.

Kwolek CJ, Jaff MR, Leal JI, et al. Results of the ROADSTER multicenter trial of transcarotid stenting with dynamic flow reversal. *J Vasc Surg*. 2015;62:1227-1235.

MRC Asymptomatic Carotid Surgery Trial (ACST) Collaborative Group. Prevention of disabling and fatal strokes by successful carotid endarterectomy in patients without recent neurological symptoms: randomised controlled trial. *Lancet*. 2004;363:1491-1502.

Narins CR, Illig KA. Patient selection for carotid stenting versus endarterectomy: a systematic review. *J Vasc Surg*. 2006;44:661-672.

North American Symptomatic Carotid Endarterectomy Trial Collaborators. Beneficial effect of carotid endarterectomy in symptomatic patients with high-grade carotid stenosis. *N Engl J Med*. 1991;325:445-453.

North American Symptomatic Carotid Endarterectomy Trial Collaborators. Benefit of carotid endarterectomy in patients with symptomatic moderate or severe stenosis. *N Engl J Med*. 1998;339:1415-1425.

Powers WJ, Rabinstein AA, Ackerson T, et al. 2018 Guidelines for the Early Management of Patients with Acute Ischemic Stroke: A Guideline for Healthcare Professionals from the American Heart Association/American Stroke Association. *Stroke*. 2018;49:e46-e110.

Ricotta JJ, Aburahma A, Ascher E, et al. Updated Society for Vascular Surgery guidelines for management of extracranial carotid disease. *J Vasc Surg*. 2011;54():e1-31.

Rosenfield K, Matsumura JS, Chaturvedi S, et al. Randomized trial of stent versus surgery for asymptomatic carotid stenosis. *N Engl J Med*. 2016;374:1011-1020.

Rothwell PM, Eliasiw M, Gutnikov SA, et al. Analysis of pooled data from the randomized trials of endarterectomy for symptomatic carotid stenosis. *Lancet*. 2003;361:107-116.

Rothwell PM, Eliasiw M, Gutnikov SA, et al. Endarterectomy for symptomatic carotid stenosis in relation to clinical subgroups and the timing of surgery. *Lancet*. 2004;363:915-924.

Simon MV, Chiappa KH, Rordorf GA, et al. Predictors of clamp-induced electroencephalographic changes during carotid endarterectomies. *J Clin Neurophysiol*. 2012;29:462-467.

13 Lower Extremity Ischemia

Lower extremity arterial disease presents on a spectrum—from asymptomatic to intermittent claudication to limb-threatening ischemia. Up to 20% of those over the age of 55 have some degree of peripheral arterial occlusive disease (PAOD). **Intermittent claudication,** or functional ischemia, of the lower extremities is the most common manifestation of PAOD. The term claudication comes from the Latin *claudicatio*, "to limp." **Limb-threatening ischemia** occurs when there is tissue loss, such as ulceration or gangrene, or ischemic rest pain. Another term used to describe this is **critical limb ischemia.** Causes may include continual progression of chronic atherosclerosis or acute processes such as plaque rupture with thrombosis, or embolism. As the term limb-threatening ischemia indicates, if treatment is not pursued, there is a high likelihood of amputation.

Patients with claudication may limp or claudicate for several reasons. The patient's calf muscles may develop cramping pain with walking. The hip and thigh muscles may cramp or tire. Walking also may be limited because of a feeling of diffuse lower extremity weakness, numbness, and heaviness. Although claudication usually is associated with vascular disease, degenerative hip disease or conditions of the spine such as spinal stenosis may cause similar symptoms that is "pseudoclaudication." Therefore, in the evaluation of lower extremity claudication, the physician must first question the underlying etiology. Is the claudication caused by arterial occlusive disease or some other problem? The history and physical exam often can answer this question (see Chapter 3). Noninvasive testing, including resting segmental pressures (e.g., ankle-brachial indices; ABI), exercise "stress" segmental pressures, accompanying pulse volume recordings (PVRs), and duplex ultrasound of the aortoiliac, femoropopliteal, and tibial segments, provide objective data to support or refute the clinical impression (see Chapter 5).

If the initial evaluation suggests arterial occlusive disease as the cause of intermittent claudication, the next question concerns how management proceeds. Which levels of the arterial system are involved? Should therapy be medical, or should a procedure such as percutaneous balloon angioplasty, stenting, or atherectomy be entertained, or should an operation be recommended? And, if surgery is chosen, what operation should be performed? If acute or limb-threatening ischemia is present, what is the likely etiology? How quickly is assessment and treatment needed?

This chapter delineates answers to these issues and gives global evaluation, diagnostic, and therapeutic insight for assessment of those with lower extremity vascular disease.

I. **PATTERNS OF DISEASE.** Vascular claudication of the lower limb generally is caused by an arterial stenosis or occlusion in two general regions. A common location of stenosis or occlusion in the **superficial femoral artery** is at the adductor canal. The other large anatomic category of claudicants has occlusive disease localized primarily to the distal abdominal aorta and iliac arteries with open distal arteries; this is termed **aortoiliac disease**. Over time, collateral branches in the groin and around the knee become well developed when occlusive disease occurs (Fig. 13.1).

Patient history, physical examination, and noninvasive segmental leg pressures and PVRs usually can identify the primary location and objectify the severity of disease. Since therapeutic decisions are influenced by the location of occlusive lesions, we categorize patients into five common patterns of peripheral arterial disease (Fig. 13.2).

A. **Aortoiliac disease (type 1 and type 2)**. Type 1, the least common pattern (10% to 15%), is limited to the distal abdominal aorta and common iliac arteries. Patients with focal aortoiliac disease are characteristically between the ages of 35 and 55, with a low incidence of hypertension and diabetes but a high frequency of heavy cigarette smoking and

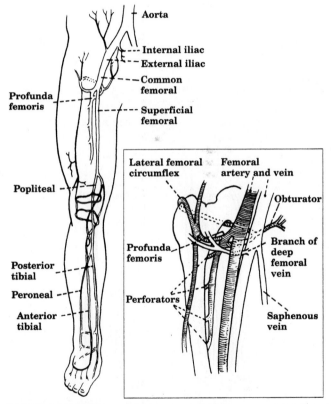

FIGURE 13.1 Arterial anatomy of the lower extremity. The most common locations of atherosclerotic occlusive disease causing claudication are the aortoiliac region and the superficial femoral artery. Enlarged drawing of the femoral region demonstrates the major collateral channels of the profunda femoris artery. Enlarged drawing of the popliteal region shows the genicular collateral network around the knee connecting the distal SFA to the infragenicular arteries.

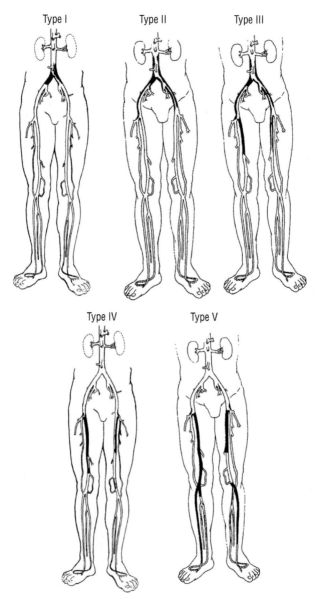

FIGURE 13.2 Patterns of arterial occlusive disease of the lower extremities. Type 1 is limited to the distal abdominal aorta and common iliac arteries. Type 2 is aortoiliac, involving the aorta, common iliacs, and also the external iliacs. Type 3 involves these areas and the femoropopliteal region. Type 4 is isolated femoropopliteal disease with preserved aortoiliac inflow and popliteal-tibial outflow. Type 5 is combined disease of the femoropopliteal and more distal tibial arteries.

hyperlipidemia. There has been an alarming increase in premature atherosclerotic aortoiliac disease in younger women (age 35 to 50) who have smoked since adolescence. These patients generally complain of proximal lower extremity claudication involving the hip and thigh muscles with progression to the calf muscles. In about 15% of such patients, however, the claudication affects only the calves. Diminished femoral pulses and femoral bruits are characteristic physical findings. Weak pedal pulses often are palpable, since the femoropopliteal system is open. Some men have the tetrad of bilateral hip and buttock claudication, impotence, leg muscle atrophy and absent femoral pulses, which is called **Leriche's syndrome.** Patients with **type 2** disease (20%) have aortoiliac atherosclerotic lesions that also involve the external iliac arteries extending to the groin. The definition of whether the patient has type 1 or 2 aortoiliac disease is made by imaging.

B. **Combined aortoiliac and femoropopliteal disease (type 3).** The majority of patients with lower extremity claudication and aortoiliac disease have combined femoropopliteal disease, which usually occurs in patients with multiple cardiovascular risk factors: smoking, hypertension, hyperlipidemia, and sometimes adult-onset diabetes mellitus. These patients usually have more incapacitating, high-grade claudication than is seen in aortoiliac or femoropopliteal disease alone or may develop more severe ischemia problems, such as rest pain, foot ulcers, or gangrene (i.e., critical ischemia).

C. **Isolated femoropopliteal disease (type 4).** Patients with isolated femoropopliteal disease generally present with calf claudication that starts after the patient walks for some time and is relieved by stopping for a few minutes. These patients are older (age 50 to 70) and have a higher prevalence of hypertension, adult-onset diabetes mellitus, and associated vascular disease of the coronary and carotid vessels than do those with aortoiliac disease. Like patients with aortoiliac disease, they frequently are cigarette smokers. They generally have good femoral pulses but no palpable popliteal or pedal pulses. Their claudication usually is improved by a supervised walking program and remains stable for long periods of time if significant proximal aortoiliac disease is not present. In fact, the following observations support initial nonoperative management: Patients over 60 years of age with superficial femoral artery occlusive disease (a) have a low likelihood of limb loss (2% to 12% in a 10-year follow-up) if followed closely on conservative treatment, (b) can expect improvement in symptoms (80%) if the initial ABI is greater than 0.6, and (c) should undergo evaluation for percutaneous treatment or reconstructive surgery if the ABI falls below 0.5. Five-year survival is 70% to 80%, and only 10% will require revascularization.

D. **Femoropopliteal-tibial disease (type 5).** These patients are at highest risk of limb loss over time. This is due to the limited long-term outcomes with revascularization treatments for disease in the tibial vessels. Furthermore, within this particular pattern of disease patients are usually older (over 65) and have a significant prevalence of diabetes mellitus, smoking, and lipid abnormalities, all of which are significant factors in disease progression. Diabetes in particular has been implicated in disease progression and is causative in infrapopliteal disease. Some within this group have classically spared aortoiliac and femoropopliteal segments with diffuse, significant tibial disease.

II. **COMMON CLINICAL SCENARIOS.** Understanding the spectrum of lower extremity ischemia and how it is classified is vital. This practical classification helps to break down and define how the limb ischemia is

Grade	Category	Clinical Description	Objective Criteria
0	0	Asymptomatic—no significant occlusive disease	Normal treadmill/stress test[a]
I	1	Mild claudication	Complete treadmill test[a]; AP after test >50 mm Hg
	2	Moderate claudication	Between categories 1 and 3
	3	Severe claudication	Cannot complete treadmill test[a]; AP after test < 50 mm Hg
		Subcritical limb ischemia No resting symptoms or tissue loss	Resting AP < 50 mm Hg, ankle or metatarsal PVR flat or barely pulsatile; TP < 40 mm Hg
		Critical limb ischemia	
II	4	Ischemic rest pain	Resting AP < 40 mm Hg, ankle or metatarsal PVR flat or barely pulsatile; TP < 30 mm Hg
III	5	Minor tissue loss— nonhealing ulcer, focal gangrene, and pedal ischemia	Resting AP < 60 mm Hg, ankle or metatarsal PVR flat or barely pulsatile; TP < 40 mm Hg
	6	Major tissue loss— extending above TM level; functional foot no longer salvageable	Same as category 5

[a]5 minutes at 2 miles per hour on a 12% incline.
AP, ankle pressure; PVR, pulse volume recording; TP, toe pressure; TM, transmetatarsal.
Adapted from Norgren L, Hiatt WR, Dormandy JA, et al. Inter-society consensus for the management of peripheral arterial disease (TASC II). *J Vasc Surg.* 2007;45(suppl S):S29A.

approached therapeutically. Chronic limb ischemia (Table 13.1) and acute limb ischemia (Table 13.2) classifications are available and reveal the spectrum of chronic disease and help define the imminent viability of the limb, respectively. **Lower limb ischemia in the great majority of cases is due to atherosclerotic disease,** but a number of other vascular diseases may also cause these symptoms (Table 13.3).

A. **Claudication** (grade I; categories 1 to 3; Table 13.1) is a reproducible, consistent pain, ache, fatigue, heaviness, numbness and/or weakness of muscle groups due to exercise-induced ischemia. Symptoms are absent at rest and abate when exercise is stopped. In general, the symptoms occur in the muscle groups one level beyond the significant disease. Thus, calf claudication alone usually indicates superficial femoral artery disease. The addition of the thigh and buttock muscles points to aortoiliac disease. Vascular claudication can usually be differentiated from other causes of leg pain, "pseudoclaudication," by careful history and examination.

	Categories of Acute Limb Ischemia						
Category	Description	Capillary Refill	Muscle Weakness	Sensory Loss	Arterial Doppler	Venous Doppler
I. Viable	Not immediately threatened	Intact	None	None	Audible	Audible
II. Threatened						
a. Marginally	Salvageable if promptly treated	Intact, slow	None	Minimal (toes) or none	Often audible	Audible
b. Immediately	Salvageable with immediate revascularization	Very slow or absent	Mild, moderate	More than toes, associated with rest pain	Usually inaudible	Audible
III. Irreversible	Major tissue loss, amputation regardless of treatment	Absent (marbling)	Profound, paralysis (rigor)	Profound, anesthetic	Inaudible	Inaudible

Adapted from Norgren L, Hiatt WR, Dormandy JA, et al. Inter-society consensus for the management of peripheral arterial disease (TASC II). *J Vasc Surg.* 2007;45(suppl S):S41A.

TABLE 3.3	Arterial Diseases Causing Claudication

Atherosclerosis (PAD)
Arteritis
Coarctation of aorta
Endofibrosis of the external iliac artery (iliac artery syndrome in cyclists)
Fibromuscular dysplasia
Peripheral emboli
Popliteal aneurysm (with secondary thromboembolism)
Adventitial cyst of the popliteal artery
Popliteal entrapment
Primary vascular tumors
Pseudoxanthoma elasticum
Remote trauma or irradiation injury
Takayasu's disease
Thromboangiitis obliterans (Buerger's disease)
Thrombosis of a persistent sciatic artery

For example, a number of elderly patients experience leg tiredness and weakness as a result of spinal stenosis. The symptoms are alleviated by bending forward and taking pressure off the spinal column, such as by leaning onto a shopping cart while walking. These patients typically have normal pedal pulses and ABIs and are best served with physical therapy and lumbar spine evaluation.

The natural history of intermittent claudication is stable in the majority of patients. Less than 5% of those with true vascular claudication will progress to amputation over many years. This being said, there are certain factors associated with advancement of PAOD to the critical point (Fig. 13.3).

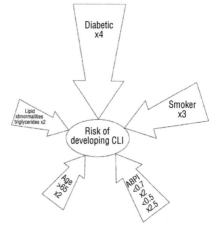

FIGURE 13.3 Influence of risk factors on the development of critical limb ischemia (CLI) in those with peripheral arterial occlusive disease (PAOD). ABPI, ankle-brachial pressure index. (From Norgren L, Hiatt WR, Dormandy JA, et al. Inter-society consensus for the management of peripheral arterial disease [TASC II]. *J Vasc Surg.* 2007;45(suppl S):S10A, with permission.)

Importantly, **intermittent claudication from atherosclerosis is a marker for systemic vascular disease,** and 10% to 15% of patients will die of associated cardiovascular morbidity within 5 years.

B. **Critical ischemia. Ischemic rest pain** in the lower extremity may be the first symptom of severe ischemia (grade II, category 4; Table 13.1). There are many causes of leg and foot pain in which arterial perfusion to the foot may be normal. These include diabetic neuropathy, arthritis, venous insufficiency, and complex regional pain syndrome. While calf pain and nocturnal leg cramps are frequent complaints to the vascular specialist, these symptoms do not indicate critical limb ischemia. Specific features suggest pain to be of ischemic origin. **Ischemic rest pain is burning and localized primarily to the forefoot below the ankle,** and the foot usually has dependent rubor and elevation pallor. Not uncommonly, patients are awoken by the pain at night and dangle their foot down for relief. Palpable pulses are absent, and Doppler signals are weak and monophasic with an ABI generally less than 0.5 (Chapter 5).

The reason ischemic rest pain is classified as limb threatening is clear. Once perfusion is so poor that rest pain develops, 95% of people will progress to limb loss within a year unless revascularization is instituted. An interesting group of patients have been identified as having "subcritical" ischemia. These patients have severe disease with no apparent symptoms, usually due to inactivity, and a resting ankle pressure less than 50 mm Hg with a toe pressure less than 40 mm Hg. Some have nonspecific symptoms in their leg with exertion, which may be attributed to the degree of their ischemia but this is usually not clear. They are at increased risk for progression to limb loss as well, but almost one-third will still have their limb at 1 year without revascularization, and with severe comorbidities medical management may be appropriate.

Ischemic rest pain usually does not occur unless the patient has at least two hemodynamically significant arterial occlusive levels of disease. Most individuals with rest pain will have one of two distinct anatomic patterns of occlusive disease that must be defined before an appropriate therapy can be selected:

1. Combined aortoiliac and superficial femoral arterial occlusive disease (type 3; Fig. 13.2)
2. Femoropopliteal arterial occlusion with distal tibial occlusive disease (type 5; Fig. 13.2)

The degree of foot ischemia depends also on the amount of collateralization that has developed.

C. **Critical ischemia. Nonhealing ulcers** of the distal foot may be the result of arterial ischemia (grade III, category 5; Table 13.1). It is also true that even with adequate arterial perfusion, ulcer healing may be prevented by infection of bone or soft tissue, pressure from improper footwear, foot malformation, or improper medical treatment. A good history and physical should provide information for sorting out the reasons for poor healing. The sensory neuropathy associated with long-term diabetes makes diabetic patients susceptible to **neuropathic foot ulcers.** Such patients may not feel the initial foot sore and therefore not present until the ulcer is deep and infected.

D. **Critical ischemia. Gangrene** is a classic sign of ischemia in the skin and subcutaneous tissue (grade III, categories 5 and 6; Table 13.1). Dry gangrene is characterized by a noninfected black eschar, whereas wet gangrene has tissue maceration and purulence.

E. **Microemboli** cause bluish, mottled spots scattered over the toes (**blue toe syndrome**), which are painful. They also may be mistaken for local traumatic bruises, and their true significance overlooked. Microemboli may originate from any point in the proximal arterial system, most commonly from the heart, aneurysms, or ulcerated plaques.

F. **Acute arterial ischemia** (Table 13.2) is characterized by the *sudden* onset of extremity pain, pallor, paresthesia, pulselessness, poikilothermia, and sometimes paralysis. If the patient has a history of claudication or previous lower extremity arterial graft, the symptoms may be caused by thrombosis of a stenotic artery, usually from acute atherosclerotic plaque rupture, or thrombosis of the arterial graft. **If the patient previously had no symptoms of peripheral vascular disease, the acute ischemia is more likely embolic.** The embolic source is usually the heart, followed distantly by more proximal atherosclerotic disease.

III. MANAGEMENT

A. **Claudication/functional ischemia.** The following principles are crucial in determining the best treatment for a patient with intermittent vascular claudication. For most patients, initial treatment is nonoperative. As mentioned, only 5% of patients with claudication will require amputation of an extremity due to progression of the disease in 5 years, most of whom continue to smoke or who have diabetes mellitus. **Lower extremity imaging can be accomplished by CTA, MRA, or duplex ultrasound. Arteriography should be viewed as an invasive intent to treat and is not necessary in the majority of patients with recent-onset vascular claudication.**

1. **Determination** of initial treatment is based on the duration, disability, and progression of the claudication. Initial management also is influenced by the patient's medical condition.

   a. **Duration.** If the leg claudication is of recent onset and is not incapacitating, a trial period of nonoperative therapy is indicated without the need for an imaging. This approach is recommended particularly for patients who are suspected of having a recent superficial femoral artery occlusion. Although they may experience sudden severe calf claudication when the artery occludes, their claudication usually improves in 6 to 8 weeks if profunda femoris arterial collaterals are well developed. In general, we prefer to follow patients with recent onset of claudication for at least 3 to 6 months to determine whether the claudication will stabilize, improve, or worsen.

   b. **Disability.** We generally ask two important questions of the patient about the disability imposed by the leg claudication: Does the leg claudication prevent normal activity, especially the performance of essential daily activities or a job? Does the claudication limit leisure activities that the patient enjoys? In our experience, the answers to these two questions are more helpful in determining patient management than is the distance the patient can walk before he or she is stopped by claudication.

   c. **Progression.** It is extremely important to determine whether the claudication is stable or progressing. Patients who have noted rapid progression of claudication over 6 months to 1 year are more likely to need arterial reconstruction than are stable claudicants. Patients with progressive claudication also are more likely to appreciate any relief that revascularization may provide.

   d. **Assessment of the patient's general medical condition** is essential for determining the proper initial management of claudication. Elective interventions for intermittent claudication should be reserved for patients who appear to have a low risk of mortality and morbidity. This assessment is discussed in detail in

Chapter 7. Patients with multiple medical problems and stable leg claudication should be followed until symptoms become incapacitating or the limb is threatened by progression to rest pain, nonhealing ulcers, or gangrene (i.e., critical limb ischemia). For example, patients with advanced chronic obstructive pulmonary disease (COPD) or heart failure are often more limited by dyspnea on exertion and their leg claudication is incidental. These patients are best managed conservatively.

2. **Nonoperative management** includes a supervised, structured walking program and smoking cessation strategy. An antiplatelet agent (e.g., 81 mg aspirin daily) and a statin are prescribed to prevent cardiovascular complications, so common in this population. Nonoperative management includes regularly scheduled follow-up assessments with noninvasive surveillance. This usually includes either ABIs or segmental pressures and PVRs. This also allows for ongoing assessment of the patient's vascular system as many people with PAOD have concomitant cerebrovascular, coronary, and aneurysmal disease.

   a. **Regular lower extremity exercise** increases metabolic adaptation to ischemia due to walking and may enhance collateral blood flow. The result is stabilization or improvement of claudication. A variety of exercise programs can alleviate claudication. A relatively simple program that has helped 80% of our patients emphasizes the following concepts:

      (1) Patients are asked to set aside a definite period and frequency for exercise in **addition** to normal daily activities (e.g., 30 minutes, 3 to 5 days per week). Exercise every day may be too much activity for many older patients; consequently, an every-other-day exercise program is ideal.

      (2) Patients are instructed to walk at a comfortable (not too fast) pace and stop for a brief rest whenever claudication becomes severe.

      (3) This walk-rest routine should be continued for 30 minutes. As the leg muscles adapt to anaerobic metabolism, the frequency and length of rest stops will decrease. After 6 to 8 weeks, most claudicants can double or triple their comfortable walking distance. In bad weather, the patient may use an indoor treadmill, walk inside a shopping mall, or use a stationary exercise bicycle.

   b. **Risk factor control.** Chapter 6 describes the important and critical cardiovascular risk factors associated with PAOD. Smoking cessation, control of hyperlipidemias, diabetes mellitus, hypertension, and weight reduction are imperative if nonoperative management is to have a maximal effect. Failure of nonoperative management in the claudicant is usually due to the inability to quit smoking and control these other factors.

   c. **Pentoxifylline** (Trental®) was the first drug approved by the U.S. Food and Drug Administration for the treatment of intermittent claudication. This rheologic agent is a methylxanthine that reduces blood viscosity by improving red blood cell membrane flexibility and inhibits platelet aggregation. Although the benefits of pentoxifylline are still debated, despite a number of clinical studies spanning decades, the medication is generally well tolerated and may play a niche role for some claudicants.

   d. **Cilostazol** (Pletal®, Otsuka Pharmaceuticals, Rockville, MD, USA) is another and more frequently used medication for intermittent claudication. It is a phosphodiesterase III inhibitor with vasodilator and antiplatelet activity. Several randomized trials have shown modest improvements in initial claudication distance and absolute claudication distance in the treated groups compared with placebo.

In our practice, pentoxifylline, 400 mg two or three times daily with meals, or cilostazol, 100 mg twice daily, have been combined with a walking program and smoking reduction for selected patients with mild to moderate claudication. If walking is improved after 6 to 8 weeks, the drug is often stopped to ascertain whether exercise and abstinence from tobacco will maintain improvement. If claudication worsens, the drug may be restarted. Common side effects of pentoxifylline are gastrointestinal upset and dizziness. For cilostazol, the most common side effects are headache and diarrhea. Cilostazol is contraindicated in those with congestive heart failure and a significant arrhythmia history. We emphasize that drug therapy with pentoxifylline or cilostazol cannot prevent the need for revascularization in patients with severe progressive claudication or critical ischemia.

3. **Indications for invasive therapy in a claudicant.** Patients must be selected carefully for percutaneous therapies or surgery for lower extremity claudication. Impairment of occupational performance and significant lifestyle limitation on a low-risk patient are reasonable indications. In this situation, it is important that a favorable anatomic situation for percutaneous or surgical reconstruction be present. The best results are obtained when the occlusive disease is localized to the aorta and iliac arteries with open distal vessels. Isolated superficial femoral artery disease with good (two or three tibial vessels continuous to the foot) runoff is also a favorable anatomic lesion for treatment. Multilevel disease can be treated in a stepwise fashion, by first addressing the inflow (most proximal level of obstruction). Patients with severe outflow disease, such as an occluded SFA or one vessel tibial runoff, may have a less favorable clinical response and lower patency rates after intervention.

The rapid advancement and use of endovascular therapies has led to readdressing the indications for intervention for claudication. In general, proponents of endovascular therapies for claudication believe that such interventions have lower associated risk to the patient and ultimately improve activity levels. In the majority of cases, endovascular therapies do not "burn bridges" for future endovascular or open surgical reconstruction. At this time, as body of evidence accumulates, we believe there is no definitive evidence that indications for intervention in claudication should be changed based solely on the availability of endovascular therapies. The remainder of this chapter emphasizes details of open surgical techniques for revascularization, as the endovascular techniques are discussed in Chapter 10.

4. **Preoperative evaluation.**
   a. The principles of assessing **operative risk** and stabilizing chronic medical problems are discussed in Chapter 7. Operative mortality for elective aortoiliac reconstruction or femoropopliteal bypass for claudication should not exceed 2% to 3%. The primary risk to life during vascular reconstructions is coronary artery disease. Significant coronary artery disease exists in at least 40% of patients with peripheral vascular disease. Mortality for endovascular therapy should be negligible as these procedures

do not require general anesthesia and tend to be shorter in duration. However, these patients may still succumb to severe cardiovascular illness, sepsis from gangrene, contrast nephropathy, or bleeding complications.

b. Before elective surgery, patients should be asked to make a commitment to **stop smoking** and to not resume tobacco use after recovery. They should be informed that the chance of graft failure approaches 30% in patients who continue to smoke regularly. Elective reconstruction for claudication in active smokers should be eschewed, but can be entertained once a significant and progressive reduction in smoking has occurred to the point of just a few cigarettes a day. Most of these individuals will quit completely after hospitalization.

c. **Lower extremity arteriography is performed only after the decision has been made to intervene with arterial reconstruction or percutaneous therapy.** In our practice, we liberally use duplex ultrasound to delineate arterial disease to aid in determining the possibility of an endovascular revascularization option prior to arteriography. CTA or MRA is particularly helpful to define (a) aortoiliac inflow disease that may make femoral access difficult and (b) patterns of disease in order to plan endovascular intervention, but can add contrast, radiation and expense, as well as delay to an evaluation. With a quality CTA, we can sometimes forego the need for invasive angiogram prior to surgical intervention, although calcified vessels obscure the true degree of stenosis and can be especially misleading in the tibial outflow vessels. Some interventionalists proceed directly to arteriography and make an on-table determination of therapeutic options. Endovascular therapy can be instituted at the same sitting as diagnostic arteriography, or delayed in a staged fashion several days to weeks later.

5. **Selection of proper procedure in aortoiliac disease.** The choice of operation or endovascular intervention for claudication depends on the general condition of the patient, the extent of the atherosclerotic process, and the experience of the surgeon/interventionalist. The preoperative arteriogram in conjunction with both resting and "stress" femoral artery pressure measurements, using techniques for distal vasodilation to unmask a stenosis, are the best determinants of which procedure to undertake in a given patient (Table 13.4). A well-trained vascular surgeon should understand the indications and limitations for the following procedures: aortoiliac endarterectomy, aortoiliac or aortofemoral bypass graft, angioplasty and stenting, and extra-anatomic reconstruction such as axillofemoral and femorofemoral bypasses.

a. **Aortoiliac endarterectomy.** In patients with occlusive disease limited to the distal aorta and common iliac arteries, **aortoiliac endarterectomy** gives excellent long-term results, provided the patient eliminates or controls his or her vascular risk factors. Endarterectomy is contraindicated in the presence of (a) aortic or iliac aneurysmal disease, (b) aortic occlusion to the level of the renal vessels, or (c) any occlusive disease in the external iliac or femoral arteries. The 5- and 10-year patency rates are 95% and 85%, respectively. However, such focal aortoiliac disease is currently treated in most patients by percutaneous balloon angioplasty and stenting with excellent results at decreased procedural risk. This has relegated endarterectomy to almost a historical setting.

TABLE 3.4	Aortofemoral Graft for Multilevel Occlusive Disease: Predictors of Success and Need for Distal Bypass

Emphasis of Evaluation	Predictors of Good AF-Only Result	Predictors of Need for Distal Bypass
Proximal disease	Absent or severely reduced femoral pulse	"Normal" femoral pulse
	Severe stenosis/occlusion (arteriogram) (positive femoral artery pressure study)[a]	Mild-moderate inflow disease (arteriogram) (negative femoral artery pressure study)
Distal disease	Good outflow tract (arteriogram)	Poor outflow tract (arteriogram)
	Index runoff resistance <0.2	Index runoff resistance ≥0.2[b]
Intraoperative	Improved pedal Doppler signals	Unimproved Doppler signals
	Normal, well-collateralized profunda	Profunda femoris artery diseased (origin ≤4 mm and no. 3 Fogarty inserted <20 cm)
Clinical	Nonadvanced ischemic symptoms (i.e., claudication, rest pain)	Advanced ischemia (necrosis/sepsis)

[a]Femoral artery pressure study. An iliac stenosis is significant when the resting pressure gradient across iliac segment is greater than 5 mm Hg or falls more than 15% after reactive hyperemia or directed injection with papaverine or nitroglycerin.
[b]Index runoff resistance = thigh-ankle pressure difference/brachial pressure.
AF, aortofemoral.
Adapted from Brewster DC, Perler BA, Robinson JG, Darling RO. Aortofemoral graft for multilevel occlusive disease: predictors of success and need for distal bypass. *Arch Surg.* 1982;117:1593-1600.

b. **Percutaneous transluminal angioplasty/stenting** is the initial interventional treatment of choice for focal arterial lesions that cause claudication (Chapter 10). While beyond the scope of this discussion, the Trans-Atlantic Inter-Society Consensus documents on the management of PAOD (TASC II [2007]) provide some anatomic framework and guidelines for revascularization (Fig. 13.4). Suffice it to say that as atherosclerotic lesions become longer, more tortuous, and completely occluded, the endovascular solutions become more difficult. Thus, a focal common iliac stenosis of less than 3 cm in length is a lesion well suited to endovascular treatment (TASC A). Endovascular recanalization of long iliac occlusions and infrarenal aortic disease, and longer severely diseased iliac lengths (TASC C and D) are also commonplace as first-line therapy, yet surgery may provide more durable long-term results. As the body of literature grows and technology advances, more complex disease is now treated endovascularly and surgery is often limited to failures of endovascular therapy.

Angioplasty results in the iliac system are enhanced by the addition of stents. Balloon-expandable stents are generally used in the common iliac where the plaque burden is usually bulky and significantly involved with calcification. The radial force of these stents is helpful in this case (Chapter 10). In the external iliac artery, self-expanding stents are generally preferred as they

TASC 2007 Classification of Aortoiliac Disease Lesions

Type A lesions
- Unilateral or bilateral stenoses of CIA
- Unilateral or bilateral single short (≤3 cm) stenosis of EIA

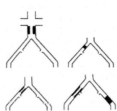

Type B lesions
- Short (≤3 cm) stenosis of infrarenal aorta
- Unilateral CIA occlusion
- Single or multiple stenosis totaling 3–10 cm involving the EIA not extending into the CFA
- Unilateral EIA occlusion not involving the origins of internal iliac or CFA

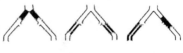

Type C lesions
- Bilateral CIA occlusions
- Bilateral EIA stenoses 3–10 cm long not extending into the CFA
- Unilateral EIA stenosis extending into the CFA
- Unilateral EIA occlusion that involves the origins of internal iliac and/or CFA
- Heavily calcified unilateral EIA occlusion with or without involvement of origins of internal iliac and/or CFA

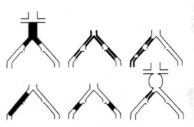

Type D lesions
- Infra-renal aortoiliac occlusion
- Diffuse disease involving the aorta and both iliac arteries requiring treatment
- Diffuse multiple stenoses involving the unilateral CIA, EIA, and CFA
- Unilateral occlusions of both CIA and EIA
- Bilateral occlusions of EIA
- Iliac stenoses in patients with AAA requiring treatment and not amenable to endograft placement or other lesions requiring open aortic or iliac surgery

FIGURE 13.4 TASC 2007 anatomic classification of aortoiliac disease lesions. Recommendations for treatment included endovascular treatment acceptable for type A, surgery superior for type D. For type B, endovascular treatment is preferred, while if a good surgical candidate, surgery is preferred for type C. The patient's comorbid condition, treatment preference after being informed, as well as the operator's experiences must be contemplated for a reasonable decision. (From Norgren L, Hiatt WR, Dormandy JA, et al. Inter-society consensus for the management of peripheral arterial disease [TASC II]. *J Vasc Surg.* 2007;45(suppl S):S49A, with permission.)

are more flexible in this variably tortuous area. Iliac stenting has a primary patency rate of 70% to 80% at 4 years. **The primary limitation of aortoiliac endovascular therapy is restenosis,** which affects 20% to 30% of patients within 3 to 5 years. Results indicate that repeated endovascular intervention may be required to achieve satisfactory, long-term relief of symptoms.

c. **Aortofemoral bypass.** A number of patients with incapacitating claudication due to diffuse, high-grade occlusive disease including the aortoiliac segments will ultimately require a **bypass graft of the aortoiliac segments** for durable relief (>5 years). Aortofemoral bypass grafts are preferred to aortoiliac bypass grafts, because not uncommonly the external iliac segment eventually becomes obliterated by progressive arteriosclerosis, albeit usually after the distal aorta and common iliac arteries. Subsequent downstream repair becomes necessary in approximately 25% to 30% of patients who are initially treated by aortoiliac bypass, compared to 10% to 15% of patients who undergo aortofemoral bypass initially. The primary patency of aortobifemoral bypass grafts is 85% to 95% at 5 years. It remains one of the most durable reconstructions in vascular surgery. In selected patients with unilateral iliac occlusive disease, unilateral aortoiliac or aortofemoral bypass grafts are occasionally performed through a retroperitoneal approach.

d. **Extra-anatomic axillofemoral or femorofemoral bypasses,** in our practice, are useful only in a very limited group of patients with severe claudication. The most suitable candidates are those with the following:

   (1) Iliac occlusion on the symptomatic lower extremity and a normal contralateral iliac artery in the case of planned femorofemoral bypass or axillary artery in the case of planned axillofemoral bypass

   (2) Previous postirradiation intestinal obstructions or fistulas that discourage intra-abdominal aortofemoral reconstruction

   (3) Known extensive postsurgical abdominal adhesions

   (4) Significant cardiopulmonary comorbidities and category 3 claudication or subcritical ischemia

   Direct aortoiliac reconstruction for claudication is preferable to extra-anatomic bypass. As such, if the patient is a candidate for direct reconstruction but has intra-abdominal contraindications, a retroperitoneal aortofemoral bypass or thoracofemoral bypass are also excellent options. When done by experienced hands, aortofemoral reconstruction is safe and, as stated, provides a very durable result in 85% to 95% of patients at 5 years. In contrast, 5-year patency for femorofemoral bypass and axillofemoral bypass for claudication ranges from 50% to 75%.

e. **Elective aortoiliac reconstruction** for occlusive disease is generally **not combined** with other nonvascular, intra-abdominal operations. For example, we favor leaving asymptomatic gallstones alone. Although the morbidity of adding cholecystectomy may be low, additional procedures do increase the risk of complications. Also, postoperative cholecystitis secondary to cholelithiasis is rare in our experience. Most postoperative cholecystitis is acalculous and occurs in patients who have been in shock and have the so-called splanchnic shock syndrome. Occasionally, however, we discover incidentally a gallbladder with cholelithiasis *and* chronic smoldering cholecystitis during operative exploration. If the aortic reconstruction goes well, we may perform cholecystectomy *after* the retroperitoneum and femoral wounds have been closed to cover the prosthetic graft.

f. **Prior to hospital admission,** complete history, physical examination, and routine diagnostic studies are performed. Baseline studies include a complete blood count, chest x-ray, 12-lead electrocardiogram (ECG), serum electrolytes, creatinine, blood sugar, liver function tests (bilirubin, aspartate aminotransferase, alkaline phosphatase, total protein, albumin), platelet count, prothrombin time (PT), partial thromboplastin time (PTT), fasting serum cholesterol and triglycerides, calcium, phosphorus, and pulmonary function tests in patients with chronic lung disease. Any cardiac testing and preoperative consultations with other specialists are arranged before admission.

(1) The patient is typed and cross-matched for 2 to 4 units of packed red blood cells for aortic operations and typed, screened, and held for femoropopliteal and extra-anatomic reconstructions. If autotransfusion is planned, arrangements are made for its availability.

(2) Generally, bowel preparation is not advised for aortic surgery. Patients are instructed to eat lightly and drink plenty of fluids to maintain hydration the day prior to surgery.

(3) An intravenous infusion of Ringer's lactated solution at 100 to 125 mL/h is started before surgery, and the night before for hospitalized patients. Elective arterial patients may have chronic intravascular volume depletion from diuretics and may have had recent contrast exposure. Adequate hydration helps to avoid intraoperative hypotension and acute kidney injury.

(4) Skin preparation includes shaving hair in the operative field as close as possible to the time of operation to minimize bacterial colonization of the shaved areas. Patients are asked to shower the night before with a chlorhexidine-based solution (Hibiclens®, Mölnlycke Health Care, Norcross, GA).

(5) Patients are instructed in deep breathing and coughing, as well as in the use of an incentive spirometer. We also teach the patient leg exercises that are used as prophylaxis against deep venous thrombosis, for stimulation of lower extremity blood flow, and for maintenance of leg muscle tone prior to ambulation.

(6) Preoperative prophylactic antibiotics are administered intravenously when the patient is called to the operating room. Generally, a first generation cephalosporin (2 g cefazolin IV) is administered and redosed if the operation is longer than 4 hours. For patients with a history of cephalosporin or severe penicillin allergy, or MRSA colonization, the patient receives IV vancomycin instead.

g. **Operative principles of aortofemoral bypass.** The complete details of operative technique are beyond the scope of this handbook. Other operative atlases describe specific techniques for arterial reconstruction in a more detailed manner. Yet, certain principles of intraoperative care do warrant emphasis here.

(1) **Patient positioning.** For a standard transperitoneal approach, the patient is kept in the supine position with the electrocautery ground beneath the buttocks. The arms generally are adducted to the sides. Ischemic heels are elevated or wrapped with a soft dressing to prevent pressure sores. For a retroperitoneal approach, the patient is rotated facing slightly right on a beanbag. The table is retroflexed at the waist level and the hips rotated back towards the left ("corkscrew" position), while the knees are flexed and supported on pillows and both arms outstretched towards the right.

(2) **Skin preparation.** The operating room should be warmed (70°F to 75°F) during the skin preparation to reduce heat loss from the patient. The skin preparation extends from the nipples to the knees for aortofemoral reconstructions and to the toes

for patients who may require an associated femoropopliteal bypass. The operative field is prepped with a chlorhexidine solution, which is superior to iodine-based scrubs to reduce risk of surgical site infection. After application of the antiseptic preparatory solution, the skin is covered with a plastic Ioban™ (3M Health Care, St. Paul, MN, USA). Although Ioban™ may not reduce the incidence of wound infection, we recommend their use to prevent contact of graft materials with the skin, which may contaminate the graft.

(3) **Systemic anticoagulation.** Heparin is used for systemic anticoagulation while the aorta and distal arteries are clamped to prevent thrombus formation. A sufficient regimen is 5,000 U or 70 U/kg bolus intravenous heparin 5 minutes prior to aortic clamping and an additional 1,000 U every 45 to 60 minutes afterwards while vessels are clamped. Although monitoring of heparin effect may not be necessary, we prefer to check an activated clotting time (ACT) before and after heparinization. An ACT of 200 to 300 seconds is adequate for most cases. Smaller additional doses of heparin (500 to 1,000 units) are given during regional irrigation of the iliac and major femoral artery branches. Reversal of heparin is optional at the termination of the procedure. In general, heparinization with the above doses does not require reversal, since the heparin effect diminishes in about 90 minutes. However, if one chooses to reverse heparinization, ACTs are the primary method used to monitor reversal with protamine sulfate (0.5 to 1.0 mg for every 100 U of heparin remaining).

(4) **Intraoperative diuretics.** Prior to aortic clamping, urine output should be maintained at 0.5 to 1.0 cc/kg/h. Even infrarenal aortic clamping diminishes renal cortical blood flow, which can be prevented in part by intravascular volume expansion with isotonic intravenous fluid. Some surgeons administer 12.5 to 25 g of the osmotic diuretic mannitol intravenously, just before clamping the aorta. In addition to improving renal perfusion, mannitol has antioxidant properties that protect the kidney from reperfusion injury and free radicals. Less frequently, furosemide, low-dose dopamine, or fenoldopam are employed as pharmacologic adjuncts to reduce renal injury.

(5) **Proximal aortic anastomosis.** Controversy exists over whether the proximal aortic graft anastomosis should be end to end or end to side (Fig. 13.5). Our experience strongly favors end-to-end aortic anastomosis. Its primary advantages are as follows:

(a) The origin of the graft is from a higher and less diseased part of the infrarenal abdominal aorta.

(b) A better hemodynamic situation, as the aortic blood flow is direct through the graft without competitive flow from the distal aorta.

(c) A more anatomic position and better retroperitoneal coverage as a segment of infrarenal aorta is resected prior to placement of the graft. The onlay or end-to-side aortic anastomosis leaves the graft protruding anteriorly. For this reason, the end-to-side graft seems more likely to adhere to adjacent bowel and cause aortoenteric fistula.

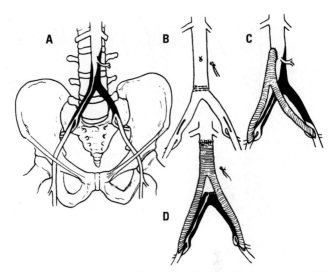

FIGURE 13.5 Types of open aortoiliac reconstruction. Aortoiliac endarterectomy **(B)** is an option for occlusive disease localized to the distal abdominal aorta and common iliac arteries. It has mostly been replaced by endovascular therapies for this focal pattern **(A)**. For aortofemoral grafting, the proximal anastomosis may be performed end to side **(C)** or end to end **(D)**. (Adapted from Darling RC, et al. Aorto-iliac reconstruction. *Surg Clin North Am.* 1979;59:565-579.)

(d) Exclusion of the diseased infrarenal and iliac segments is achieved, and this may reduce the possibility of later atheroembolization.

Situations where an end-to-side is preferable relate to renal and gut perfusion and are as follows:

- When there are accessory renal arteries supplying significant parenchyma from the infrarenal aorta.
- A large inferior mesenteric artery (IMA) is present and antegrade flow in the IMA is desired for adequate colon perfusion.
- When significant disease is mainly located in the external iliac arteries. In this situation, antegrade pelvic blood flow to the hypogastric arteries is best preserved to avoid pelvic ischemia.

(6) **Distal anastomosis** in aortofemoral bypass has a significant influence on graft patency. The leading cause of late aortofemoral graft failure is loss of outflow and this can be minimized if the correct distal configuration is chosen. There are five methods of distal anastomosis (Fig. 13.6).

Type 1 anastomosis to the common femoral artery is preferred for patients with widely patent profunda femoris and superficial femoral arteries.

Type 2 anastomosis carries the graft onto the proximal superficial femoral artery and is recommended when the orifice of the superficial femoral artery is stenotic but the distal arteries and profunda femoris artery are otherwise normal.

Type 3 anastomosis (known as profundaplasty) carries the graft onto the profunda femoris artery and is recommended for

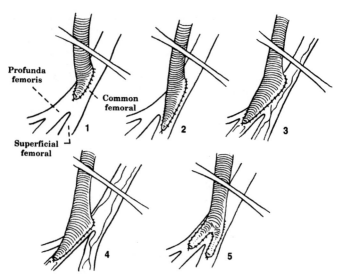

FIGURE 13.6 Types of femoral anastomosis for aortofemoral bypass grafts: (*1*) type 1 anastomosis to the common femoral artery; (*2*) type 2 anastomosis, in which the graft is carried onto the proximal superficial femoral artery; (*3*) type 3 anastomosis, in which the graft is carried onto the profunda femoris artery; (*4*) type 4 anastomosis, involving only the profunda femoris artery; (*5*) type 5 anastomosis, involving a patch angioplasty of both the superficial and deep femoral arterial orifices. (Adapted from Darling RC, et al. Aortoiliac reconstruction. *Surg Clin North Am.* 1979;59:565-579.)

patients with extensive superficial femoral artery disease or occlusion. In most patients, the profunda femoris artery is of adequate diameter (3 to 4 mm) and length (15 to 20 cm) to maintain aortofemoral graft flow and perfuse the leg via collaterals.

Type 4 anastomosis is done only to the profunda femoris artery. It is necessary when the common femoral and superficial femoral arteries are extensively obliterated.

Type 5 anastomosis splits the hood of the graft to patch proximal stenoses of both the superficial femoral and the profunda femoris arteries.

The need for concomitant distal bypass in conjunction with aortofemoral bypass occurs in some 17% to 20% of cases, but these are in the scenario of limb-threatening ischemia and will be discussed subsequently.

(7) **Revascularization of the inferior mesenteric artery (IMA),** by either bypass or reimplantation, should be performed when a large (>3.5 to 4.0 mm) IMA is present. Also, if the IMA is patent but shows poor back bleeding at the time of aortic reconstruction, or an IMA pressure is transduced at ≤40 mm Hg, strong consideration to IMA reimplantation should be given, because this indicates poor collateralization from the superior mesenteric artery (Chapter 16; Figs. 16.1 to 16.3).

(8) After completing the femoral anastomoses, **Doppler signals** are auscultated in the groins with a sterile probe. Also, the feet

are examined for expected flow in the pedal vessels. Absence of Doppler signals should prompt investigation of the bypass for evidence of thrombosis or kinking, distal emboli down the leg, or technical issues at an anastomosis. Intraoperative angiography may be necessary if the reason for poor flow cannot be elucidated. **As a general rule, the patient should not leave the operating room with absent Doppler signals in the foot.**

6. **Femoropopliteal bypass** for stable claudication is being performed less frequently now than it was in the past. Long-term follow-up of patients with leg claudication from a solitary superficial femoral artery occlusion indicates that nonoperative treatment often stabilizes the problem. In addition, progression of proximal aortoiliac disease may lead to poor inflow to a femoropopliteal bypass and eventual hemodynamic graft failure, often within 5 years. Therefore, patients who undergo femoropopliteal bypass for claudication alone should have a good anatomic situation, which includes normal aortoiliac inflow, a patent popliteal artery above the knee with two- or three-vessel runoff, and good quality saphenous vein. All evidence continues to suggest autogenous saphenous vein remains superior to all other graft materials for durability of a femoropopliteal bypass. However, use of Dacron or ePTFE prosthetic for above-knee femoropopliteal bypass for claudication remains accepted. Endovascular therapies are also reducing the number of femoropopliteal bypasses performed. Hybrid procedures may be used to treat both the aortoiliac inflow with endovascular techniques such as iliac angioplasty and stenting with concomitant femoropopliteal bypass grafting. Alternatively, iliac disease may be treated by endovascular means in one setting, with staged femoropopliteal endovascular intervention or surgical bypass. **Due to reduced durability compared to above-knee reconstructions, below-the-knee femoropopliteal or femorotibial bypasses should be limb salvage procedures, and rarely should they be used to treat claudication alone.**

7. **Femoropopliteal percutaneous endovascular intervention** for functional lower limb ischemia is now commonplace. Purported benefits of endovascular SFA intervention include decreased morbidity and mortality, no incisions, no need for and preservation of autogenous conduit, decreased hospital stay and resource utilization, and, finally, less social and family stress. Further, evidence suggests that there is a limited downside to endovascular therapy in that recurrent endovascular intervention is possible and surgical options and distal targets are not compromised.

Similar to aortoiliac disease, information from the TASC II (2007) documents has delineated the treatment opinions (endovascular vs open) based on anatomic classification of femoropopliteal disease (Fig. 13.7). Endovascular therapy appears appropriate for more focal, simple (TASC A) lesions. The more lengthy, calcified, and recurrent a stenosis or occlusion (TASC D) is, the less amenable it is to endovascular therapy.

Some debate has centered on superiority of primary stenting in the SFA. With the advent of nitinol alloy stent engineering, it appears now that when using these self-expanding stents, restenosis, objective ankle pressure improvements, and clinical success are superior to angioplasty alone at 1 year. Even using nitinol stents, primary patency of SFA interventions is roughly 50% to 60% at 3 years. Assisted primary patency has been shown to be improved compared to this, and

TASC 2007 Classification of Femoropopliteal Disease Lesions

Type A lesions

• Single stenosis ≤10 cm in length
• Single occlusion ≤5 cm in length

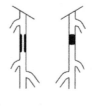

Type B lesions

• Multiple lesions (stenoses or occlusions),
  each ≤5 cm
• Single stenosis or occlusion ≤15 cm not
  involving the infrageniculate popliteal artery
• Single or multiple lesions in the absence of
  continuous tibial vessels to improve inflow
  for a distal bypass
• Heavily calcified occlusion ≤5 cm in length
• Single popliteal stenosis

Type C lesions

• Multiple stenoses or occlusions totaling
  >15 cm with or without heavy calcification
• Recurrent stenoses or occlusions that need
  treatment after two endovascular
  interventions

Type D lesions

• Chronic total occlusions of CFA or SFA
  (>20 cm, involving the popliteal artery)
• Chronic total occlusion of popliteal artery
  and proximal trifurcation vessels

FIGURE 13.7 TASC 2007 anatomic classification of femoropopliteal lesions. Recommendations for treatment include endovascular results acceptable for type A, surgery superior for type D. For type B, endovascular treatment is preferred, while if a good surgical candidate, surgery is preferred for type C. The patient's comorbid condition, treatment preference after being informed, as well as the operator's experiences must be contemplated for a reasonable decision. (From Norgren L, Hiatt WR, Dormandy JA, et al. Inter-society consensus for the management of peripheral arterial disease [TASC II]. *J Vasc Surg.* 2007;45(suppl S):S51A, with permission.)

the overwhelming majority of recurrent procedures necessary are also endovascular. Therefore, some feel that this type of therapy is comparable to prosthetic femoropopliteal bypass overall. Moreover, the impact and indications for directional atherectomy, laser atherectomy, ePTFE covered stents, drug-eluting stents, drug-coated balloons, reentry devices, and embolic protection devices in the SFA are still under investigation. Antiproliferative drugs such as paclitaxel, when applied to a balloon or stent, have promising results in the prevention of restenosis within the couple years after intervention.

B. Critical/limb-threatening ischemia.

1. **Prompt recognition** of the signs of critical limb ischemia and timely initiation of therapy are necessary if the limb is to be saved. The initial patient evaluation, therefore, must determine whether the patient needs emergent treatment or a less emergent diagnostic workup. This determination is based primarily on the patient history and physical examination supplemented by the results of noninvasive vascular tests and radiologic studies. In general, decompensation of long-standing ischemia due to atherosclerosis is less emergent than acute ischemia, due to significant collateral development in the former.

   A number of diagnostic tests are available to quickly determine the best treatment plan for the threatened limb. Tests should be selected to provide the maximum amount of information with the minimum amount of discomfort and delay for the patient, who often is experiencing considerable pain.

   a. **Noninvasive vascular testing.** Continuous wave Doppler, ABIs and PVRs are simple yet accurate methods to determine criteria for ischemic rest pain and the likelihood of healing (see Chapter 5). Ischemic rest pain generally is associated with a Doppler ankle pressure below 35 mm Hg in nondiabetics (ABI of 0.3 to 0.4) and below 55 mm Hg in diabetics. Ischemic rest pain is unlikely when ankle pressures exceed 55 mm Hg in the nondiabetic and 80 mm Hg in the diabetic. Foot ulcers that are not infected and not associated with osteomyelitis have a favorable chance of healing if the ankle pressure is above 65 mm Hg in the nondiabetic and above 90 mm Hg in the diabetic. Ankle and forefoot PVRs that are less than 5 mm or flat, predict ischemic rest pain and poor tissue healing. Toe pressures of less than 20 to 30 mm Hg are also associated with advanced ischemia. A minimal TP suggesting adequacy for healing is 40 mm Hg. Resting supine transcutaneous oxygen (Tco_2) measurements of less than 20 to 30 torr are indicative of severe ischemia, especially if forefoot Tco_2 levels fall to less than 10 torr with leg elevation.

   b. **Plain radiograph** of the bone underlying an ulcer may show signs of osteomyelitis, including bone rarefaction, periosteal elevation, and new bone formation. A bone scan or MRI is indicated when osteomyelitis seems likely but a plain radiograph is negative. Bone changes may not be apparent until osteomyelitis has been active for 2 to 3 weeks.

   c. **Cultures** and **Gram stains** can be obtained of purulent wounds to identify residing organisms, and histologic stains also may reveal fungi. Routine cultures of open foot wounds and ulcers are not advised, as colonization is ubiquitous.

   d. An **ECG** is essential when arterial embolism is suspected, as atrial fibrillation is a common underlying condition. For cases in which intermittent arrhythmia is suspected, a continuous ECG monitor (Holter) may be used.

   e. An **echocardiogram** should be done as part of the diagnostic workup for arterial embolism that may originate from the heart. The echocardiogram may reveal a diseased valve or mural thrombus. Transesophogeal echocardiography (TEE) is more sensitive than transthoracic echo and is indicated if cardioembolism is highly suspected.

   f. **Duplex ultrasound** of the aortoiliac segment also should be performed in the evaluation of thromboemboli, since emboli may be shed from a thrombus in an abdominal aortic aneurysm or significant occlusive disease can be identified. A **CTA** of the abdomen with lower extremity runoff will also reveal this pathology, in addition to the location and extent of the thromboembolus, but requires contrast dye, radiation, and cost that ultrasound does not. If a femoral or popliteal aneurysm is suspected as a result of physical examination, ultrasound is an accurate method to confirm peripheral aneurysms that also may act as the source of emboli or acute thrombosis. A CT scan of the thoracic aorta may also be necessary, as this segment can be diseased and lead to embolism.

g. **Arteriography** remains the definitive method to delineate the exact level of arterial occlusion and to define vascular anatomy before selecting a proper intervention (i.e., thrombolysis, other percutaneous therapies, or surgical revascularization). Contrast angiography with digital subtraction techniques can generally visualize distal tibial or plantar arch vessels. In the operating room, a sterile Doppler probe can be used to localize a tibial or pedal artery before surgical incision. Although the presence of a patent pedal arch on arteriography was once considered predictive of success for femorodistal bypass, additional studies have reported reasonable patency rates and limb salvage in patients in whom the pedal arch appears absent or diseased.

h. Studies for hypercoagulability (Chapter 19) should be analyzed in patients who present with atypical arterial thrombosis. This group includes young adults (age 20 to 40 years) with arterial occlusive disease and other individuals with recurrent arterial thromboembolism.

2. **Management** may begin after it has been determined **whether the patient has acute or decompensated chronic limb ischemia**. In our experience, the following principles provide the best chance of limb salvage. The general dictum of treatment is that **acute ischemia** of class IIb requires an immediate trip to the angiography suite or operating room for evaluation and treatment. Class III ischemia should usually be treated with primary amputation as the chance of recovering a functional limb is nil. With lesser degrees of ischemia, individualization of diagnosis and treatment is recommended.

a. **Acute limb ischemia** is usually caused by a thromboembolus, popliteal aneurysm thrombosis, or a sudden arterial or bypass graft occlusion. Thrombosis of a chronic arterial stenosis may cause temporary pain, pallor, and paresthesia, but usually it does not progress to paralysis. In this situation, the acute symptoms often resolve because of previously developed collateral vessels.

(1) **Immediate treatment** should include systemic heparinization (5,000 to 10,000 units IV, then 1,000 units/h adjusted to maintain the APTT to twice baseline, usually 60 to 90 seconds) to prevent further propagation of thrombus. If leg pain is severe, a narcotic may be administered while further tests are arranged.

(2) **Initial diagnostic tests** should include routine blood counts, electrolytes, glucose, and baseline coagulation studies (PT, PTT, and platelet count). An ECG should be done to check for atrial fibrillation and any sign of acute myocardial infarction.

Continuous wave Doppler may be used to localize the level of obstruction and record ankle pressures. Absence of arterial signals at the ankle almost always means that urgent surgical intervention will be necessary (class IIb or III ischemia; Table 13.2). If the ankle has monophasic Doppler signals and the foot has sensation and movement (class I or IIa), 2 to 3 hours may be allowed for workup, initial therapy and heparinization, and observation. If the leg does not improve during this time, urgent surgical intervention will generally be necessary.

(3) **An emergency arteriogram or CTA** usually is performed to determine the location of the arterial occlusion as well as the inflow and outflow on either side. Arteriography can be performed in a radiographic suite or the operating room. However, arterial exploration in the operating room can be undertaken immediately if the acute occlusion is clearly an embolus. Intraoperative arteriograms can be performed if necessary. Time is important in acute arterial occlusion, as irreversible nerve and muscle damage may occur within 6 hours.

(4) **The choice of procedure** for an acute arterial occlusion will depend on the underlying etiology. **Thromboembolectomy** with Fogarty balloon catheters is the operation of choice for thromboemboli. Thrombectomy of the femoral or iliac arteries can be accomplished through a femoral arteriotomy, often with local anesthetic and minimal sedation in frail, elderly patients. A popliteal embolus should generally be extracted through a popliteal arteriotomy, so that each tibial artery may be checked for clot. Passing a catheter from the groin will not clean out all of the tibial arteries. Extracted thromboemboli should be sent for pathologic examination, as occasionally arterial tumor embolism will be the first manifestation of an atrial myxoma or other vascular tumor. After embolectomy, the patient should be continued on heparin, followed by long-term oral anticoagulant such as warfarin or a Factor Xa inhibitor.

Bypass grafting of an arteriosclerotic occlusion of the iliac or superficial femoral artery may occasionally be necessary to salvage the acutely ischemic leg. In another example, a few seriously ill cardiac patients who are dependent on a transfemoral intra-aortic balloon assist device will develop limb-threatening ischemia. An emergency femorofemoral bypass may be necessary if the balloon must remain in place for cardiac support. Another difficult situation to deal with is acute popliteal aneurysm occlusion. Classically, operative bypass has led to 40% to 50% limb loss in these patients. The addition of preoperative thrombolytic therapy both to open the distal outflow and to allow a better distal target evaluation has reduced this to about 10% to 20%.

If the acute arterial ischemia is caused by a bypass graft occlusion, **catheter-based thrombolytic therapy can be effective** using pulse spray with subsequent drip therapy (e.g., 0.5 to 1 mg/kg tPA) for 12 to 24 hours via a percutaneous thrombolytic catheter or in combination with mechanical thrombectomy devices (Chapter 10). Some degree of systemic heparinization either intravenously or via the arterial sheath should accompany this process. Following successful thrombolysis, an arteriogram may reveal the cause of the occlusion (e.g., distal anastomotic stenosis, proximal inflow disease, or graft pathology or kinking). Once the cause is identified, it can be treated with either endovascular means (e.g., angioplasty/stent) or surgery (e.g., jump graft to patent distal vessel).

This same approach can also be used for treatment of acute native arterial occlusions, such as that mentioned above for popliteal aneurysm thrombosis. Data evaluating the use of thrombolysis in arterial occlusions are mixed and confusing, but with lower grade acute ischemia and significant thrombus burden, thrombolysis may be beneficial. Possible benefits include the opening and improvement of outflow, identification of a focal culprit lesion amenable to a less-invasive endovascular procedure, or influencing the level of distal anastomosis required with surgical bypass and thus affecting durability of the reconstruction. The trade-off is a higher likelihood of bleeding complications. Not uncommonly, the limb appears to clinically deteriorate temporarily with drip thrombolytic therapy as thrombus becomes unstable, and particles embolize. This usually improves with continued lysis, but close observation is required.

b. **Chronic critical limb ischemia** is usually associated with combined arteriosclerotic occlusive disease of the aortoiliac region, femoropopliteal segment, and/or distal tibial arteries.

(1) **Foot protection** from further injury is the first order of care. The heel should be protected from pressure sores by a soft gauze pad secured with a gauze roll, **not** tape. The heels themselves should either be elevated off of the bed surface or placed in egg crates or commercially made vascular "boots" (e.g., Rooke® boot, Osborn Medical, Centennial, CO). Lambswool or gauze should be placed between the toes to prevent "kissing" ulcers caused by toes and toenails rubbing against one another. A lanolin-based lotion should be applied daily to the foot to keep the skin soft and prevent cracking, especially over the heel. If pressure bothers the foot, bed sheets may be draped over a footboard (Fig. 13.8). Elevating the head of the bed 6 inches may relieve ischemic pain by the effect of gravity on arterial perfusion. We do not recommend so-called metal bed cradles or tents, as a patient may inadvertently abrade the lower leg or foot against the metal frame, causing skin ulceration.

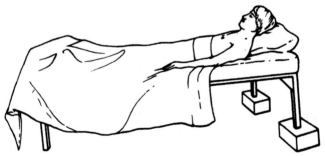

FIGURE 13.8 Bed position for patients with ischemic rest pain of the lower extremity. The head of the bed is elevated 6 inches to improve arterial perfusion of the pedal circulation by gravity. Sheets are draped over a footboard to alleviate pressure on the feet and either lambswool or gauze placed between the toes and egg-crate or Rooke boots used to protect the heels.

(2) **Local infection** should be controlled before insertion of synthetic bypass grafts. Local debridement and drainage of infected foot/toe tissue and parenteral antibiotics should precede graft procedures by several days. Otherwise, graft infection may occur in the groin, where lymphatics may be laden with bacteria. Deep foot space infection is a particular problem in the diabetic population. If sepsis is present, urgent amputation is indicated. If the patient is not toxic, drainage/debridement may be attempted. Large heel ulcers or significant areas of tissue loss may ultimately lead to amputation, regardless of blood flow.

(3) **Arteriography and other imaging** were discussed earlier.

(4) The **choice of operation or percutaneous procedure** depends on the location of the occlusive disease and the condition of the patient.

   (a) **Combined severe aortoiliac and femoropopliteal occlusive disease** should be treated by inflow correction of the aortoiliac disease as described above. For those with rest pain, aortoiliac inflow correction may be all that is needed. Long-term limb salvage will be accomplished in most patients with multilevel occlusive disease by aortofemoral bypass or aortoiliac endovascular intervention alone (i.e., treatment of inflow disease).

      When significant femoropopliteal disease is also present, determining which patients will need simultaneous femoropopliteal revascularization is not easy. Preoperative factors that suggest a combined procedure is indicated are extensive below-the-knee femoropopliteal-tibial occlusions combined with tissue loss and an ankle pressure below 30 mm Hg. Modest inflow disease suggest that correction of inflow alone will not suffice for tissue healing. Also, a poorly formed profunda may not supply adequate flow to the lower leg in the presence of significant SFA disease. If the profunda orifice accepts a 4-mm probe and a no. 3 Fogarty balloon can be advanced at least 20 cm, the profunda is adequately developed. In high-risk patients, extra-anatomic axillofemoral or femorofemoral bypass may be used as an inflow procedure when endovascular solutions are not feasible.

   (b) **Occlusive disease of the common femoral artery, profunda orifice, and superficial femoral artery** orifice may be managed by endarterectomy, profundaplasty, or iliofemoral bypass bifurcation reconstruction. Profundaplasty is most likely to succeed when (a) aortoiliac inflow is normal, (b) the distal profunda femoris artery is normal and has developed collateral pathways to the popliteal artery, and (c) the popliteal artery is patent with at least two- or three-vessel runoff. The profunda-popliteal collateral index and the low thigh to ankle gradient pressure index have been described to assist with this decision; however, this anatomic situation is very rare, so we seldom use profundaplasty as the sole operation for limb salvage. Indeed, patients with this disease pattern usually require a bypass to a distal target potentially in conjunction with some type of common femoral or profunda femoris revascularization. Currently, endovascular therapies in the common femoral and femoral bifurcation are not as effective or durable as in other anatomic sites.

(c) **Femoropopliteal artery occlusion** can be managed by bypass grafting or percutaneous treatments. When performing femoropopliteal bypass for limb salvage, we prefer greater saphenous vein (GSV) for conduit, which is superior to synthetic bypass. Greater saphenous vein above-knee femoropopliteal bypasses have an 80% primary patency over 5 years. Below the knee, this is roughly 70%. Should adequate GSV be unavailable, we use prosthetic conduit. Others espouse arm vein and spliced vein segments as femoropopliteal bypass constructs. Each of these has benefits and disadvantages. Another option is cryopreserved allogenic vein graft, but results using cryopreserved vein have been disappointing and it is expensive. They are seldom used except in cases with high infection risk and no autologous vein.

Current synthetic choices for femoropopliteal bypass are Dacron and polytetrafluoroethylene (PTFE) and heparin-bonded PTFE. In the above-knee position, ePTFE primary and secondary patency is 55% to 65% and 60% to 70% at 5 years, respectively. These grafts provide excellent long-term patency when the distal anastomosis is above the knee, but poorer patency is observed in below-the-knee bypasses. In a prospective randomized comparison of autologous saphenous vein to expanded PTFE grafts, primary patency of vein was clearly superior to PTFE for infrapopliteal bypass (49% vs 12% at 4 years). However, there was no significant difference in limb salvage (vein vs PTFE, 57% vs 61%). **In summary, bypass patency decreases with anastomoses below the knee and with use of prosthetic grafts. Overall limb salvage rates exceed bypass patency rates, probably because the foot wounds heal in the interim while perfusion is good.**

As described above, percutaneous SFA interventions such as transluminal angioplasty and stenting are now performed routinely with comparable early and mid-term results to surgical bypass. The effectiveness of percutaneous treatments depends on a number of variables, including the extent and location of disease, degree of calcification, presence of diabetes, and smoking status.

(d) The most challenging group of patients who require operation for limb salvage have **severe type V disease of the femoropopliteal and tibial levels.** Acceptable long-term patency (50% to 60% at 5 years) and excellent limb salvage rates (50% to 73% at 5 years) may be achieved by femorotibial, femoroperoneal, and pedal bypass grafts using GSV. Multi-segment femorodistal occlusive disease also has been successfully treated by sequential anastomoses of a vein graft to several patent segments. Adequate GSV is generally believed to be at least 3.5 mm in diameter when distended and without sclerotic segments or stenoses. **Patency of femoral-infrapopliteal vein bypasses is comparable for each tibial artery and is similar in diabetics and nondiabetics.** Standard choices for lower extremity bypass with vein are: reversed, non-reversed in situ, or non-reversed, translocated vein graft. The technique of reversed saphenous vein grafting involves the harvest of the vein from its subcutaneous bed, and it is reversed in flow direction for the bypass, such that the valves do not obstruct the flow of pulsatile blood.

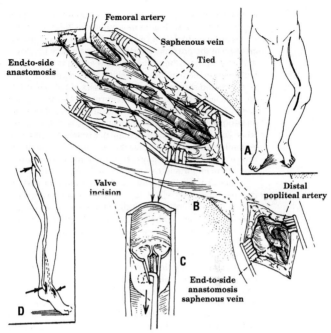

FIGURE 13.9 Technique of in situ saphenous femoropopliteal and tibial bypass grafting. **(A)** Greater saphenous vein may be exposed through one or two long incisions along the medial aspect of the thigh and calf. **(B)** Saphenous vein is left in its natural bed. Its valves are cut with special instruments "valvulotomes." **(C)** Its branches are tied to prevent arteriovenous fistulas. Proximal anastomosis is made to the common femoral or superficial femoral artery, and distal anastomosis is constructed to the distal popliteal artery or to the tibial or peroneal branches. **(D)** Long bypasses to the level of the ankle are possible by this technique. Incisions may also be limited to the groin and the level of distal anastomosis with side branches and vein defects identified with angioscopy, arteriography, duplex ultrasound, and continuous wave Doppler. Side branches may then be ligated with small incisions or embolized via a distal side branch.

Several factors have rejuvenated enthusiasm for in situ **saphenous vein bypass grafting** after its original description in 1962 (Fig. 13.9). Proponents claim a higher use of smaller veins, a lesser degree of endothelial damage, better size match at the anastomoses, and improved hemodynamics. However, similar early and late patency rates for in situ versus reversed infrapopliteal bypasses (1-year, 87% to 90%; 3-year, 82% to 85%; and 5-year, 77% to 85%) have been shown in several studies. During in situ bypass, the saphenous vein is left in its native bed in the subcutaneous tissue and the valves are lysed with a valvulotome. Identification of venous defects as well as ligation of large side branches to prevent problematic arteriovenous fistulas is required. Several techniques to accomplish these are described.

Another good option for distal vein bypasses with targets at or below the trifurcation is nonreversed, translocated GSV. After harvest from its native bed, the vein is distended and valvulotomes passed, similar to the technique for in situ bypass. However, with a nonreversed, translocated graft the vein is distended either by vein solution or with blood flow after creation of the proximal anastomosis, but before placing the graft in the tunnel. Pulsatile blood flow assists in finding problem areas on the vein that need side branch ligation, repair, or resection and splicing. Usually two passes of the valvulotome are sufficient. The benefit of a nonreversed, translocated vein is for graft-artery size match at both the proximal and distal anastomoses, when a subcutaneous graft is not desired, or when anatomic or lateral subcutaneous tunneling is preferred. Regardless of the vein construct used, careful preparation of the vein and the meticulous technique of anastomosis are likely more important than position of the vein graft.

Because a vein remains the best conduit for early and late patency, extra effort to obtain a suitable vein seems justified. These options include the contralateral leg vein, arm veins, lesser saphenous veins, spliced vein-segment grafts, and shorter bypasses using less vein (e.g., SFA-tibial, popliteal-tibial, or tibiotibial bypasses).

Techniques of vein adjunct at the distal anastomosis when using prosthetic below the knee include **Taylor patch, Linton patch, Miller cuff, and St. Mary's boot** (Fig. 13.10). These emphasize a long arteriotomy and placement of a cuff of vein using one of these techniques between the prosthetic and the target arteriotomy. These are known to improve results of prosthetic-distal bypass by improving the compliance mismatch at the anastomosis. Although all of these conduit alternatives are generally not viewed as the first option, they represent reasonable choices when GSV is not available. But remember, tibial level revascularization using alternative autogenous reconstructions provides better long-term results than those based on prosthetic. Reports detail patencies of 50% to 60% at 4 years versus 30% to 40%, respectively.

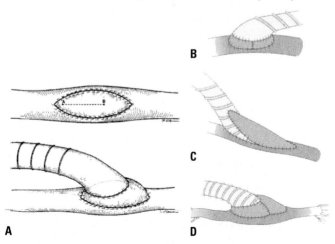

FIGURE 13.10 Types of vein adjuncts at the distal anastomosis of infrageniculate prosthetic bypass grafts. **(A)** Linton patch, **(B)** Miller cuff, **(C)** Taylor patch, **(D)** St. Mary's boot. These adjuncts help to alter shear stresses at the distal anastomosis and improve patency.

Conduit selection is seldom this concrete, and the entire clinical picture, goal of revascularization, and status of the patient must be considered. Likewise, the proper selection of a distal target to maximize the patency, limb salvage, and potential success of the bypass graft is important and depends upon many factors. The availability of conduit, outflow, degree of limb threat (rest pain vs ulceration vs gangrene), as well as collateralization, all play a role. In general, for critical limb ischemia, the best tibial (anterior or posterior) is chosen as they are in direct continuity with the foot's arterial arches. The peroneal artery is appropriate if (a) the tibial arteries are diffusely diseased, (b) rest pain or minimal tissue loss is present, (c) conduit will not allow a more distal bypass, and (d) there are well-developed collaterals from the distal peroneal branches to the pedal/plantar arteries and arches.

Endovascular therapies in the infrageniculate popliteal and tibial level can be accomplished in concert with or without percutaneous intervention in the SFA. Similar to other lower extremity territories, long occlusions and more complex disease are less likely to have a durable result. Treatment of critical limb ischemia with endovascular methods in the popliteal-tibial region remains a considerable challenge. Results of angioplasty and stenting alone are mixed, and generally over half fail in 1 year. However, limb salvage results generally exceed patency of an intervention, probably because in the duration that the intervention is patent, the foot wound heals. Limb salvage rates have exceeded 80% at several years' follow-up. Reporting standards have also varied, with the initial infrapopliteal TASC criteria from 2000 later modified to include more complex disease in lower TASC categories. Techniques such as atherectomy have comparable results and may be preferred for more calcified lesions, but the precise role or any advantage in therapy remains to be determined.

(e) Patients presenting with **significant tissue loss or gangrene of the foot** deserve special mention. Attempts to salvage such a limb may require an extended hospitalization, significant effort at wound and foot care, and considerable expense. However, limb salvage is possible in 70% at 1 year and 60% at 3 years, but generally only about 30% at 5 years after surgery. Successful revascularization results in lower costs than does primary amputation.

In patients over 80 years of age, limb salvage is comparable to younger groups, with a 3-year survival of about 50% and a limb preservation rate of 70%. Consequently, data support an attempt at arterial reconstruction in most elderly patients with critical limb ischemia. Nonetheless, the individual patient as a whole should be considered. Those with significant comorbidities, dementia, or neurologic degenerative disorders with minimal or no ambulation may be considered for primary amputation.

Primary amputation is appropriate when gangrene extensively involves the forefoot and heel. Whether a failed below-knee femoropopliteal bypass changes the level of amputation depends on numerous factors, but generally an unsuccessful reconstruction does not alter final amputation level.

    (f) **Lumbar sympathectomy** alone is not sufficient to salvage limbs that are at risk. However, relief of rest pain has been achieved when the preoperative ankle-brachial index is relatively high (i.e., >0.35) or for pain relief with microembolic phenomenon. Results are not favorable when tissue necrosis is present. It is not considered a treatment option for critical limb ischemia except in very rare cases.

    (g) **Intraoperative duplex or angiography** has also been advocated and used as immediate evaluation of the technical success of lower extremity revascularizations. It is easy to use in most vascular practices and may assist in the identification of technical errors, residual graft defects, and clamp site injuries requiring attention.

3. **Preoperative preparation.** Lab tests for limb salvage cases are the same as those outlined for claudication previously. Skin preparation should include the abdomen and both legs, as the opposite leg vein is occasionally explored. A prophylactic antibiotic with good gram-positive skin coverage should be given prior to the incision. In those with tissue loss, gangrene, or diabetic foot infection, broad-spectrum antibiotics, such as vancomycin and an extended spectrum penicillin derivative, should be used.

4. **Patient positioning.** Most lower extremity arterial revascularizations are performed with the patient supine. The heels must be protected from pressure sores by elevating the calves on soft towels or placing soft pads on the heels. The feet are typically prepped sterilely as well, and covered with a clear bowel bag or towel, to allow for assessment of Doppler signals at the completion of the case. Open or gangrenous foot wounds are covered with impermeable dressing and therefore kept out of the surgical field.

5. **Surgical exposure.** Certain features of surgical exposure facilitate performing the bypass graft anastomoses and prevent postoperative wound complications.

    a. The incisions for exposure of the **GSV** must be made directly over the vein. There is a tendency to bevel the incision and bring it too far anterior to the course of the vein, which results in skin flap necrosis. Leaving skin bridges along the saphenous vein harvest site may also alleviate skin flap necrosis. Some advocate subcutaneous, endoscopic vein harvest.

    b. The **above-knee popliteal artery** can be exposed through a medial distal thigh incision going over the top edge of the sartorius muscle and beneath the adductor magnus tendon. **Three noteworthy anatomic features are present at the adductor magnus tendon: the superficial femoral artery becomes the popliteal artery, the supreme (descending) geniculate artery (an important collateral) originates from the proximal popliteal artery, and the saphenous nerve becomes superficial.** Injury to the nerve can result in bothersome chronic leg neuralgia.

    c. The **below-knee popliteal artery** is exposed via a medial proximal leg incision. The medial head of the gastrocnemius muscle is retracted inferiorly. The popliteal vein and tibial nerve are medial and posterior to the artery. Extensive exposure of the popliteal artery may require detachment of the semimembranosus and semitendinosus muscle tendons. Insertions of the semitendinosus, gracilis, and sartorius muscles form the **pes anserinus (foot of a goose)** on the medial surface of the tibia.

    d. Occasionally, the entire popliteal artery requires exposure for repairs, such as for a popliteal aneurysm (Fig. 13.11). This

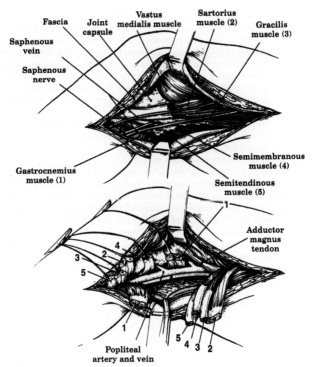

FIGURE 13.11 Medial approach to the popliteal artery. The saphenous nerve should be gently retracted to minimize postoperative saphenous neuralgia. Division of the medial knee tendons and medial head of the gastrocnemius muscle provides clear popliteal artery exposure with minimal morbidity. Most patients have a single great saphenous vein, although an accessory saphenous vein may be present. Tendons can be reapproximated with minimal morbidity, and this exposure can be limited to either the above-knee or below-knee aspects.

exposure also allows for ligation of feeding collaterals into the aneurysm sac. Divided tendons can be anatomically reattached at the conclusion of the operation. Such an extensive exposure appears to increase postoperative leg edema but does not result in knee instability in most patients.

For focal mid–popliteal artery aneurysms or for popliteal artery entrapment, a posterior approach from a longitudinal knee incision provides excellent exposure without cutting normal tendons.

8. The **tibioperoneal trunk and proximal posterior tibial artery** can be exposed through the medial knee approach by detaching the soleus muscle at its arch on the posterior table of the tibia. Placing a right-angled instrument through the foramen for initial dissection is helpful. Exposure of the proximal **anterior tibial artery** generally requires a separate anterior lateral leg incision, which is made one fingerbreadth lateral to the anterior edge of the tibia and carried 8 to 10 cm distally. The artery is located

in the groove between the anterior tibialis and extensor digito-rum longus muscles and can be approached the length of the leg in this groove. The **peroneal artery** can be approached from the medial side by extending dissection behind the tibia and over the posterior tibial vessels or laterally with a fibular resection.

   f. Bypasses can also be taken to the **pedal arteries** (Fig. 13.12) in select patients. The most common pedal artery for distal anas-tomosis is the dorsalis pedis followed by the common and lateral plantar arteries. Incisions are directly over the pedal artery, and, upon completion, the skin only is closed with interrupted per-manent fine filament sutures. This decreases local tissue trauma in ischemic foot tissue.

6. **Preparation of the saphenous vein.** Endothelial damage during prep-aration of saphenous vein is an important factor in graft failure. Optimum preparation includes gentle dissection of the vein, care-ful ligation of side branches away from the vein wall, minimal warm ischemic time if the vein is removed from the leg, and limited dis-tention. Gentle dilation of the vein can be achieved with vein solu-tion. Immersion of the vein in solution should not occur until ready for bypass and may minimize endothelial damage. We use 500 cc Ringer's lactate with 10,000 units heparin and 120 mg papaverine. If splicing of segments is necessary after removing inadequate areas, the ends should be beveled and fine suture (7-0) should be used to create a widely open anastomosis.

7. **Distal arterial control** can be accomplished with minimal damage to the arteries by using Yasargil clips. Alternatively, a pneumatic thigh tourniquet can be applied after the proximal anastomosis is performed. The tourniquet is inflated to 300 mm Hg after the lower limb is wrapped tightly for exsanguination with an elastic Esmarch bandage while the leg is elevated. This is particularly useful when the arterial system is highly calcified and infrageniculate control with clamps unsavory.

8. **Anastomotic technique** should emphasize a long gentle anastomotic angle to minimize turbulence. Distal popliteal and tibial arterial anastomoses are constructed more accurately under low-power mag-nification. If prosthetic bypass is performed to tibial vessels, the use of a **vein adjunct** as mentioned previously may reduce intimal hyper-plasia at the distal anastomosis and improve patency. Polypropylene permanent suture should be used. Size and strength of the suture should be chosen as appropriate for the size and amount of disease in the area. Generally, running anastomoses are used. Sometimes, when the target vessel is small or in an enclosed area where vision is difficult, we use several interrupted, horizontal mattress sutures at the toe of the anastomosis, securing them after placement and using a limb of the lateral-most suture to run the remaining portion. This improves accuracy and splays the distal hood of the graft and prevents a bunching of the graft toe, which may become a nidus for intimal hyperplasia. Another helpful technique, particularly when the target vessel is fragile, is to place both the heel and a toe suture prior to beginning the anastomotic suture line. This assures proper length and distributes tension along the arteriotomy.

9. **Wound closure** is a critical component of lower extremity revascu-larization. We prefer dissolving sutures in several layers. Running sutures on deeper layers may be prone to bunching and inaccurate closure, although interrupted sutures are more time-consuming. Skin is closed with a subcuticular closure and Steri-Strips. It is important

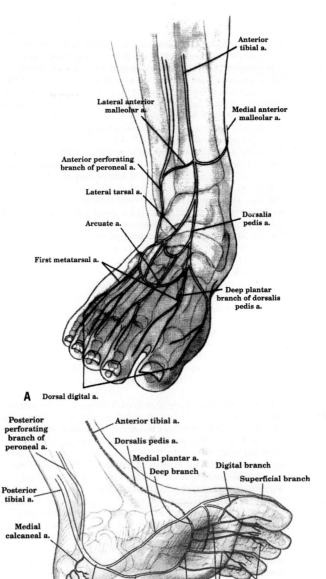

FIGURE 13.12 Anatomy of the pedal arteries. **(A)** Dorsum of foot, **(B)** Plantar surface of foot. (Adapted from Gloviczki P, Bower TC, Toomey BJ, et al. Microscope-aided pedal bypasses is an effective and low-risk operation to salvage the ischemic foot. *Am J Surg.* 1994;168:76-84.)

to reapproximate the skin edges and not pull so much on this stitch to bunch skin with tension. This leads to skin edge ischemia and necrosis with skin breakdown. This may be a pathway for infection, or at least poor wound healing in these patients with poor skin to begin with. Interrupted nylon stitches are used for re-do skin closures, usually in a vertical mattress fashion with eversion and approximation of the skin edges. It is important to ligate lymphatic vessels to avoid a lymph leak, and hemostasis must be good to prevent hematoma. Lymphatic leaks or hematomas can lead to wound breakdown and devastating infections. Loose dressings of gauze wraps should be used, and tape should be avoided.

10. **Associated amputations.** Some patients require an amputation after lower extremity arterial bypass or endovascular revascularization to remove necrotic tissue present before surgery. This is usually foot-based when revascularization is attempted for limb salvage. Whether amputations should be done simultaneously with arterial reconstruction or staged afterward is debatable. Certainly, infected lesions or abscesses need debridement and drainage prior to grafting. Superficial dry gangrene may autoamputate after foot circulation is improved. Thus, we normally wait several days after arterial reconstruction to perform necessary digital or partial foot amputations. This time allows better demarcation of the proper amputation level and perfusion to supply tissue with antibiotics and a granulation process to begin. Although this has been our general approach, we do combine revascularization with toe or forefoot amputations in select patients.

C. **Postoperative care.** Despite multiple medical problems and sometimes extensive operations, most patients who undergo aortic or lower extremity arterial reconstruction for occlusive disease can expect a reasonably uncomplicated recovery if certain principles of care are followed. The postprocedural care for endovascular intervention is described in Chapter 10.

1. **Initial stabilization** after aortic reconstructions should be done in an intensive care or step-down setting where vital signs, urine output, ECG rhythm, and respiratory status can be monitored continuously for 12 to 24 hours. On arrival to the recovery area, the patient's blood pressure, heart rate, and rhythm should be checked, and arterial blood gas is drawn for analysis. If the patient is intubated, ventilator settings should be adjusted after review of the initial blood gas. A plan for extubation should be established.

After these vital functions have been stabilized, additional baseline tests may be obtained, including a portable chest x-ray to check endotracheal tube position and to ensure adequate lung expansion. In addition, formal 12-lead ECG should be compared with the preoperative ECG for any evidence of myocardial ischemia or rhythm changes. Cardiac isoenzymes should be sent for study if intraoperative myocardial ischemia or arrhythmia was detected; however, in general, routine cardiac enzymes are unnecessary. Blood also should be sent for measurement of hematocrit, serum electrolytes, blood sugar, PT/PTT, and platelet count.

After lower extremity revascularization, patients should remain under intensive observation for at least 6 to 12 hours. Similar laboratory evaluations should be accomplished. It is during this immediate postoperative period that most early graft occlusions occur. Hourly checks of pedal pulses with Doppler signal confirmation should be made. Absence or diminution in Doppler flow should prompt rapid assessment by the vascular team. Early bypass occlusion often results in severe acute ischemia, due to loss of collateral flow from surgical dissection, clot propagation distally, and dependence on the bypass for limb perfusion. Prompt heparinization and graft thrombectomy/revision is necessary for limb salvage.

Most patients are prescribed antiplatelet therapy, usually aspirin, which in femoropopliteal grafts with good outflow is appropriate. DVT prophylaxis with either low molecular weight or unfractionated heparin is ordered until the patient is ambulatory. We occasionally will use low-dose intravenous heparin (300 to 500 units per hour) in addition to aspirin for the first 24 to 48 hours after surgery for complex or prolonged tibial reconstructions, or those requiring intraoperative revision. Long-term anticoagulation in combination with low-dose aspirin (81 mg) is sometimes used for below-knee synthetic grafts or marginal quality vein grafts, revision grafts to the tibial arteries, or those with poor runoff (one or fewer vessels in continuity to the ankle). However, there are no conclusive data that anticoagulation is superior to antiplatelet therapy for graft maintenance postoperatively, and combined therapy increases risk of any bleeding in the long term.

2. **Fluid management** must be meticulous, as many vascular patients have significant heart disease and will not tolerate fluid overload. A few guidelines for fluid administration should make fluid management easy.

   a. Patients leave the operating room after large amounts of fluid have been given. Most of this fluid is sequestered in interstitial spaces and will remain there until it is slowly mobilized and excreted in 48 to 72 hours. In addition, inappropriate secretion of antidiuretic hormone results in sodium and water retention. Therefore, postoperative fluids should be limited to about 80 mL/h (1 mL/kg body weight per hour) of 5% dextrose in half normal saline with 20 to 30 mEq potassium per liter. When needed, the rate of intravenous fluid can be increased or bolus fluid given.

   b. Some patients are cold and vasoconstricted when they arrive in the recovery area. As they rewarm and vasodilate, additional fluid may be necessary, indicated by decreased urine output, low filling pressures, and tachycardia. If the hemoglobin is less than 8 g/dL or hematocrit less than 25%, packed red blood cells should be transfused. Otherwise, volume replacement may be made with a bolus (5 to 10 mL/kg of a balanced salt solution, e.g., Ringer's lactated solution).

   c. When patients begin to mobilize excess fluid on the **2nd or 3rd postoperative day,** maintenance intravenous rates may need to be reduced or stopped. If the patient is edematous and urine output has not increased, a small dose (10 to 20 mg) of furosemide may initiate a good diuresis.

3. **Postoperative pulmonary care** is critical after extubation and is discussed in Chapter 8.

4. **Pain management** is a key component to early ambulation, pulmonary care, and gastrointestinal function. Epidural anesthesia that provides analgesia for 2 to 4 days after abdominal operations is an excellent method. Standard narcotic-based therapy is also used. See Chapter 8.

5. **Antibiotics** should be continued for 24 hours postoperatively unless otherwise indicated.

6. After aortic bypass, **diet** with liquids is initiated with presence of bowel sounds and flatus, and advanced as tolerated. Nasogastric tube decompression is necessary if the patient develops abdominal distension, nausea, and ileus. Ileus can result from extensive lysis of adhesions or dissection of the duodenum. Narcotics also slow bowel motility. Appetite after aortic reconstruction usually is poor, and patients generally do not resume normal caloric intake for several weeks. A weight loss of 5 to 10 pounds is not uncommon in the first month following surgery. Patients with lower extremity bypass can resume a normal diet the same day as surgery.

7. **Wound care** requires special attention, since local infection may rapidly extend to a prosthetic graft or cause a bacteremia that could seed the graft surface. Initial dressings should be removed on the first postoperative day. If the wound is sealed, no further dressing is needed, but a simple gauze covering may be helpful to protect groin wounds and absorb sweat. If serosanguineous fluid is leaking from the wound, a sterile gauze dressing should be applied until the drainage stops. Lymph leaks from groin incisions may be treacherous, since infection of the deeper inguinal lymphatics may also infect an adjacent graft. Prolonged lymph leakage increases the risk of bacterial invasion of the perigraft lymphatics and may result in an early prosthetic graft infection. Most minor lymph leaks will resolve in 3 to 5 days. If a groin lymph leak is copious and not decreased or closed in 3 to 5 days, wound exploration, ligation of culprit nodes or lymph vessels, and reclosure are done.

8. The proper time to **ambulate** a patient after aortic or other peripheral arterial reconstruction is another controversial area. Proper timing is individualized with consideration of the following.

   a. Many patients after aortic reconstruction are not hemodynamically stable for 24 to 48 hours, and tachycardia with swings in blood pressure is not well tolerated. Incisional pain may also contribute to tachycardia and hypertension. Furthermore, within 48 to 72 hours, mobilization of fluid expands intravascular volume, placing additional stress on the heart. If hemodynamically labile patients attempt to ambulate before tachycardia is controlled and fluids are mobilized, they may experience myocardial ischemia. Myocardial infarction occurs most commonly on the 3rd postoperative day.

   b. If the patient has an inguinal lymph leak, it is most likely to stop if lower extremity activity is curtailed by bed rest. Since ambulation may be delayed, we insist that patients perform leg exercises (flexion and extension of calf and thigh muscles) for at least 5 minutes every hour. These exercises improve venous emptying from calf muscles and are prophylaxis for deep venous thrombosis. The leg exercise also increases blood flow to the legs and consequently through any graft. Finally, these exercises help maintain leg muscle tone prior to ambulation. In our experience, delayed ambulation in some patients has not increased either pulmonary complications or venous thromboembolism, provided coughing, deep breathing, appropriate mechanical and pharmacologic DVT prophylaxis, and footboard exercises are performed routinely. No pneumatic compression devices should be placed on legs after an infrageniculate bypass.

   c. **Edema** can be a problem after revascularization and is multifactorial owing to lymphatic trauma, reperfusion, and dysfunctional vasoregulation. However, usually, after 2 to 4 days it is manageable. When not ambulatory, the patient should be supine with the leg elevated. If reconstruction is above the knee, compression hose may be helpful. Infrageniculate and pedal bypass may require longer periods of leg elevation as tissue loss and incisions may be compromised by significant edema. Prolonged sitting is to be avoided. Not uncommonly, edema after lower extremity revascularization may last for several weeks to months, and fitted graded compression hose and elevation are useful.

9. After **endovascular procedures** involving an intervention for lower extremity occlusive disease, standard care usually involves maximal antiplatelet therapy including aspirin and clopidogrel. Similar to open reconstruction, certain infrageniculate interventions may warrant anticoagulation, but this is not well defined. Patients with manual pressure used for hemostasis after sheath removal should remain supine for 6 hours. If a closure device is used, we have them remain supine for 2 to 4 hours, barring problems. Monitoring of the revascularization is similar to those mentioned above for open operation. We obtain duplex ultrasound and pressure studies on lower extremity endovascular interventions in follow-up in order to assess patency and physiologic improvement. Patients are usually able to be discharged the same day, unless foot sepsis or other medical conditions require inpatient care.

IV. **POSTOPERATIVE COMPLICATIONS.** Early graft-related complications following operations for lower extremity occlusive disease affect about 3% to 5% of patients. Late complications such as anastomotic aneurysm, graft thrombosis, or graft infection are more common, involving approximately 10% of patients. We focus here on the recognition of such complications and the principles of management.

A. **Early graft-related complications**

1. **Hemorrhage** from an arterial graft anastomosis is manifested by a groin or leg hematoma in femoral or popliteal anastomoses and shock in aortic or iliac anastomoses. Treatment is early reoperation, evacuation of the hematoma, and suture control of the bleeding site. Failure to follow this approach may result in infection of the hematoma, pseudoaneurysm formation, or death.

Postoperative hemorrhage usually occurs in two patterns. In the first and most common form, bleeding occurs within 24 hours from the vein graft or an anastomosis. Early repair and hematoma evacuation usually do not lead to graft failure or infection. The second pattern of postoperative hemorrhage is rare and occurs from 3 to 28 days after operation and in most cases is caused by early and aggressive graft infection. Hemorrhage usually occurs at the proximal or distal anastomosis in conjunction with signs of local infection and possibly systemic sepsis. These patients are at greater risk of eventual limb loss.

2. **Early thrombosis** may be the result of a technical error at the anastomosis, an embolus, or inadequate runoff to maintain graft flow. Also, inadequate inflow may be the result of clamp injury or unrecognized disease on preoperative imaging. Other causes of early thrombosis may include graft kinking, poor vein conduit, extrinsic muscle or tendon compression, or an intimal flap. Occasionally, early graft thrombosis is due to a previously undiagnosed hypercoagulable condition. Routine perioperative vascular monitoring of the reconstruction (see Chapter 8) should recognize thrombosis or compromised inflow or

outflow before severe ischemia occurs. Proper management of early graft thrombosis includes anticoagulation, operative reexploration, thromboembolectomy, and graft revision. It often also includes operative arteriography. In our experience, the long-term prognosis of early graft failure has been poor, even if the graft is successfully reopened.

3. **Infections** of bypass grafts were classified by **D. Emerick Szilagyi who described three grades of infection: grade I, superficial involving the skin and dermis; grade II, involving the subcutaneous and fatty tissue but not the graft; and grade III, involving the graft** (Table 13.5). This grading system has important implications for the management of early infections involving arterial reconstructions. Early infections are usually due to virulent organisms and are very morbid complications. Grade I infections can be managed with close observation, local wound care, and antibiotics, while grade II infections require opening and irrigation in the operating room. Grade III infections may lead to anastomotic hemorrhage or graft erosion, and therefore graft removal with extra-anatomic bypass is the preferred method of management.

4. **Colon ischemia** may affect 1% to 5% of patients who undergo aortic reconstruction for occlusive disease and is more common than that associated with aneurysm repair. It usually affects the left or sigmoid colon. Ischemia may result from IMA ligation, low cardiac output states and/or inadequate collateral blood flow from the superior mesenteric or internal iliac arteries. Very rarely, it has been reported after lower extremity bypass due to ligation of common femoral artery branches, which can supply the pelvis in patients with diffuse occlusions of their mesenteric and internal iliac arteries. Superficial mucosal or muscularis ischemia usually causes transient diarrhea and resolves spontaneously without mortality. Late colon stricture may occur. Transmural colon ischemia will progress to bowel perforation, sepsis, and death in at least 70% of cases.

Clinical manifestations vary with the severity of ischemia. Bloody diarrhea, lower abdominal pain, and unexplained fluid requirements or sepsis suggest colon ischemia. Flexible lower endoscopy may reveal changes of patchy hemorrhage, edema, congestion, or pallor. More severe signs include ulceration and mucosal sloughing. Mild cases need bowel rest, antibiotics, and hydration until the

TABLE 13.5	Clinical Classification of Infection Associated with Arterial Reconstruction	
Grade	Clinical Description of Infection	Management
I	Involving only the skin and dermis	Local wound care and antibiotics
II	Extending into subcutaneous and fatty tissue but not the graft	Exploration and washout of the wound in the operating room
III	Graft involved in the infection	Exploration and washout of the wound with graft removal and establishment of alternative route perfusion

Source: Szilagyi DE, Smith RF, Elliott JP, Vrandecic MP. Infection in arterial reconstruction with synthetic grafts. *Ann Surg.* 1972;176:321-333.

diarrhea resolves. When there is any clinical decline or presentation with fluid requirements and sepsis or if symptoms and signs persist, resection of necrotic colon with formation of a colostomy is necessary. Any bowel movement within 48 hours of aortic reconstruction should prompt flexible sigmoidoscopy. Routine use of IMA reimplantation during aortic reconstruction is debated. The potential mitigating effect of IMA revascularization on the incidence of colon ischemia is not clear. Many individuals with aortoiliac occlusive disease have an occluded IMA negating need for reconstruction. If the IMA is patent, then the factors mentioned previously, such as an enlarged IMA or associated internal iliac and SMA disease, should be scrutinized and reimplantation considered.

5. **Compartment syndrome of the leg** is caused by prolonged acute ischemia (>6 hours) before revascularization. After restoration of perfusion, edema forms within the calf muscles. Since these muscles are enveloped in fixed fascial compartments, swelling leads to increased pressure within the compartments leading to myonecrosis and permanent nerve damage. The anterior compartment is most susceptible to this ischemic syndrome. The earliest clinical signs are leg pain with sensory deficits on the dorsum of the foot and weakness of toe dorsiflexion. Treatment is fasciotomy. Prophylactic fasciotomy should be considered for all cases of acute arterial ischemia in which revascularization is delayed beyond 4 to 6 hours.

6. **Femoral nerve injury** may occur after groin operations, especially in repeat procedures or extensive dissections of the profunda femoris artery. The injury may not be apparent until the patient tries to ambulate and discovers that he or she cannot extend at the knee because of quadriceps weakness. Treatment requires a flexible knee brace. Many femoral nerve apraxias will resolve in 3 to 6 months. Sensory deficits such as numbness and paresthesias are much more common than motor ones and may be related to inflammation, edema, and hematoma surrounding the cutaneous femoral nerve branches.

7. **Early complications after endovascular reconstruction** involve access site problems, early thrombosis, and rarely perforation. Acute pseudoaneurysm, local groin hematoma, retroperitoneal bleeding, acute site thrombosis with limb ischemia or thromboembolism, arteriovenous fistula, and closure device infection are all described access site complications. In general, the more complicated the procedure and the more anticoagulation required, the higher the incidence of these site problems. Access technique is crucial and when performed poorly may lead to dissection, intimal flaps, and lacerations. Overall they occur in 1% to 10%. Acute thrombosis at the endovascular intervention site may occur due to arterial dissection, incomplete therapy with residual stenosis, treatment of more complex lesions such as long-segment occlusions, as well as diseased inflow or outflow vessels.

B. **Late graft-related complications** are not uncommon and occur in about 20% of patients who undergo aortic reconstructive procedures for occlusive disease, and roughly 30% of those with reconstructions below the inguinal ligament.

1. **Gastrointestinal hemorrhage,** especially hematemesis, in a patient who has ever received a prosthetic aortic graft must raise the suspicion of a rare but life-threatening complication, an **aortoenteric fistula**, and may occur years after the initial operation. Although the initial hemorrhage ("herald bleed") may stop and not recur for days, untreated aortoenteric fistulas eventually lead to hemorrhage and death. Therefore, such patients should be resuscitated and undergo

emergency diagnostic studies. CT scan will show proximity of the duodenum to the graft, often with perigraft inflammation or abscess. Endoscopy can be helpful to rule out other sources of bleeding. If the source of hemorrhage is located in the stomach or duodenal bulb, appropriate therapy is instituted. Occasionally, graft material can be seen eroding into the duodenum, but nonvisualization of graft material on endoscopy does not exclude aortoenteric fistula.

Unstable patients with diagnosis of aortoenteric fistula must undergo emergent laparotomy. Classically, repair of aortoenteric fistulas requires closure of the intestine and removal of the adjacent graft with extra-anatomic bypass (e.g., axillobifemoral bypass). If gastrointestinal hemorrhage is minor, and the patient stabilizes, a less hurried operation can be accomplished. Graft-enteric erosion that is not associated with local abscess and gross infection can be successfully managed with in situ graft replacement, bowel repair, and omental coverage of the new graft in 85% of patients. Alternatively, stable patients can undergo axillobifemoral bypass followed by staged laparotomy, graft resection, and duodenal repair.

2. **Chronic aortic or lower limb graft infection** may present as an aortoenteric fistula, femoral pseudoaneurysm, groin abscess, frank sepsis, or a chronically draining sinus tract. Most infections of aortic prostheses originate in the groin and are commonly caused by *Staphylococcus*. Although infection may originate at one anastomosis, it rarely remains localized, and spreads along the perigraft plane to eventually involve the entire graft. CT scan or high-resolution ultrasound may show poor incorporation of the graft or perigraft fluid collections.

Sometimes the diagnosis of infection is difficult. Infections may be indolent, with no visible fluid collections, negative blood cultures, no fever, and no leukocytosis. An arteriogram or CTA should be done to define the involved anatomy and an indium white blood cell scan may demonstrate the infected site. Although removal of a focally infected segment of graft may succeed in eliminating infection, resolution of many graft infections will require extraction of the entire prosthesis and an extra-anatomic bypass. Putting off or limiting operations often allows a local infection to spread, and eventually life-threatening graft hemorrhage or sepsis may occur. Graft preservation may be considered if (a) the infection does not involve a body cavity, (b) the graft is patent, (c) the anastomoses are not involved by gross infection, and (d) the patient is not physiologically septic. These situations still typically require operative washout(s), muscle flap coverage, and often use of a negative pressure wound therapy device such as the VAC® (KCI, San Antonio, TX).

Patients with infected abdominal aortic grafts have discouraging 30-day and 1-year survival rates of 70% to 80% and 40% to 50%, respectively. Staged revascularization (i.e., axillofemoral bypass) followed by infected graft removal in 24 to 48 hours is the classically described treatment of aortic graft infection. The term sequential treatment is used when extra-anatomic revascularization precedes graft removal and aortic stump oversewing at the same sitting. Mortality is lower when a new remote revascularization precedes removal of an infected abdominal aortic graft or treatment of an aortoenteric erosion or fistula. These approaches substantially reduce major amputation from 40% when graft removal precedes revascularization to 5% to 10% when the extra-anatomic bypass is done first. When extra-anatomic revascularization precedes removal of an infected graft, subsequent infection of the new bypass has been rare.

In recent years, in situ reconstruction of the aorta with femoral vein grafts (neo-aorto-iliac systems), rifampin-soaked prosthetic grafts, or allogenic aortic homografts have added another therapeutic option. In general, in situ reconstruction is appropriate for more indolent infections where the patient is stable. More aggressive infections with virulent organisms and sepsis require extra-anatomic reconstruction and graft removal.

3. **Graft thrombosis** that occurs within a few weeks to months of operation often is the result of a technical problem in graft placement or anastomosis. Graft stenosis or occlusion after this time, but before 2 years, is generally due to myointimal hyperplasia. After 18 to 24 months, graft failure is caused by atherosclerotic progression.

Failed aortofemoral grafts are usually due to loss of outflow and limb thrombosis. Treatment usually involves limb thrombo-embolectomy or thrombolysis with some sort of outflow procedure. Reoperations to maintain patency of failing or thrombosed aortofemoral grafts succeed in nearly 80% of patients and result in long-term limb preservation in 60% to 70%. Operative mortality for revision of femoral anastomotic problems is 1% to 2%.

Special discussion about lower extremity graft failure is warranted. Increasing evidence documents that alterations in the vein graft itself may also lead to graft thrombosis. Mills and colleagues have emphasized that 10% to 15% of reversed saphenous vein grafts develop significant inflow, intrinsic graft, or outflow stenosis at a mean follow-up of 2 years. The peak incidence of early hemodynamic graft failure occurs within 12 months of graft implantation. Intrinsic graft stenoses cause the majority of failures (60%). These lesions are usually focal intimal hyperplasia distributed equally at the proximal and distal anastomoses. The remaining causes are inflow failure (13%), outflow failure (9%), muscle entrapment (4%), and hypercoagulable conditions (4%).

If these vein graft alterations are detected before graft thrombosis occurs, successful repair and long-term patency can be accomplished. Results are much poorer after thrombosis occurs. **Late cumulative vein graft patency is 75% to 80% for revised grafts, but only 5% to 15% for thrombosed grafts at 5 years. Thus, emphasis is on detecting failing grafts before they occlude.** Periodic reevaluation (every 3 to 6 months for 2 years; then annually if normal) should focus on any recurrent symptoms, such as return or progression of claudication, and objective signs of a failing graft. These signs include reduced segmental pressures and a 0.15 fall in the ankle-brachial pressure index. Important duplex ultrasound criteria predicting graft failure are now defined, and duplex should also be accomplished at these times (Chapter 5). Specifics include an increased peak systolic velocity across a stenotic area (two to three times the normal graft velocity), plus a decrease in peak systolic flow velocity to less than 45 cm/s in the graft beyond the area of stenosis. Collectively, these duplex findings and clinical warning signs may be an indication for arteriography to define correctable lesions before graft thrombosis occurs (Table 13.6).

When lesions intrinsic to vein grafts are found on surveillance, treatment may include balloon angioplasty or open revision. While improved outcomes with surveillance of prosthetic grafts are not as conclusive, many still proceed with a surveillance program. One reason for this is that when prosthetic grafts occlude, they are associated with loss of outflow, whereas with vein grafts this is less frequent. Thus, if a culprit lesion is noted, treatment can be important.

T A B L E

TABLE 3.6	Graft Surveillance Criteria			
Category	High-Velocity Criteria		Low-Velocity Criteria	ΔABI
I. Highest risk	PSV > 300 cm/s or Vr > 3.5 or EDV > 100 cm/s	and	PSV < 45 cm/s or	>0.15
II. High risk	PSV > 300 cm/s or Vr > 3.5	and	PSV > 45 cm/s and	<0.15
III. Intermediate risk	200–300 cm/s PSV or Vr > 2.0	and	PSV > 45 cm/s and	<0.15
IV. Low risk	PSV < 200 cm/s or Vr < 2.0	and	PSV > 45 cm/s and	<0.15

Duplex surveillance criteria for vein bypass grafts of the lower extremities. Category I may be admitted for heparinization with expedited angiography ± revision. Category II should have elective arteriography ± revision. Category III should have intensified surveillance (every 3 months) and Category IV is considered appropriate for continued standard surveillance.
PSV, Peak systolic velocity; EDV, end diastolic velocity; cm/s, centimeters per second; Vr, velocity ratio = PSV in stenosis/PSV of normal proximal area.

When infrainguinal bypasses fail, reoperative surgery can achieve limb salvage in about 50% of patients. As mentioned previously, directed thrombolytic therapy of graft thrombosis can be helpful in certain acute circumstances. There is suggestion that thrombolytic therapy can improve limb outcomes and limit the magnitude of surgical revision if graft thrombosis is less than 14 days old. This comes at an apparent increased risk of stroke, embolism, and bleeding. Once a graft is occluded for several weeks, surgical thromboembolectomy is performed or a new bypass graft is inserted. Some patients may benefit from an attempt at complex endovascular therapy on the native vessels, particularly if suitable conduit is not available.

4. **Anastomotic pseudoaneurysm** occurs most frequently at the common femoral artery. The causative factors are complex and include atherosclerotic deterioration of the artery and anastomotic disruption due to inadequate suturing, infection, graft dilation, and suture deterioration. Clinically, asymptomatic anastomotic aneurysms of less than 2.5 cm may be safely followed by observation. However, large false aneurysms or symptomatic aneurysms should be electively repaired before they are complicated by thrombosis, distal emboli, or rupture. Most late groin pseudoaneurysms are degenerative in nature. However, an infection must be clearly ruled out. One must be prepared to treat a graft infection when taking on reoperation for pseudoaneurysm.

5. **Sexual dysfunction** in men following aortoiliac operations may be manifested by impaired or absent penile erection and retrograde ejaculation after otherwise normal coitus. This may occur in up to some 25% of men. Previously normal sexual function may be altered by the interruption of preaortic sympathetic fibers, the parasympathetic pelvic splanchnic nerves, or the internal iliac artery flow. It is obvious that the surgeon must know whether any sexual dysfunction

existed before surgery. If impotence is a significant problem to the patient postoperatively, he may be referred to a urologist for evaluation and treatment.

6. **Spinal cord ischemia** following operations on the abdominal aorta is rare, occurring in less than 0.5%. It is considered unpredictable. However, it can be emphasized that the problem appears to occur in patients in whom internal iliac artery perfusion was impaired, when atheromatous embolism is evident, and when early postoperative hypotension or low cardiac output may further compromise marginal spinal cord perfusion.

7. **Late complications of endovascular reconstructions** of the lower extremities center around intervention site restenosis, thrombosis, and failure, as well as progressive stenosis of the access site. The main drawback to iliac stenting is restenosis. There is some evidence that the main limitation of SFA intervention is restenosis allowing later percutaneous reintervention without negative consequences on the distal outflow and loss of surgical options. Some refuting data exist, however, and there is no clinical equipoise to date. Tibial intervention is hindered by a high frequency of restenosis and thrombosis, despite satisfactory limb salvage rates.

Surveillance has also become part of the postprocedure protocol for lower extremity endovascular interventions. As mentioned earlier, study of SFA angioplasty and stenting and iliac interventions has suggested that assisted primary patency for these procedures is significantly enhanced with repeat intervention. This makes the argument to surveil compelling. While criteria indicating significant restenosis are less well understood compared to vein grafts, these are active areas of study.

Selected Readings

Brewster DC. Current controversies in the management of aortoiliac occlusive disease. *J Vasc Surg.* 1997;25:365-379.
Classic article describes best practices and controversies in open aortic bypass grafting that remain valid in current practice.

Dake MD, Ansel GM, Jaff MR, et al. Paclitaxel-eluting stents show superiority to balloon angioplasty and bare metal stents in femoropopliteal disease: twelve-month Zilver PTX randomized study results. *Circ Cardiovasc Interv.* 2011;4:495-504.
Paclitaxel-coated stents improved one-year patency of stents in the SFA by reducing restenosis.

Dorigo W, Pulli R, Castelli P, et al.; Propaten Italian Registry Group. A multicenter comparison between autologous saphenous vein and heparin-bonded expanded polytetrafluoroethylene (ePTFE) graft in the treatment of critical limb ischemia in diabetics. *J Vasc Surg.* 2011;54:1332-1338.
Modern registry of heparin-bonded ePTFE bypass versus autologous vein. Vein bypasses have better patency, but acceptable results for limb salvage were achieved with prosthetic.

Ferris BL, Mills JL, Hughes JD, et al. Is early postoperative duplex scan surveillance of leg bypass grafts clinically important? *J Vasc Surg.* 2003;37:495-500.
Standardizing the process of postoperative lower extremity vein graft surveillance.

Giles KA, Pomposelli FB, Hamdan AD, et al. Infrapopliteal angioplasty for critical limb ischemia: relation of TransAtlantic InterSociety Consensus class to outcome in 176 limbs. *J Vasc Surg.* 2008;48:128-136.
Several year outcomes of tibial angioplasty for limb salvage stratified by original TASC criteria.

Hirsch AT, Haskal ZJ, Hertzer NR, et al. ACC/AHA guidelines for the management of patients with peripheral arterial disease (lower extremity, renal, mesenteric, and abdominal aortic). *J Am Coll Cardiol.* 2006;47:1239-1312.

Collaborative document summarizes the diagnostic workup, medical and interventional treatment of lower extremity disease, as well as additional vascular pathology.

How TV, Rowe CS, Gilling-Smith GL, et al. Interposition vein cuff anastomosis alters wall shear stress distribution in the recipient artery. *J Vasc Surg.* 2000;31:1008-1017.

Technical article regarding the fluid dynamics at anastomoses and use of vein cuffs.

Lo RC, Darling J, Bensley RP, et al. Long-term outcomes following infrapopliteal angioplasty for critical limb ischemia. *J Vasc Surg.* 2013;57:1455-1464.

One- to 5-year outcomes in patients undergoing tibial interventions, in which half were performed in conjunction with proximal intervention.

Mills JL, Fujitani RM, Taylor SM. The characteristics and anatomic distribution of lesions that cause reversed vein graft failure: a five-year prospective study. *J Vasc Surg.* 1993;17:195-206.

Mid-term bypass failure is often as a result of myointimal hyperplasia as described in this study.

Mwipatayi BP, Thomas S, Wong J, et al.; Covered Versus Balloon Expandable Stent Trial (COBEST) Co-investigators. A comparison of covered vs bare expandable stents for the treatment of aortoiliac occlusive disease. *J Vasc Surg.* 2011;54:1561-1570.

Patency of covered iliac stents was superior to that of bare metal stents for TASC C and D lesions in this multicenter trial.

Raptis S, Faris I, Miller J, Quigley F. The fate of the aortofemoral graft. *Eur J Vasc Endovasc Surg.* 1995;9:97-102.

The natural history of aortobifemoral bypass grafting, including long-term complications and adjuvant operations, is defined in this series of 301 patients.

Society for Vascular Surgery Lower Extremity Guidelines Writing Group; Conte MS, Pomposelli FB, Clair DG, et al. Society for Vascular Surgery practice guidelines for atherosclerotic occlusive disease of the lower extremities: management of asymptomatic disease and claudication. *J Vasc Surg.* 2015;61:2S-41S.

Up-to-date guidelines from the Society for Vascular Surgery on medical and interventional management of lower extremity claudication.

Stewart KJ, Hiatt WR, Regensteiner JG, Hirsch AT. Exercise training for claudication. *N Engl J Med.* 2002;347:1941-1951.

Physiology of exercise training for claudication is explained.

TransAtlantic Inter-Society Consensus Working Group II. Inter-society Consensus for the Management of Peripheral Arterial Disease (TASC II). *J Vasc Surg.* 2007;45(suppl S):S5-S67.

Comprehensive document summarizes the clinical data for the diagnosis and treatment of lower extremity occlusive disease and specifies often-utilized "TASC classifications."

Tinder CN, Chavanpun JP, Bandyk DF. Efficacy of duplex ultrasound surveillance after infrainguinal vein bypass may be enhanced by identification of characteristics predictive of graft stenosis development. *J Vasc Surg.* 2008;48:613-618.

Duplex surveillance is important for lower extremity bypass, particularly "higher risk" bypasses.

Veith FJ, Gupta SK, Ascer E, et al. Six-year prospective multicenter randomized comparison of autologous saphenous vein and expanded polytetrafluoroethylene grafts in infrainguinal arterial reconstructions. *J Vasc Surg.* 1986;3:104-114.

Data on patency and limb salvage rates for vein versus PTFE lower limb bypass.

White JV, Rutherford RB, Ryjewski C. Chronic subcritical ischemia: a poorly recognized stage of critical limb ischemia. *Semin Vasc Surg.* 2007;20:62-67.

Small series examined the natural history of patients with asymptomatic but objectively severe chronic limb ischemia.

14 Aneurysms and Aortic Dissection

Management of arterial aneurysms and aortic dissection requires an understanding of natural history, diagnosis, and treatment options. Over the last 30 years, these options have changed dramatically with the development of endovascular techniques. **Despite these changes, the best results continue to follow carefully planned elective treatment before complications of rupture, thrombosis, or embolism occur.** The contrast in mortality between elective (2% to 4%) and ruptured abdominal aortic aneurysm (AAA) repair (30% to 70%) remains one of the most striking examples of the importance of early recognition and proper treatment of these diseases.

Aortic dissections are a commonly encountered degenerative disease of the aorta, which are distinctly different from aortic aneurysms. This chapter focuses on the natural history, diagnosis, and management of aneurysms and aortic dissections. The hemodynamics of aneurysms are discussed in Chapter 1. Chapter 3 outlines the initial physical evaluation, and Chapter 5 outlines several useful diagnostic tests that may be used to diagnose and follow these conditions.

ABDOMINAL AORTIC ANEURYSM

I. **EPIDEMIOLOGY.** During the past 40 to 50 years, the incidence of AAAs has increased significantly. This is attributed to increased detection with the use of ultrasound and computed tomography (CT) and an aging population. The rising incidence has been tenfold for small AAAs (<5 cm), while the incidence for larger aneurysms has increased by a factor of 2. Small aneurysms account for 50% of all recognized AAAs, an important consideration given that much of the uncertainty surrounding appropriate management concerns aneurysms less than 5.5 cm.

II. **NATURAL HISTORY AND THE EVOLUTION OF EVIDENCE-BASED APPROACH.** Aortic aneurysms are a disease of the elderly largely diagnosed in the sixth and seventh decades of life. As many as 20% of patients with an AAA have a family history of aortic aneurysm. The expansion rate of AAAs is 2 to 3 mm per year and increases as the aneurysm enlarges. Twenty percent of aneurysms expand at a rate of more than 4 mm per year, while 80% grow at a slower pace. **Importantly, active cigarette smoking has been shown to be associated with an increased expansion rate and has been identified as an independent risk factor for aneurysm rupture.**

The natural history of AAA is expansion and rupture, an outcome that is related directly to aneurysm diameter. Less commonly, enlarging aneurysms may erode into the vena cava resulting in an **aortocaval fistula**, or into the intestine presenting as gastrointestinal bleeding (i.e., **aorto-enteric fistula**). These concepts are controversial, not because of the risk associated with open surgery, but because experts have debated the size at which repair should occur. Initially, aneurysms greater than 6 cm were considered appropriate for elective repair. Autopsy studies in the 1970s

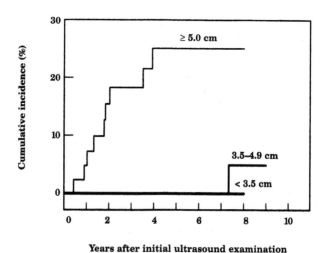

FIGURE 14.1 Cumulative incidence of rupture of abdominal aortic aneurysms according to the diameter of the aneurysm at the initial ultrasound examination. (From Nevitt MP, Ballard DJ, Hallett JW Jr. Prognosis of abdominal aortic aneurysms: a population-based study. *NEJM.* 1989;321:1009-1014, with permission.)

and 1980s suggested that even small aneurysms (4 to 5 cm) could rupture, which resulted in a more aggressive approach to repair. **Population-based studies in the 1990s showed that rupture risk did not increase until aneurysm diameter reached 5 cm** (Figs. 14.1 and 14.2). Rupture risk for small (<5 cm) AAAs was shown to be approximately 1% per year, 5% to 10% per year for medium-sized (5 to 7 cm) AAAs, and at least 10% to 25% per year for large (7 cm) AAAs (Table 14.1). **The U.K. Small Aneurysm and Aneurysm Detection and Management (ADAM) trials** were prospective randomized studies

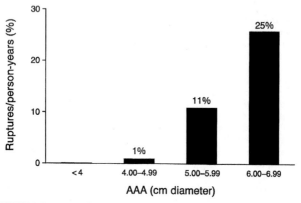

FIGURE 14.2 Rupture risk of abdominal aortic aneurysm (AAA) per year for size diameter. (From Reed WW, Hallett JW Jr, Damiano MA, et al. Learning from the last ultrasound: a population-based study of patients with abdominal aortic aneurysm. *Arch Int Med.* 1997;157: 2064-2068, with permission.)

TABLE 14.1	Estimated Annual Rupture Risk of AAA

AAA Diameter (cm)	Rupture Risk (%/y)
<4	0
4–5	0.5–5
5–6	3–15
6–7	10–20
7–8	20–40
>8	30–50

looking for survival benefit in early open repair of aneurysms between 4 and 5.4 cm. Findings from these trials confirmed the population-based studies of the 1990s, while showing no benefit to early open repair of aneurysms between 4 and 5.4 cm. Several caveats from these studies are worth noting. First, safe observation of aneurysms between 4 and 5.4 cm includes ultrasound every 3 to 6 months, which many feel is unrealistic for some patients. Second, in both studies, two-thirds of patients in the "observation" group crossed over to eventual open repair once their aneurysms reached 5.5 cm during the study period. **Finally, in this era of endovascular aneurysm repair (EVAR), it is important to remember that both the U.K. Small Aneurysm and the ADAM trial compared observation to early open aneurysm repair and not to EVAR.** What makes this relevant is that the mortality associated with open repair in these two trials was 5.8% and 2.7%, respectively, which is higher than for EVAR. **However, later comparison of surveillance and EVAR was done in the PIVOTAL and CESAR trials. They again showed that there was no survival or aneurysm-related mortality benefit to early repair with EVAR compared to surveillance in aneurysms under 5 to 5.5 cm.** Similar to the open trials, of those surveilled, 50% to 60% required repair during the 36 months after entry due to growth.

In 1997 the U.S. Food and Drug Administration (FDA) approved the first device for EVAR. Nearly two decades later, the expanded use of this procedure seems to have had a positive impact on the mortality associated with AAA repair. Information from the Medicare database reveals the number of AAA repairs in the United States had increased over this period (just over 90,000 per year). The percentage of AAAs treated with EVAR increased substantially to over 75% of repairs. While the operative mortality of open aneurysm repair remained roughly 5%, EVAR's operative mortality was less than 1.5%, showing this less invasive approach has reduced the overall mortality associated with AAA repair; something that had not been possible in this country for decades. From these decades of clinical study, one can be assured that nearly all AAAs that rupture have enlarged to over 5 cm in diameter. While rupture deaths have decreased in the EVAR era, still today 70% of patients with ruptured AAA are unaware of the diagnosis until the day of rupture. This statistic has been used as an important rallying cry for those advocating for the wider use of ultrasound screening to detect AAAs in targeted populations. Recently, the USPSTF and Medicare recommended screening in certain populations, most prominently, men over age 65 who have ever smoked. Screening has now been shown to reduce aneurysm-related mortality, all-cause mortality, and rupture rates in surveilled populations. Identifying the proper timing and extent of screening remains to be fully defined.

Most recently, our understanding of aneurysm repair was bolstered by the longer-term results of the EVAR-1, and DREAM trials, as well as some mature experiences in EVAR. All have shown that secondary interventions with EVAR are significantly more common than with open repair, and thus the need for ongoing surveillance and close monitoring is critical. Moreover, beyond the 8-year mark after repair in the EVAR-1 trial, all-cause mortality and aneurysm-related mortality were less in those undergoing open repair. Today, it is evident that EVAR decreases operative mortality at the cost of reintervention and later events, thus making patient selection and determination of patient longevity vital in repair considerations.

III. INDICATIONS FOR OPERATION

A. **A practical approach using aneurysm diameter.** Currently in our practice, patients with asymptomatic AAAs less than 5 cm are followed with ultrasound. For these patients, CT scans are typically not obtained and aneurysm repair is not recommended unless part of a clinical trial or if the most recent measurement confirms rapid expansion (i.e., more than 6 mm in 6 months or more than 1 cm in 1 year). Aneurysms less than 5 cm may occasionally be repaired as part of treatment for symptomatic aortoiliac occlusive disease with open (e.g., aortobifemoral bypass) or endovascular techniques.

Good-risk patients with aneurysms between 5 and 5.4 cm receive a contrast-enhanced aortic CT to define the size, shape, and extent of the aneurysm. Such patients are provided a summation of our clinical understanding of aneurysm observation versus repair, open and EVAR. Patients are made aware that although it is safe to observe aneurysms less than 5.5 cm, close surveillance will be required and it is likely that within 1 to 3 years the aneurysm will expand and repair will be required. Repair of asymptomatic aneurysms between 5 and 5.4 cm is not rushed and is strongly influenced by individual patient factors, such as medical comorbidity (e.g., risk of anesthesia), ability to commit to close surveillance, candidacy for EVAR, and level of patient anxiety regarding the aneurysm. **If these individual factors weigh in favor of repair, good-risk patients with AAAs between 5 and 5.4 cm are offered an operation either open or EVAR.** Finally all good-risk patients who present with an aneurysm of 5.5 cm or larger receive a contrast-enhanced aortic CT and are offered repair, open or EVAR, in an expeditious manner. A caveat in this is women, and smaller individuals whose aneurysms may be relatively larger compared to their body stature may be considered for a repair threshold of 5 cm.

For high-risk patients, older patients or those with more limited life expectancy and aneurysms greater than 5 cm, we defer to less invasive EVAR if aneurysm morphology permits. If such high-risk patients are not standard, infrarenal endovascular candidates, we may delay open operation until the aneurysm expands to 6 cm or becomes symptomatic. Today, most of these patients are considered for fenestrated endovascular repair (FEVAR) if the aneurysm is morphologically suitable.

B. A less common but more urgent indication for AAA repair is evidence of **peripheral emboli** in the lower extremities of patients with aneurysms.

C. **Urgent aneurysm repair is also indicated for patients with a known aneurysm that has become tender or is associated with abdominal or back pain.** These patients should be hospitalized and considered to have a symptomatic aneurysm, even though their vital signs may be normal and their abdominal symptoms nonspecific.

D. **Patients with ruptured aneurysms and shock should be taken directly to the operating room for resuscitation and operation.** With now decades of experience, improved devices, hybrid operating room development, and contemporary "on-the-shelf" endovascular inventories, use of endovascular ruptured repair (i.e., rEVAR) is an option that has become fully viable. Outcomes assessment for EVAR versus open repair in rupture is interesting. Medicare data and some observational studies suggest significant reduction in operative mortality with rEVAR, while three prospective, randomized trials (AJAX, IMPROVE, and ECAR) have indicated no survival benefit, either with rupture treatment or in the longer term.

IV. **PREOPERATIVE EVALUATION.** The preoperative evaluation for an elective AAA should define the size and extent of the aneurysm, associated medical risks, and associated vascular disease.

A. **Size and extent of AAA.** The reliability of the abdominal exam to detect and measure an AAA is poor. Information from the ADAM trial showed that the accuracy of the physical exam to detect an aneurysm in an individual with an abdominal girth of 38 inches or more was around 50%. The simplest and least expensive test to diagnose and measure an AAA is ultrasound. Measurement of the anterior-posterior diameter is more accurate than the transverse diameter, reliably measuring to within 2 to 3 mm. Ultrasound is also the favored method to follow changes in aneurysm diameter over time (i.e., aneurysm surveillance).

Although some prefer routine CT scan for patients with suspected or known small AAAs, this imaging modality costs more than ultrasound and carries morbidity associated with contrast administration and radiation. In our practices, contrast-enhanced aortic CT is reserved for aneurysms that are greater than 5 cm, tortuous and beyond the accuracy of ultrasound, or in which repair is actively, or in which repair is actively being planned. In addition to assessing the size of an AAA, a common reason to obtain a CT is anatomic evaluation for EVAR (Fig. 14.3). **In this regard, CT assesses the following characteristics of the proximal aortic and distal iliac artery seal or landing zones where the endograft is fixed, thereby excluding the aneurysm from flow and pressure:**

1. **The diameter and length in relation to branch arteries (e.g., renal and internal iliac arteries)**
2. **The degree of circumferential calcification and/or thrombus**

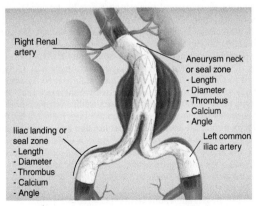

FIGURE 14.3 Evaluation for endovascular aneurysm repair (EVAR) includes evaluation of the landing or seal zones of the endograft, which include the aortic neck below the renal arteries as well as the iliac arteries. These zones of endograft fixation are evaluated for their length, diameter, degree of thrombus, degree of calcification, and degree of angle or tortuosity. If any one of these four variables or a combination of one or more is unfavorable, the likelihood of an effective seal is reduced and the aneurysm should not be considered a candidate for tradiaional, infrarenal EVAR. Depending on the experience of the institution, somewhere between 50% and 75% of AAAs are anatomic candidates for EVAR.

3. **The degree of tortuosity or angle of the neck, aneurysm, and iliac arteries**
4. **The length of aneurysm in relation to the aortic bifurcation and branch arteries**

   In addition, an aortic CT is indicated when a juxtarenal, suprarenal, or thoracoabdominal aneurysm is suspected. One must remember that CT scan may occasionally overestimate the diameter of an aneurysm because the measurements are made perpendicular to the body axis, which introduces some error if the aorta is tortuous. **This error can now be corrected for by use of modern CT software, which allows for maximum intensity projection (MIP) reconstructions and calculations referred to as center line measurements of aneurysm length and diameter.**

B. **Aortography** is not reliable for determining aneurysm diameter, as luminal thrombus obscures the outer limit of the aneurysm wall. Aortography prior to aneurysm repair, open or endovascular, should be used selectively for the following criteria:

1. Decreased peripheral pulses or symptoms of lower-extremity claudication
2. Poorly controlled hypertension or renal insufficiency indicating renal artery occlusive disease
3. Suprarenal or thoracoabdominal aortic aneurysms (TAAs) requiring delineation of visceral and intercostal arteries
4. Symptoms of intestinal ischemia suggesting visceral artery occlusive disease
5. Suspected horseshoe kidney with multiple renal arteries on ultrasound or CT

   Although once commonplace, aortography prior to EVAR or open repair is now rarely necessary because of the high quality of dynamic, spiral, contrast-enhanced aortic CT. One or more of these criteria for preoperative aortography are present in fewer than 10% of patients with AAA, making this invasive preoperative test uncommon. Many times these features may be delineated on fine-cut aortic CT, and a plan to address them in either a staged or simultaneous manner to the aneurysm repair is made.

C. **Medical risks.** Most medical comorbidities can be detected by the performance of a thorough history and physical exam, both of which are outlined in more detail in Chapters 3 and 6. As many as 50% of patients with AAAs have some degree of coronary artery disease. Evidence-based guidelines offered by the American Heart Association (AHA) and the American College of Cardiology (ACC) regarding evaluation prior to AAA repair are outlined in Chapter 7. These guidelines include recommendations for preoperative cardiac testing and selective preoperative cardiac revascularization. **In the context of these guidelines, traditional open aortic aneurysm repair is categorized as a high-risk procedure (see Table 7.5) because of the need for an abdominal or retroperitoneal incision and cross-clamping of the aorta.** Endovascular aneurysm repair should be considered an intermediate risk procedure (see Table 7.5) as it may be done under regional or local anesthesia, does not require aortic cross-clamp, and is now performed percutaneously in many cases. In our experience, adherence to the AHA/ACC Clinical Guidelines contributes to a low elective operative mortality for open (3% to 4%) and endovascular (<2%) AAA repair.

   A more aggressive approach to AAA repair in older or high-risk patients has been advocated by some. EVAR now clearly offers an option that is safer for many of these patients although they must still be carefully selected and treated by an experienced anesthesia and endovascular team. Under these conditions, EVAR in high-risk patients can now be accomplished with an operative mortality of less than 5%. If not repaired, many of these high-risk patients with larger AAAs will succumb to aneurysm rupture.

D. **Associated vascular disease. Approximately 10% of patients with an AAA will have associated carotid occlusive disease in the form of an asymptomatic carotid bruit or symptoms such as TIA or stroke.** In our practice, these patients undergo carotid duplex to determine the significance of the carotid disease (Chapter 5). Patients with symptomatic carotid stenoses undergo expeditious treatment of the carotid prior to AAA repair even if the aneurysm is large. In these cases, the timing of the AAA repair depends on the size of the aneurysm and, unless it is quite large (>7 cm) or symptomatic, the aneurysm repair is performed a week or two after treatment of the symptomatic carotid. Patients with asymptomatic carotid stenoses may undergo elective AAA repair prior to carotid endarterectomy. Exceptions to this are patients with asymptomatic unilateral preocclusive stenosis or bilateral high-grade stenoses, in which case it is reasonable to treat the carotid prior to AAA repair. However, patients with symptomatic or large aneurysms (>7 cm) should undergo AAA repair without delay for carotid surgery. Overall, the risk of perioperative stroke from carotid occlusive disease during AAA repair is low, and clinical evidence supporting preoperative carotid treatment is lacking.

V. **PREOPERATIVE PREPARATION FOR ELECTIVE AAA REPAIR IS NOW OCCUPIED MOSTLY BY STUDY OF AORTIC CT RECONSTRUCTIONS IN CONSIDERATION OF EVAR.** Suitability for EVAR, type of endograft, and specific endovascular approach all require significant consideration and planning. To this end, it is our practice to have more than one set of eyes evaluate the aortic CT prior to final decisions regarding EVAR. This is productive when in the form of discussion within our vascular and endovascular surgery groups, but may also be accomplished with experienced radiologists or even trusted clinical specialists employed by industry. Careful evaluation of the aortic CT in these forums helps the endovascular specialist anticipate and plan for "trouble spots" during EVAR before starting the case. This type of disciplined preoperative preparation before EVAR maximizes the likelihood of a successful treatment and minimizes the chances of a misguided endovascular attempt.

VI. **MANAGEMENT OF A RUPTURED ANEURYSM.** As noted, EVAR has been utilized to treat ruptured AAAs, but in many institutions, without advanced endovascular programs, management remains emergent open repair. The key to successful management of a ruptured AAA with open or endovascular techniques is expeditious movement of the patient to the operating room. While most patients who are candidates for rEVAR will tolerate prompt CTA for quick planning, delay in the emergency or radiology departments often results in deterioration and death from hemorrhage.

Traditionally, only about half of patients with a ruptured AAA who arrive at the hospital were discharged alive. More recent analyses suggest this may be slowly improving. Factors predicting poor outcome or death are profound shock, cardiac arrest (need for CPR), preexisting cardiac or renal disease, and technical complications during the operation. Several factors, however, can enhance the likelihood of survival for a patient with a ruptured AAA.

A. **Rapid transport.** Patients with suspected AAA rupture should be transported or transferred rapidly to a hospital prepared for aneurysm patients, where a surgical team should be waiting for assessment and resuscitation. An operating room should be readied as the patient arrives.

B. **Resuscitation** should include two large-bore (14 or 16 gauge) intravenous lines, a nasogastric tube, and a Foley catheter. Blood should be typed and cross-matched for packed red blood cells. Crystalloid solutions are acceptable for initial volume administration; however, emergency release type O negative or cross-matched blood and fresh frozen plasma should be given at a 1:1 ratio to patients with evidence of shock (i.e., component blood therapy). **In a strategy referred to as *permissive hypotension*, blood pressure should be maintained only to a level to support urine output and mental status.** Systolic pressures of 90 to 100 mm Hg are adequate if the patient is awake with some urine output. Inotropic agents, vasopressors, and overuse of crystalloid with the goal of achieving a normal blood pressure will worsen the situation by causing hemorrhage before bleeding can be controlled in the operating room.

If available, a rapid autotransfusion device (i.e., cell saver) should be set up in the operating room. Arterial and central venous lines can be placed and prophylactic antibiotics administered in the operating room.

C. **Accurate diagnosis.** If the patient has no previous diagnosis of AAA or the diagnosis is in question, ultrasound in the emergency department is the most expeditious method to determine the presence or absence of AAA. If the patient has shown no evidence of hemodynamic compromise, or if EVAR is an option at the institution, an aortic CT scan should be considered. An ECG should also be performed to rule out acute myocardial infarction.

D. **Immediate operation.** A patient who has had hemodynamic compromise (e.g., syncope or shock) and has a pulsatile abdominal mass or a known AAA should be taken directly to the operating room. Performance of a contrast aortic CT in this setting is risky and should only be directed by an experienced endovascular surgeon who is present and who is considering emergent EVAR for ruptured AAA.

E. **Temperature control.** Patients with a ruptured AAA and shock become hypothermic quickly. Those with a body temperature below 33°C develop capillary leak syndrome necessitating more volume, manifest a diffuse coagulopathy, and slip suddenly into life-threatening cardiac arrhythmias. The three useful means of preventing hypothermia are **(a) warming the operating room to 70°F to 80°F before the patient arrives, (b) using the Bair Hugger warming tent over the upper thorax and head, and (c) use of high-volume, countercurrent warming infusing systems for all administered intravenous fluids.**

F. **Aortic control can be obtained by open aortic clamping or with insertion of a large compliant aortic occlusion balloon from a femoral or brachial artery sheath.** Since blood pressure can decrease precipitously with induction of anesthesia, the patient should be prepped, and the necessary arterial sheaths and occlusion balloons positioned prior to the patient being anesthetized. If open repair is pursued, a midline incision is the most common approach. Sometimes, the retroperitoneal approach may be chosen. If the retroperitoneal hematoma is massive, initial aortic control should be gained by compression or clamping of the aorta at the diaphragm (Fig. 14.4). In many patients, however, the aorta can be clamped below the renal arteries. At this site, care must be taken to avoid injury to the duodenum and left renal vein. Rarely, a patient with multiple prior abdominal operations may need a left thoracotomy for initial aortic clamping. Prior to clamping, mannitol (25 g) may be given as a diuretic and free-radical scavenger.

G. **Anticoagulation.** Administration of heparin during ruptured AAA repair may be problematic. If the patient is hypothermic and in shock, a coagulopathy may already exist. On the other hand, lower-extremity thrombosis is not uncommon during ruptured AAA repair. Consequently, smaller systemic doses of heparin (2,500 to 3,000 units) or regional administration of heparin into the iliac arteries may decrease lower-extremity thrombosis.

H. Assessing limb and vital organ perfusion. Lower-extremity perfusion must be assessed before leaving the operating room. This can be achieved by palpating pulses, listening for Doppler signals, or by using calf plethysmographic pulse waveforms. If a significant thrombus or embolus is suspected to either lower extremity, thromboembolectomy should be performed using a Fogarty catheter. In these instances, removal of the thrombus or embolus and restoration of flow to the extremity is best

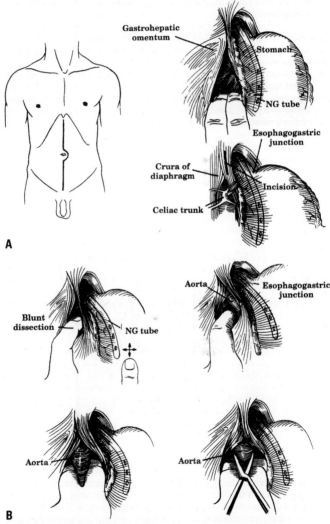

FIGURE 14.4 (A, B) Supraceliac aortic clamping is useful for large ruptured abdominal aortic aneurysms and huge retroperitoneal hematomas that obscure the proximal aneurysm neck at the renal level. *NG,* nasogastric. (The Mayo Foundation, with permission.)

achieved by exposure and opening of the femoral artery of the affected leg as opposed to attempts from the abdomen.

Likewise, the colon should be inspected for viability. If questionable, intravenous fluorescein can be given and the bowel inspected with a Wood's lamp. When the abdomen is massively distended, a tight primary closure may cause abdominal compartment syndrome and compromise renal or visceral perfusion. In such instances, the abdominal fascia should not be closed and the abdominal contents covered with a temporary abdominal closure. Delayed closure of the fascia can be accomplished in 48 to 72 hours when patient physiology and abdominal edema have improved.

VII. **TECHNICAL ASPECTS OF AAA REPAIR.** The following section briefly reviews some of the technical aspects involved with open and endovascular aneurysm repair (Fig. 14.3).

A. **Open aneurysm exposure may be performed through a midline or left retroperitoneal approach** (Fig. 14.5). Both exposures have certain advantages, and use of one over the other tends to be specific to the institution or surgeon. Those who prefer a midline incision and the inframesocolic transperitoneal approach cite the excellent exposure of the entire aneurysm—both

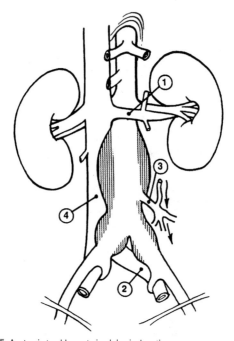

FIGURE 14.5 Anatomic trouble spots in abdominal aortic aneurysm exposure. (1) The left renal vein or one of its branches (left renal lumbar, gonadal, or adrenal) may be injured during exposure of the aneurysm neck, especially with ruptured aneurysms. In 5% of cases, the left renal vein lies posterior to the aorta and may be injured in any attempt to encircle the proximal aorta for control. (2) The common iliac veins are usually adherent to the iliac arteries and may be injured during dissection. (3) The inferior mesenteric artery should be ligated on or within the aneurysm sac to avoid ligation of critical collateral vessels from the marginal artery of Drummond. (4) Dissection of the aneurysm sac from the vena cava is usually unnecessary.

renal arteries and both iliac arteries. The disadvantage of the transperitoneal approach is the open exposure of the bowel contents and a larger, more painful incision. The retroperitoneal exposure is touted by some to be less painful, improve postoperative respiratory mechanics, and to produce less physiologic stress because it avoids exposure of the bowel contents, which remain in the peritoneal sack. The disadvantage of retroperitoneal exposure is that it provides limited exposure of the right renal and common iliac arteries, which may be particularly important in some cases.

For aneurysms that extend to the renal arteries, transperitoneal exposure of the renal arteries and suprarenal aorta may be facilitated by division of the left renal vein, leaving the adrenal and gonadal veins as outflow for the left kidney. Another alternative is extensive mobilization of the left renal vein by division of the adrenal, gonadal, and lumbar branches, allowing the vein to be retracted up or down to expose the suprarenal aortic segment. Those who advocate the retroperitoneal approach point out that this exposure facilitates visualization of the suprarenal aortic segment without manipulation of the left renal vein, as the left kidney including the left renal vein is reflected up with the peritoneal contents away from the aorta. After isolation of the proximal and distal clamp sites, intravenous heparin (100 unit/kg) and occasionally mannitol (25 g) is administered and allowed to circulate for 5 minutes.

B. **Flow through the aneurysm is arrested by proximal and distal clamping.** This should be confirmed by palpating the aneurysm to assure the absence of pulsatility. Once this is confirmed, the aneurysm is opened, the layered mural thrombus removed, and the back-bleeding lumbar arteries suture ligated. Attention is also given to the inferior mesenteric artery, which most often has back bleeding into the open aneurysm sac. Depending upon the degree of bleeding from the inferior mesenteric artery (IMA) and surgeon preference, the IMA may either be ligated or temporarily occluded until the graft has been sutured in place and perfusion to the lower extremities reestablished. The prosthetic graft is sutured to the normal proximal aortic neck inside the aneurysm sac after the proximal aneurysm has been cut down to allow formation of a good sewing ring **(Creech technique)**. This sequence of steps from clamping, opening the aneurysm, occluding back-bleeding vessels, and suturing in a graft in the bed of the aneurysm to restore antegrade flow is referred to as **endoaneurysmorrhaphy.** In cases where the duodenum is adherent to the AAA **(e.g., inflammatory aneurysm)**, we do not dissect it from the aneurysm but attempt to work around it. If infection is suspected, the aneurysm should be cultured and completely excised. After the graft is in place, the clamps removed, and flow restored, perfusion to the colon is assessed and in most cases the inferior mesenteric artery may then be ligated. In instances where normal circulation to the bowel may not be present, such as a previous colon resection, the inferior mesenteric artery may be implanted onto the prosthetic graft.

C. **Retroperitoneal coverage** of the graft should be completed using the aneurysm sac to separate the graft from the intestine. If this is not done, the intestine, especially the duodenum, can adhere to the graft years later and result in an aortoenteric fistula.

D. **EVAR was introduced by Parodi in the early 1990s and is now the operative approach for the majority of AAAs treated in the United States.** EVAR involves the passage of self-expandable, covered stents (i.e., stent grafts) into the aorta through the femoral arteries. Precise positioning of the stent graft below the renal arteries and in the desired iliac "landing zones" is achieved using fluoroscopy and contrast arteriography. As the stent graft is fixed at normal arterial segments at the proximal infrarenal aorta (i.e., neck) and the iliac arteries, the AAA is excluded from flow and, therefore, arterial pressure. If appropriate fixation and seal is achieved, flow and pressure go through the graft, allowing the walls of the AAA to be depressurized and in many cases decrease in size and "shrink" or "heal" around the graft. Constructs of EVAR include bifurcated devices into both iliac arteries, or more rarely, aorto-uni-iliac grafts used in conjunction with a femoral to femoral bypass and iliac occlusion in some way to prevent retrograde flow into the aneurysm. Proximal endograft components may have bare, suprarenal fixation stents.

Incomplete positioning or sealing of the aneurysm sac following endograft placement results in endoleak (Fig. 14.6). Endoleaks are categorized into four main groups according to their cause and may not be significant depending upon the category. **Type I endoleaks** result from failure of primary graft-artery seal points at the aortic neck or iliac arteries and are generally considered a technical failure of endograft placement. Examples of type I endoleak include failure to achieve a seal at the proximal aortic neck below the renal arteries resulting in antegrade flow around the deployed stent into the aneurysm sac (Ia); failure to achieve seal at the iliac distal seal zone resulting in back flow into the sac (Ib); or back flow into the sac around an iliac occlusion device (Ic). Type I endoleaks leave the aneurysm fully pressurized and should be corrected in the operating room. **Type II endoleaks** represent back bleeding into the aneurysm sac from the inferior mesenteric artery (IIa) or patent lumbar arteries (IIB). Type II endoleaks are present at the conclusion of up to 25% of EVAR cases and are not immediately treated, as most do not pressurize the aneurysm sac and will resolve over time. Type II endoleaks are only relevant if they persist and if the aneurysm sac does not decrease in diameter, or continues to expand, over a period of 1 to 2 years. In these

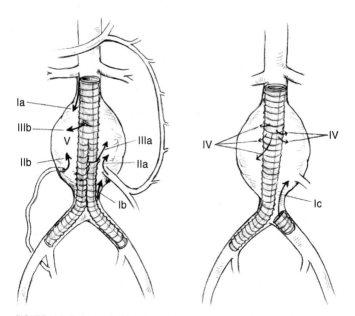

FIGURE 14.6 Endoleak. Endoleak types after endovascular abdominal aortic aneurysm repair. (From Eliason JL, Upchurch GR Jr. Endovascular abdominal aortic aneurysm repair. *Circulation.* 2008;117(13):1738-1744.)

cases, type II endoleaks can be treated with the endovascular technique of coil embolization. **Type III endoleaks** represent flow into the aneurysm sac from junction points in the modular bifurcated endografts (IIIa) or disruptions of the graft material (IIIb). Like type I leaks, type III leaks are viewed as a technical failure of the endograft and should be corrected when they are identified or soon thereafter, as the aneurysm sac remains pressurized. **Type IV endoleaks** represent flow into the aneurysm sac from porosity in the graft material itself. Type IV endoleaks are uncommon and are treated individually depending on their appearance on imaging studies (e.g., CTA or aortography) and whether or not the aneurysm sac is decreasing in diameter. **Type V endoleak** is given the term "endotension," which implies sac pressurization and growth without a radiographically identified endoleak.

Although EVAR is successful, with a 98% technical success rate, and studies show lower morbidity and mortality with its use compared to open repair, it does have drawbacks. Specifically, as noted above, following EVAR, patients require more graft surveillance and even reintervention than patients who have undergone open repair. The follow-up of endografts is necessary to assess aneurysm size and the presence or absence of endoleaks. This follow-up regimen includes contrast-enhanced CT scans, which can lead to detrimental effects on renal function over years of surveillance. The use of contrast CT scans to follow endografts has been reduced in recent years with increased reliance on duplex ultrasound. Recent studies have shown that 25% of patients who have undergone EVAR will require some graft-related reintervention at 5 years, compared to 2% of patients who have undergone open repair. Nearly all these interventions are performed with endovascular techniques and include treatment of endoleaks.

VIII. **CONCURRENT INTRA-ABDOMINAL DISEASE**. As a rule, we prefer not to combine elective AAA surgery with other intra-abdominal procedures that could be safely postponed. Therefore, if the coexisting pathology does not have an urgent need to be treated (e.g., asymptomatic gallstones), we proceed with the planned aneurysm repair, open or EVAR.

If the coexisting disease process has urgency, such as the case of gastrointestinal or genitourinary malignancy, we then consider the size of the AAA and whether it can be treated with EVAR. If the AAA is 5.5 cm or larger and EVAR is an option, we proceed with endovascular repair quickly, allowing full focus on treatment of the urgent malignancy or other disease process in the weeks that follow. If the aneurysm is 5 to 5.4 cm or is not an endovascular candidate and the coexisting process has urgency, we defer treatment of the AAA until after the other pathology has been addressed. This is especially the case in instances where the other disease process is symptomatic, such as cholelithiasis, cholecystitis, or an obstructing colon cancer. In these cases, we follow the aneurysm closely in the perioperative period with ultrasound or even CT, as there have been anecdotal reports of aneurysm expansion following abdominal operations for other reasons.

On the rare occasion when intra-abdominal pathology is encountered during open AAA repair, the aneurysm repair should proceed as planned in almost all cases. This is particularly the case when the aneurysm is greater than 5.5 cm. Even in cases where pathology is incidentally noted or palpated in the bowel or solid organs, the open aneurysm repair should be completed and the findings noted in the operative dictation. Appropriate consultation, imaging, and endoscopy should be made in the early postoperative period in such cases. The only exception to this rule may be in a patient with an aneurysm less than 5.5 cm in whom an obstructing colon cancer is encountered at the time of open AAA repair. In such a case, it would be reasonable to leave the aneurysm untreated and turn focus to the obstructing colon cancer, recognizing that the aneurysm would require close observation in the perioperative period.

IX. **POSTOPERATIVE COMPLICATIONS.** Early postoperative complications include cardiac or respiratory dysfunction, postoperative bleeding, and renal insufficiency (Chapters 7 and 8). Graft-limb thrombosis or lower-extremity embolization can lead to lower-extremity ischemia requiring urgent intervention. **Colon ischemia occurs in 1% to 2% of AAA repairs and usually manifests in the early postoperative period as a bloody bowel movement.** In these cases, urgent lower endoscopy is indicated to make the diagnosis of colon ischemia and to allow appropriate treatment, such as broad spectrum antibiotics, aggressive resuscitation, or return to the operating room for removal of nonviable colon. Aortoenteric fistula, anastomotic aneurysm, prosthetic graft infection, and sexual dysfunction are complications seen in the later postoperative period.

X. **LONG-TERM FOLLOW-UP.** Long-term survival following elective AAA repair is 70% to 80% at 5 years and 50% at 10 years, which is less than that in age-matched controls without AAA. As discussed above, long-term survival in those who are candidates for both types of repair is similar between EVAR and open repair with more aneurysm-related problems and reduced long-term survival starting at the 8- to 10-year mark postrepair. Many times, older and less fit patients are more likely to undergo EVAR, and this may be irrelevant but has implications for patient selection. One of the most important factors in long-term survival of patients following AAA repair is the presence or absence of coronary heart disease. Patients with clinically evident heart disease have a decreased survival of 50% at 5 years and only 30% at 10 years. Although less common than cardiac morbidity, stroke affects 5% of patients at 5 years and 10% at 10 years following aneurysm repair.

  Late graft-related complications following AAA repair include graft limb occlusion, graft infection, and anastomotic aneurysm. These long-term complications are less frequent following open AAA repair (0.5% to 1% per year) than following EVAR (up to 5% per year). Additionally, up to 25% of patients will develop aneurysmal dilation of the aorta proximal to the AAA repair over time. Although these aneurysms in the paravisceral or thoracic aorta are often small, their incidence along with that of graft-related complications confirms the need to periodically check patients who have undergone AAA repair.

  Specifically, we evaluate patients twice in the first year after open AAA repair and annually thereafter. The evaluation includes a physical exam of the femoral and popliteal arteries, a duplex ultrasound of the aortic graft, and a chest x-ray. If no other concerns are present, contrast CT scan of the aorta is obtained every 5 years following open AAA repair. **Postoperative surveillance following EVAR is changing with an increased reliance on duplex ultrasound compared to contrast CT scan.** In our practice, patients who have undergone an uncomplicated EVAR receive one contrast-enhanced CT scan and an aortic duplex in the month following the procedure. If there is no endoleak, we repeat the duplex in 6 months and the CT scan at the 1-year mark following EVAR. Without evidence of endoleak and aneurysm growth, annual duplex scan can be performed with CT scan every 2 to 3 years in these patients. In those with renal dysfunction, noncontrast CT is used along with duplex. If the 1-month postoperative CT shows a type II endoleak, the CT is repeated at 6 months, to assess for enlargement of the aneurysm or endoleak closure. Identification of a type I or III endoleak or aneurysm enlargement

(>3 mm) is an indication for a formal aortogram to more thoroughly evaluate the endograft and the dynamics of the aneurysm and consideration for secondary intervention. Most endoleaks and graft-related complications following EVAR can be treated with endovascular techniques.

JUXTARENAL/SUPRARENAL ABDOMINAL ANEURYSM

Aneurysms of the abdominal aorta may be more extensive. Juxtarenal aneurysms are those in which the neck of the aneurysm is short and its length is 10 mm or less from the renal arteries. Suprarenal aneurysms involve at least one renal artery origin. These may be approached via midline or retroperitoneal/thoracoabdominal incisions. Aortic control requires clamping in the supraceliac aorta or in the "renovisceral" segment among these arteries. Proximal graft reconstruction may require beveling of the aortic graft and/ or renal or visceral artery bypasses. In more complex cases, renal preservation with cold, crystalloid-based solutions as discussed below with thoracoabdominal aneurysm may be used. Open repair of these aneurysms can be accomplished with very similar outcomes to infrarenal open AAA repair.

Fenestrated or branched endovascular grafts (F/BEVARs) along with "chimney, periscope, sandwich, or snorkel: CHIMPS," techniques to repair these aneurysms are now an everyday reality, and their use is now widespread. These provide the ability to extend the proximal seal zone into more healthy aorta. F/BEVAR technology incorporates scallops to preserve branch flow, and fenestrations for stents to be placed into renovisceral vessels in an endograft construct individually built based upon patient anatomy (Fig. 14.7). CHIMPS

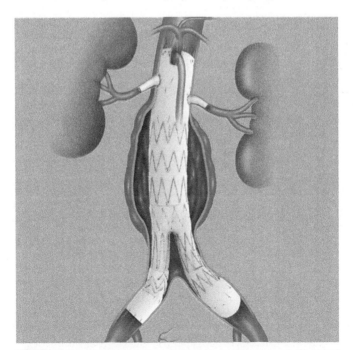

FIGURE 14.7 Fenestrated endovascular graft. Fenestrated endovascular repair of juxtarenal aneurysm with bilateral renal artery fenestrations and covered renal stents as well as an SMA scallop to provide proximal seal in the aorta above a juxtarenal aneurysm.

is performed by placing parallel grafts into the renal and visceral vessels next to the aortic graft component. Work is being done to create an endovascular construct for these types of aneurysms, which is more generalizable and perhaps someday "on the shelf." The operative and long-term results of these endovascular repairs for juxtarenal and suprarenal aneurysms are taking shape. Their technical success is over 95% although the need for reintervention can approach 25% to 30% at 5 years. Aneurysm-related mortality, a marker of adequate longer-term aneurysm treatment, is low.

THORACOABDOMINAL AORTIC ANEURYSM

TAA is defined as simultaneous aneurysm involvement of the thoracic and abdominal aortic segments. TAAs represent less than 10% of degenerative aortic aneurysms and are classified based on a scheme reported by E. Stanley Crawford (Fig. 14.8). Natural history data on TAAs reveal a negligible rupture risk for aneurysms less than 4 cm. In contrast, 5-year rupture risk is nearly 20% for TAAs between 4 and 6 cm and 33% for those greater than 6 cm. Therefore, the threshold for open repair has traditionally been an aneurysm diameter of 6 cm in healthy patients or for aneurysms that have expanded 1 cm in a year's time. Open repair of TAAs was the only option for treatment until 2005, when the FDA approved a commercially available thoracic aortic stent graft. The role of thoracic endovascular aneurysm repair (TEVAR) in the treatment of thoracic aortic aneurysms (TA) has now become clearer with TEVAR, providing superior operative outcomes compared to thoracotomy and open repair. Aneurysm-related mortality long-term is low. However, introduction of endovascular techniques as a less invasive option to repair thoracoabdominal aneurysms (TAA) has generated considerable enthusiasm. Experience grows rapidly particularly in centers of excellence with FDA-approved investigational device exemptions (IDEs). The developmental limitations have included appropriate branch/fenestrated graft designs for durable renovisceral perfusion and limiting spinal cord ischemia (Fig. 14.9). Operative results and midterm outcomes in expert hands are impressive and reasonable. More will be learned of this technique in the next few years.

I. **PREOPERATIVE EVALUATION.** In addition to history and physical, a contrast-enhanced dynamic CT scan of the aorta is required. Because of the tortuosity of the thoracic aorta, it is important that measurements of diameter be made perpendicular and not tangential to the aortic centerline axis. Accurate measurements can best be obtained using axial centerline software with 3D reconstructions, which allows for sizing of diameter and assessments of length within the aneurysm. Although contrast aortography was historically mandatory prior to TAA repair, advances in CT imaging have allowed this invasive preoperative test to be performed selectively. One indication proposed by some for preoperative aortography is localization of the great radicular artery (i.e., **artery of Adamkiewicz**), which is felt to be useful in decreasing the risk of perioperative spinal cord ischemia. Even this has been largely abandoned with the continued evolution and detail in spiral CTA and MRA. This artery arises from a T_9 to T_{12} intercostal artery in 75% of patients and is the main blood supply to the anterior spinal artery. The utility of preoperative localization of this artery in reducing the incidence of cord ischemia has not been universally accepted, and most groups rely on other perioperative adjuncts to avoid this often devastating complication.

II. **OPERATIVE PRINCIPLES.** The open operative approach to TAA follows one of two distinct methods: (a) **clamp-and-sew** with adjuncts used to

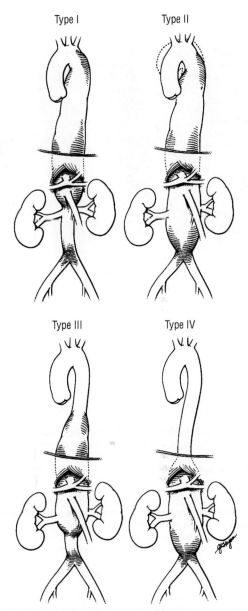

FIGURE 14.8 Crawford classification of thoracoabdominal aortic aneurysms. (From Crawford ES, Crawford JL, Safi HJ. Thoracoabdominal aortic aneurysms: preoperative and intraoperative factors determining immediate and long-term results of operations in 805 patients. *J Vasc Surg*. 1986;3:389-404, with permission.)

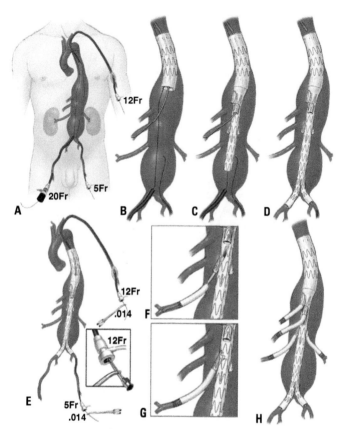

FIGURE 14.9 Total endovascular repair of a thoracoabdominal aneurysm using a branched endograft with covered stents into the renovisceral arteries. Bilateral femoral and left axillary accesses are used. (From Darling RC, Ozaki CK. *Master Techniques in Surgery: Vascular Surgery: Arterial Procedures.* Philadelphia: Wolters Kluwer Health; 2016, with permission.)

minimize end-organ ischemia or (b) **distal aortic perfusion with sequential clamping** of the graft. Both use a left thoracoabdominal approach, and the choice is influenced by the experience of the surgical, anesthesia, and intensive care teams. The renovisceral segment can be sewn into the graft as a patch with a left renal bypass, or individual grafts from the aortic graft can be used. Most larger volume centers dealing with TAA have transitioned to distal perfusion as operative results have been shown to be superior with this strategy. Operative death, paraplegia, and hemodialysis rates of 5% or less each are described. The following are adjuncts used individually or together during TAA repair to reduce morbidity (Fig. 14.10).

A. **Distal aortic perfusion** is achieved with left atrial to femoral artery bypass utilizing a Bio-Medicus pump (Medtronics, Minneapolis, MN, USA). This technique provides distal perfusion to the lower extremities, pelvis, and renovisceral arteries during aortic graft placement and may benefit the

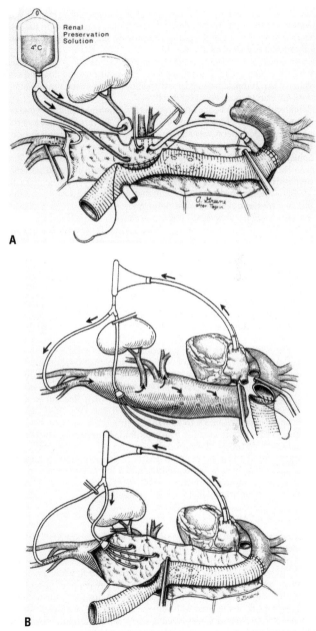

FIGURE 14.10 Strategies for open thoracoabdominal aneurysm repair. **(A)** Clamp-and-sew with inline mesenteric shunting, renal cold perfusion, and spinal cord hypothermia. **(B)** Distal aortic perfusion with sequential clamping and renovisceral perfusion and motor-evoked potential-guided intercostal reconstruction.

heart by unloading the left ventricle during aortic cross-clamp. When working within the renovisceral segment, individual perfusion catheters from the arterial line of the pump can provide simultaneous perfusion to other renal and visceral arteries.

B. **Regional spinal cord hypothermia** (mean 26°C) using an epidural catheter with infusion of cold saline reduces the metabolic rate and demand of the spinal cord. Temperature and pressure may be monitored simultaneously with a separate intrathecal catheter.

C. **Cerebrospinal fluid drainage** improves perfusion pressure of the spinal cord when pressure is greater than 10 to 15 cm H_2O. This technique is commonly used perioperatively and for 1 to 3 days following the operation.

D. **Renal cooling.** Direct application of ice and infusion of renal preservation solution (4°C lactated Ringer's with mannitol and methylprednisolone) into the renal artery after opening the aorta reduces local metabolic demands and stimulates diuresis. Warm blood perfusion from the Bio-Medicus pump can also be used with distal aortic perfusion.

E. **In-line mesenteric shunting.** After performance of the proximal anastomosis, an arterial perfusion catheter is placed from the proximal graft to the celiac or superior mesenteric artery ostia. This allows prograde, pulsatile perfusion to the viscera while the remainder of the graft is being placed. This is largely an adjunct used with clamp-and-sew technique.

III. **POSTOPERATIVE COURSE.** Operative mortality of TAA repair averages 4% to 8% but is much higher in urgent or emergent cases. Other factors that are associated with higher morbidity and mortality are preoperative renal dysfunction (Cr 1.8 mg/dL), intraoperative hypotension, intraoperative transfusion requirements, the development of postoperative spinal cord ischemia, and hypothermia (<35°C).

   Respiratory failure is the most common complication following TAA repair (15% to 40%). Risk factors are active smoking, baseline pulmonary disease, and division of the phrenic nerve during thoracoabdominal exposure. The incidence of **spinal cord ischemic complications** ranges from 4% to 16% in large series following all types of TAA. This can be as high as 30% in patients with extensive type I and II TAA (Fig. 14.8). **Renal failure** can be expected in 5% to 20% of patients following TAA repair and increases the risk of mortality nearly tenfold. A survival of 55% to 75% at 5 years can be expected following elective TAA repair with cardiac events representing the leading cause of death. Rupture of another aneurysm accounts for 3% to 5% of late deaths, and a later aortic event or graft-related complication may occur in up to 18% of surviving patients, emphasizing the importance of lifelong aortic surveillance.

AORTIC DISSECTION

Dissection is a common vascular catastrophe affecting the aorta and is distinct from degenerative aneurysms. Dissection results from an aortic defect that allows a false lumen to form between the intima and adventitia. The DeBakey classification of aortic dissection includes types I and II, which involve the ascending aorta, and type III, which involves only the descending aorta (Fig. 14.11). The Stanford classification includes type A, involving the ascending aorta, and type B, involving only the descending aorta. Complications of dissection include aortic valve insufficiency, aneurysm formation, aortic rupture, and coronary, cerebral, visceral, renal, or peripheral ischemia.

I. **PREOPERATIVE EVALUATION.** Aortic dissections present as tearing chest or back pain in patients between the ages of 50 and 70 years. A history

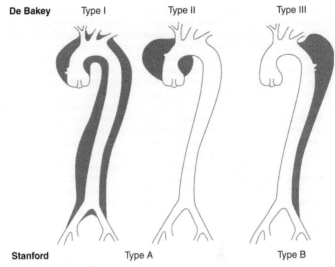

FIGURE 14.11 Classifications of aortic dissection. (From Herzog E. *Cardiac Care Unit Survival Guide*. Philadelphia: Wolters Kluwer Health; 2013, with permission.)

of hypertension is present in 80% to 90% of patients. The physical exam should be mindful of branch arteries from the aorta, which may be rendered ischemic by the dissection plane. End-organ ischemia can present in the coronary, cerebral, visceral (i.e., mesenteric or renal), or extremity distribution. Initial diagnostic tests should include an EKG and chest radiograph, but the diagnosis of aortic dissection is made by contrast-enhanced dynamic aortic CT. Gadolinium-enhanced MRA has also been found to be effective in most institutions but generally takes considerably longer to obtain than CT. Contrast aortography is generally reserved for individuals in whom an intervention is planned and not simply as a diagnostic modality.

II. **MANAGEMENT. A critical initial step in the management of aortic dissection is to decrease the mean arterial pressure and contracting force of the heart.** This is achieved foremost with intravenous beta-blockade. Sodium nitroprusside can be useful as a secondary agent but only after the patient has been started on a beta-blocker and stabilized, so as not to cause untoward vasodilation with a compensatory increase in heart rate and contractility. Nearly all patients with dissections involving the ascending aorta (DeBakey, types I and II; Stanford type A) require emergent surgery to prevent nearly uniform death from cardiac tamponade, coronary ischemia, or aortic regurgitation with acute heart failure. This involves replacement of the ascending aorta and sometimes the aortic valve via a median sternotomy in order to abolish direct false lumen flow. Today, if the dissection is a DeBakey type I and there is concern for later further aortic intervention procedures, replacing all or part of the aortic arch potentially including either a graft sewn to the distal aortic arch and everted into the descending aorta (elephant trunk technique) or even the placement of a thoracic endograft retrograde through the open sternotomy while on hypothermic circulatory arrest (frozen elephant trunk) may facilitate later endovascular descending aortic repair by providing a proximal landing zone. Open repair is also simplified in this scenario as an aortic graft can be sewn to either the everted open graft or the end of the placed endograft. Type A dissection is a serious medical condition that even when treated surgically carries up to a 20% in-hospital mortality. **DeBakey type III or Stanford type B dissections can be managed medically in the acute setting 90% of the time.** Intervention in the acute phase, mostly consisting of TEVAR-based approaches, and rarely today open surgery via a left thoracoabdominal approach are reserved for the 5% to 10% of patients who develop complications of dissection. **Complications from type B dissections that constitute indication for immediate intervention include development of end-organ ischemia (malperfusion), aortic rupture, and refractory or recurrent pain.** Open surgery in the acute phase carries a very high mortality (30%) which is why medical therapy is so important. When dissections become complicated, a "complication-specific" approach should be used. TEVAR to cover the proximal entry tear with stenting into renovisceral vessels and sometimes infrarenal stenting to augment true lumen flow is key. This approach has reduced mortality to 5% to 10% in complicated type B dissection. Should lower extremity ischemia be a problem, a femoral to femoral bypass is also an option depending on dissection anatomy.

III. **POSTOPERATIVE COURSE.** Patients with Stanford A dissections have a higher likelihood of death in the first 24 to 48 hours after onset than patients with Stanford B dissections if not surgically corrected. Stanford A dissections carry an operative mortality of approximately 10% to 20%. A 5-year survival of 75% to 85% exists in patients who leave the hospital alive following type A dissection with 15% to 25% needing another aortic intervention. The story of type B dissection is a bit more controversial. Most patients are treated medically and do well. However, 40% develop aneurysmal degeneration of the dissected aorta over time, leading to another intervention. Predictors of this aneurysmal formation are related to initial aortic size, persistent false lumen flow, and entry tear morphology. This leads to the current hot topic regarding endovascular treatment of "uncomplicated" type B dissection early in its course to allow the aorta to essentially heal or remodel. The INSTEAD and ADSORB trials, as well as the International Registry of Aortic Dissection (IRAD), have shown survival benefit with this approach. Long-term survival has been improved to 75% to 80% over 5 years with intervention compared to 50% to 60% without.

FEMORAL ARTERY ANEURYSM

True femoral artery aneurysms (FAAs) usually are found in male patients who have AAAs and/or aneurysms of the popliteal artery. In contrast to AAAs, the natural history of femoral artery is not expansion and rupture but rather distal embolization and thrombosis, which occur in about 30% of FAAs. In these instances, patients present with acute limb ischemia requiring urgent intervention. For these reasons, elective surgical repair is warranted in most cases when FAAs are discovered. This is particularly true if the FAA is greater than or equal to 3.5 cm or there is a large thrombus burden.

I. **PREOPERATIVE EVALUATION.** Because the majority of patients with FAAs will have an associated AAA or popliteal artery aneurysm, the preoperative evaluation must include careful palpation of the abdominal aorta and popliteal arteries. Duplex ultrasound of these areas is also indicated as a more sensitive test to detect concurrent aneurysm disease. In general, contrast arteriography is indicated prior to operative intervention to define distal runoff and delineate involvement of the profunda femoris and superficial femoral arteries. In reality, similar anatomic detail may now be obtained in certain institutions with contrast-enhanced CTA or even MRA in combination with duplex ultrasound.

II. **OPERATIVE PRINCIPLES.** Three factors govern the choice of operation for common FAAs: (a) location of the origin of the profunda femoris artery, (b) patency of the superficial femoral artery, and (c) patency of the aneurysm itself.

A. In **type 1 FAAs** in which the profunda femoris orifice is distal to the aneurysm and all vessels are patent, the simplest and most successful repair is a vein or synthetic graft interposition for the resected aneurysm.

B. In **typo 2 FAAs**, the profunda femoris arises from the aneurysmal sac. We cannot overemphasize the importance of **maintaining patency of the profunda femoris when such aneurysms are repaired.** In most instances, such aneurysms are resected and an interposition graft (vein or prosthetic material) is sewn to the superficial femoral artery. A small side-arm graft is then constructed to the profunda femoris artery.

C. When the superficial femoral artery is **chronically occluded,** it is ligated and an end-to-end anastomosis of the graft to the profunda femoris artery is performed.

III. **POSTOPERATIVE FOLLOW-UP.** After FAA repair, patients should be followed annually. Duplex ultrasound is an ideal method to monitor grafts and to discover other aneurysms. Newly discovered aneurysms of the abdominal aorta or popliteal arteries should be corrected as indicated.

POPLITEAL ARTERY ANEURYSMS

Like other peripheral aneurysms, popliteal artery aneurysms have a natural history of embolization and thrombosis. In a recent study by the Mayo Clinic, 60% popliteal artery aneurysms undergoing repair presented with symptoms (39% chronic ischemia and 21% acute limb ischemia), while 40% were asymptomatic. Large popliteal artery aneurysms may also present as a pulsatile mass behind the knee, which may obstruct the popliteal vein or compress the tibial nerve. Popliteal aneurysms at greatest risk for thromboembolic events have three characteristics that guide indications for elective repair: (a) size greater than 2 cm, (b) intraluminal thrombus on duplex, and (c) decreased pedal pulses or evidence of distal embolization indicating symptoms and compromised runoff.

I. **PREOPERATIVE EVALUATION.** Like patients with FAAs, these patients must be carefully examined for other aneurysms, especially in the aortoiliac location. In the same series from Mayo, approximately 50% of patients had bilateral popliteal aneurysms, 50% had AAAs, and almost 10% had aneurysms in the thoracic or paravisceral aorta. Preoperative imaging of the extremity should define not only the location and extent of the PAA but also delineate the below-the-knee runoff. Special consideration should be given to the condition of the superficial femoral artery and the distal runoff in order to plan an effective operative approach. This information can be obtained with contrast arteriography of the extremity. However, with the increasing sensitivity of CTA and MRA in some institutions, these modalities may be combined with duplex to provide all the necessary preoperative anatomic information in some situations.

II. **OPERATIVE PRINCIPLES**. The preferred surgical treatment for popliteal artery aneurysms is the medial approach, which allows exposure of the above- and below-the-knee popliteal artery. This approach allows proximal and distal ligation of the aneurysm followed by greater saphenous vein bypass. **One should not be fooled into assuming that the distal superficial femoral artery will be a normal artery suitable as an inflow vessel.** In up to two-thirds of cases, the superficial femoral artery above the knee is diseased and not suitable for inflow. Therefore, origination of the vein bypass must come from the common femoral artery in the groin in these cases.

Historically, simple ligation and bypass of the aneurysm from the medial approach has been effective in treating popliteal artery aneurysms. There is some evidence that ligation alone results in continued pressurization and even expansion of the popliteal aneurysm from patent side branches feeding into the ligated aneurysm. Some practitioners now advocate opening the aneurysm after ligation to oversew any back-bleeding vessels to eliminate this possibility. In about 15% of cases, a posterior approach to the popliteal artery aneurysm is used and is particularly useful for large aneurysms causing symptoms of compression. This approach, which is performed through a single incision with the patient prone, allows for more complete decompression of the aneurysm and popliteal space. In these cases, larger aneurysms should be opened, the thrombus removed, and a portion of the sac resected to prevent compressive symptoms from the mass effect of the aneurysm.

Popliteal artery aneurysms that present with acute thrombosis and acute limb ischemia are best treated with an attempt at preoperative catheter-directed thrombolysis. If initiated early enough after the onset of symptoms, this preoperative adjunct significantly increases the chance of a successful surgical reconstruction in the ensuing 24 to 48 hours. Catheter-directed thrombolysis is described in Chapter 10 and involves placement of an infusion catheter (i.e., soaker hose) into the thrombosed aneurysm and outflow and administration of a thrombolytic agent such as TPA. This technique improves the infrapopliteal outflow and has decreased the limb-loss rate associated with thrombosed popliteal artery aneurysm from 30% to 10%.

Endovascular treatment of popliteal artery aneurysms using a self-expanding covered stent is also an option. In fact, in select groups of patients, the short- and mid-term success of this technique appears acceptable. However, its broad application is limited by yet-to-be-defined anatomic criteria of the femoral and popliteal arteries and established long-term effectiveness. Runoff should be reasonable with at least two patent and stenosis-free tibial arteries. Currently, the standard treatment for popliteal artery aneurysms is open repair, and the endovascular approach is reserved for select patients who are not good operative candidates.

III. **POSTOPERATIVE FOLLOW-UP**. Patients treated for popliteal artery aneurysms should be reevaluated annually, not only to assess the bypass with duplex but also to check for the development of aneurysms elsewhere in the arterial system.

Selected Readings

Abdominal Aortic Aneurysm

Aneurysm Detection and Management (ADAM) Veterans Affairs Cooperative Study Group. Immediate repair compared to surveillance of small abdominal aortic aneurysms. *NEJM*. 2002;346:1437-1444.

British Society for Endovascular Therapy (BSET) and the Global Collaborators on Advanced Stent-Graft Techniques for Aneurysm Repair (GLOBALSTAR) Registry. Early results of fenestrated endovascular repair of Juxtarenal aortic aneurysms in the United Kingdom. *Circulation.* 2012;125:2707-2715.

Blankensteijn JD, de Jong SE, Prinssen M, et al. (Dutch Randomized Endovascular Aneurysm Management (DREAM) Trial Group. Two-year outcomes after conventional or endovascular repair of abdominal aortic aneurysms. *NEJM.* 2005;352:2398-2405.

Cao P, De Rango P, Verzini F, et al. Comparison of surveillance versus aortic endografting for small aneurysm repair (CESAR): results of a randomised trial. *Eur J Vasc Endovasc Surg.* 2011;41:13-25.

Conrad MF, Crawford RS, Pedraza JD, et al. Long-term durability of open abdominal aortic aneurysm repair. *J Vasc Surg.* 2007;46:669-675.

Haulon S, Amiot S, Magnan PE, et al. An analysis of the French multicentre experience of fenestrated aortic endografts. *Ann Surg.* 2010;251:357-362.

Ouriel K, Clair DG, Kent KC, et al. Endovascular repair compared with surveillance for patients with small abdominal aortic aneurysms. *J Vasc Surg.* 2010;51:1081-7.

Patel R, Sweeting MJ, Powell JT, et al. Endovascular versus open repair of abdominal aortic aneurysm in 15-years' follow-up of the UK endovascular aneurysm repair trial 1 (EVAR-1): a randomized controlled trial. *Lancet.* 2016;388:2366-2374.

Patel VI, Lancaster RT, Conrad MF, et al. Comparable mortality with open repair of complex and infrarenal aortic aneurysm. *J Vasc Surg.* 2011;54:952-959.

Powell JT, Sweeting MJ, Blankensteijn J, et al. Meta-analysis of individual patient data from EVAR-1, DREAM, OVER, and ACE trials comparing outcomes of endovascular or open repair for abdominal aortic aneurysms over 5-years. *BJS.* 2017;104:166-178.

Schermerhorn ML, Buck DB, O'Malley AJ, et al. Long-term outcomes of abdominal aortic aneurysm in the Medicare population. *N Engl J Med.* 2015;373:328-338.

Schermerhorn ML, Bensley RP, Giles KA, et al. Changes in abdominal aortic aneurysm rupture and short-term mortality 1995–2008: a retrospective, observational study. *Ann Surg.* 2012;256:651-658.

Tsai S, Conrad MF, Patel VI, et al. Durability of open repair of juxtarenal abdominal aortic aneurysms. *J Vasc Surg.* 2012;56(1):2-7.

U.K. Small Aneurysm Trial Participants. Mortality results for randomised controlled trial of early elective surgery or ultrasonographic surveillance for small abdominal aortic aneurysms. *Lancet.* 1998;352:1649-1655.

Van Beek SC, Conijn AP, Koelemay MJ, et al. Endovascular aneurysm repair versus open repair for patients with a ruptured abdominal aortic aneurysm: a systematic review and meta-analysis of short-term survival. *Eur J Vasc Endovasc Surg.* 2014;47:593-602.

Van Beek SC, Vahl A, Wisselink W, et al. Midterm reinterventions and survival after endovascular versus open repair for ruptured abdominal aortic aneurysm. *Eur J Vasc Endovasc Surg.* 2015;49:661-668.

Van Schaik TG, Yeung KK, Verhagen HJ, et al. Long-term survival and secondary procedures after open or endovascular repair of abdominal aortic aneurysms. *J Vasc Surg.* 2017;66:1379-1389.

Thoracoabdominal Aortic Aneurysm

Clouse WD, Marone LK, Davison JK, et al. Late aortic and graft-related events after thoracoabdominal aneurysm repair. *J Vasc Surg.* 2003;37:254-261.

Coselli JS, LeMaire SA, Preventza O, et al. Outcomes of 3309 thoracoabdominal aortic aneurysm repairs. *J Thorac Cardiovasc Surg.* 2016;151:1323-1338.

Estrera AL, Sandhu HK, Charlton-Ouw KM, et al. A quarter century of organ protection in open thoracoabdominal repair. *Ann Surg.* 2015;262:660-668.

Guillou M, Bianchini A, Sobocinski J, et al. Endovascular treatment of thoracoabdominal aortic aneurysms. *J Vasc Surg.* 2012;56:65-73.

Lancaster RT, Conrad MF, Patel VI, et al. Further experience with distal aortic perfusion and motor-evoked potential monitoring in the management of extent I-III thoracoabdominal aneurysms. *J Vasc Surg.* 2013;58:283-290.

Latz CA, Patel VI, Cambria RP, et al. The durability of open surgical repair of type IV thoracoabdominal aneurysm. *J Vasc Surg.*

Latz CA, Cambria RP, Patel VI, et al. The durability of open surgical repair of type I-III thoracoabdominal aneurysm. *J Vasc Surg* (in press).

Mastracci TM, Eagleton MJ, Kuramochi Y, Bathurst S, Wolski K. Twelve-year results of fenestrated endografts for juxtarenal and group IV thoracoabdominal aneurysms. *J Vasc Surg*. 2015;61:355-364.

Oderich GS, Ribeiro M, de Souza LR, et al. Endovascular repair of thoracoabdominal aortic aneurysms using fenestrated and branched endografts. *J Thorac Cardiovasc Surg*. 2017;153:S32-S41.

Patel VI, Ergul EA, Conrad MF, et al. Continued favorable results with open surgical repair of type IV thoracoabdominal aortic aneurysms. *J Vasc Surg*. 2011;53:1492-1498.

Wynne MM, Acher C, Marks E, et al. Postoperative renal failure in thoracoabdominal aortic aneurysm repair with simple cross-clamp technique and 4°C renal perfusion. *J Vasc Surg*. 2015;61:611-622.

Peripheral Artery Aneurysm

Diwan A, Sarkar R, Stanley JC, et al. Incidence of femoral and popliteal artery aneurysms in patients with abdominal aortic aneurysms. *J Vasc Surg*. 2000;31:863-869.

Eslami M, Rybin D, Doros G, et al. Open repair of asymptomatic popliteal artery aneurysm is associated with better outcomes than endovascular repair. *J Vasc Surg*. 2015;61:663-669.

Golchehr B, Zeebregts CJ, Reijnen MMP, et al. Long-term outcome of endovascular popliteal artery aneurysm repair. *J Vasc Surg*. 2018;67:1797-1804.

Jones WT III, Hagino RT, Chiou AC, et al. Graft patency is not the only clinical predictor of success after exclusion and bypass of popliteal artery aneurysms. *J Vasc Surg*. 2003;37:392-398.

Lawrence PF, Harlander-Locke MP, Oderich GS, et al. The current management of isolated femoral artery aneurysms is too aggressive for their natural history. *J Vasc Surg*. 2014;59:343-349.

Leake AE, Avgerinos ED, Chaer RA, et al. Contemporary outcomes of open and endovascular popliteal artery aneurysm repair. *J Vasc Surg*. 2016;63:70-76.

Renal Artery Diseases

Vascular providers are frequently asked to assess and provide recommendations for patients with different forms of renal artery disease. **From renal artery aneurysms to fibromuscular dysplasia (FMD) to atherosclerotic renovascular disease (ARVD), conditions affecting the renal vasculature have a range of pathophysiology and natural history. Regardless of etiology, all forms of renal artery disease have two main clinical end points of concern; one related to elevation of the patient's blood pressure (i.e., refractory and sometimes severe hypertension) and the other pertaining to deterioration of renal excretory function.**

Renal artery disease, either from ARVD or FMD, is the most common cause of secondary hypertension, and some degree of renal artery stenosis is present in 1% to 5% of patients with the condition. Some community-based screening programs have found that the incidence of ARVD is as high as 7% in patients over the age of 65 years. Of patients referred to a vascular lab with a history of vascular disease and or concerns for renal artery occlusive disease, about 25% will have ARVD identified on duplex; a frequency that increases in those taking two or more blood pressure medications. In the context of all patients with hypertension, ARVD is the cause in only about 5% of cases. While this seems low, the increasing number of Americans with hypertension (approximately one-third of population) makes the prevalence of this disease process important, especially given the aging nature of the U.S. population.

For most patients undergoing initial evaluation of high blood pressure, an extensive workup of the renal arteries (i.e., duplex ultrasound, contrast angiography, or magnetic resonance angiography [MRA]) is *not* indicated. Because the incidence of renal vascular hypertension is low, providers should initially encourage a healthier lifestyle (i.e., exercise, weight reduction), attempt to reduce other risk factors or contributors (i.e., initiate smoking cessation program and better control of diabetes), and optimize the use of one or two basic antihypertensive medications.

Medications that block the renin-angiotensin system—either conventional angiotensin-converting enzyme inhibitors (ACE inhibitors) or angiotensin-II receptor blockers (ARBs)—are among a group of first-line agents to be used in hypertensive patients. The combination of these medications with a beta-receptor blocker (i.e., beta-blocker) or a calcium channel blocker is effective in treating hypertension in the majority of patients, even those with mild and moderate degrees of renal artery occlusive disease. HMG-CoA reductase inhibitors, also known as statins, have also been shown to have a beneficial effect in hypertensive patients and are frequently used as part of "best medical management" of this condition.

The challenge arises when patients require more than 2 to 3 medications to control hypertension or they have deterioration of renal function or decrements in kidney size. In these cases, the provider must identify those patients who will benefit from intensification of medical management versus those in whom diagnostic imaging and some type of renal artery revascularization may be indicated. In the past, clinical decision-making for this more complex group of patients was based mostly on uncontrolled and often single-center studies performed in the 1990s and early 2000s. However, in recent years, several prospective, randomized, multicenter studies have been completed that examine the mid- and long-term outcomes of patients treated with best medical management alone or in combination with renal artery revascularization (i.e., stenting or open revascularization). The results of these larger and more rigorous studies afford good information for providers and patients as to what can be expected in the mid- and long term following these different therapeutic approaches.

Although it is intuitive that progressive ARVD (i.e., worsening of renal artery stenosis) can accelerate hypertension and kidney injury, what is been shown in experimental animal studies and in more recent clinical trials is that simply restoring vessel patency is not enough to normalize blood pressure and recover kidney function. Kidney injury resulting from ARVD is now known to be a complex interaction between oxidative stress injury and activation of inflammatory cells that results in chronic, and often irreversible, fibrosis of the renal parenchyma. In this context, improving or normalizing renal artery patency with an intervention may not reverse the damage or provide clinical improvement.

This understanding of the disease process has resulted in a paradigm shift *away* from simply treating the arterial stenosis with an endovascular or open procedure. Instead, therapeutic strategies have shifted toward optimizing cardiovascular risk factors and medical management in most patients. Future therapies are being developed to target cell-based functions that may allow regeneration of vascular, glomerular, and tubular structures within the kidney to stabilize or recover. There remains a role for endovascular and open revascularization in pediatric patients with congenital renal artery conditions, patients with FMD, and a small percentage of patients with ARVD. However, compared to 10 to 15 years ago, the interventional approach today is more selective.

This chapter reviews the pathophysiology of renal artery disease as well as diagnostic and therapeutic options. Indications for initiating a more comprehensive diagnostic workup are presented as are the basic technical approaches to diagnostic and therapeutic procedures. Finally, this chapter reviews several multicenter, prospective studies that have been completed since the previous edition of this handbook.

I. **RENIN-ANGIOTENSIN SYSTEM.** In order to manage renovascular hypertension, one must review the relationship of the kidney to blood pressure control. By adjusting sodium and water retention and through the release of vasoactive factors, the kidney functions as an endocrine organ helping maintain blood pressure through several mechanisms. A hemodynamically significant obstruction or stenosis of the renal artery (renal artery stenosis or RAS) or an overall decrease in blood volume decreases flow to the kidney. This decrement in flow is "viewed" by the kidney as hypovolemia or hypotension, and it initiates a response from the kidney that involves release of local and circulating factors. **More specifically, baroreceptors in the juxtaglomerular apparatus of the kidney detect decreases in renal blood flow and respond by releasing the enzyme renin. Renin cleaves the serum globulin angiotensin I, forming the vasoactive peptide angiotensin II, which increases renal blood flow by several mechanisms.** Angiotensin II stimulates adrenal release of aldosterone, causes systemic vasoconstriction, and exerts an antidiuretic, antinatriuretic action on the kidney (i.e., fluid or volume retention). Angiotensin II also causes vasoconstriction of the efferent arterioles of the juxtaglomerular apparatus, decreasing flow out of this system and producing a subsequent increase in pressure.

The result is sodium and water retention, expansion of extracellular fluid volume, and an increase in systemic blood pressure. One effective class of medications used to treat hypertension includes drugs that inhibit conversion of angiotensin I to angiotensin II (ACE inhibitors) or directly block the angiotensin II receptors (ARBs).

II. **DIAGNOSTIC EVALUATION OF THE RENAL ARTERIES SHOULD BE PERFORMED ONLY IN APPROPRIATE CLINICAL CIRCUMSTANCES.** As was noted previously, 5% of patients with hypertension have some form of renal artery disease resulting in a functional renal artery stenosis. This association occurs more often in hypertensive children and young adults, who more commonly have congenital conditions such as aortic coarctation, congenital renal artery stenosis, or FMD. In this population of young individuals with hypertension, diagnostic evaluation of the renal arteries is warranted early in their evaluation to look for unusual, congenital abnormalities or FMD.

In contrast, elderly adults are most commonly affected by essential hypertension, and routine diagnostic evaluation of the renal arteries is not necessary early in the course of their workup. In these cases, even though older patients are at risk for atherosclerosis and renal artery disease, initiation of one or two medications along with lifestyle and risk factor modification is usually effective in reducing blood pressure. A thorough history and physical exam should be performed, and routine lab tests, including serum creatinine and creatinine clearance, should be performed. If there is no indication from the history, physical exam, or lab testing that the renal arteries are involved, basic medical management (e.g., one or two medications) may be initiated without diagnostic evaluation of the renal arteries. If this strategy, which includes lifestyle (i.e., exercise and weight loss) and risk modification (i.e., smoking cessation), is not effective at achieving a desirable blood pressure within 3 to 6 months, then diagnostic evaluation of the renal arteries should be more strongly considered.

The preferred diagnostic test to identify and measure renal artery disease differs among groups and institutions. However, initial evaluation should begin with a noninvasive test such as duplex ultrasound, CTA, and MRA. Because duplex spares the nephrotoxic effects of contrast needed to perform CTA and MRA, it is the favored initial test in most cases (Chapter 5). Invasive renal arteriography should not be used as an initial diagnostic test but should be reserved for cases in which an intervention is planned. Angiography may be indicated in unusual cases in which one or more of the noninvasive studies are inconclusive or discordant (i.e., show different findings). In special instances in which open revascularization is planned, contrast arteriography may be performed to provide precise anatomic information prior to the operation (i.e., preoperative imaging or pressure measurement).

A. **Screening tests. Duplex ultrasound is the primary noninvasive test of choice in screening for renal artery disease.** Renal duplex requires the patient to fast in order to reduce the amount of bowel gas interference. Evaluation of the renal arteries with duplex also requires an experienced vascular technologist and about 45 minutes of time (Chapter 5). Another noninvasive option for evaluation of the renal arteries is gadolinium-enhanced MRA. MRA has the advantage of imaging the entire aorta and branch vessels and can often provide very clear and 3D-reconstructable images. MRA is especially useful in cases of renal artery aneurysms and FMD. Quality of MRA can be institution-specific, and some vascular specialists see MRA as overestimating the degree of renal artery occlusive disease. MRA is also relatively expensive and is not always tolerated by patients who may be claustrophobic.

In our practices, MRA is most often used to confirm duplex imaging that provides conflicting or equivocal results. Like MRA, CTA of the renals provides clear and 3D-reconstructable images of the aorta, main renal arteries, and renal hilum. Unfortunately, the contrast needed to achieve such imaging carries some nephrotoxic effect and often precludes use of this imaging modality. We rarely use CTA to image just the renal arteries in the setting of suspected renovascular hypertension and save this modality for patients with renal artery aneurysms or congenital abnormalities in younger patients who have normal renal function.

B. **Catheter-directed arteriography carries the risk of contrast material and should be reserved for cases when an intervention is planned or when noninvasive studies are inconclusive or in disagreement. Renal arteriography may also be used to provide detailed imaging and or pressure measurements prior to open revascularization in patients with congenital condition involving the aorta and its branch vessels, including the renal arteries.** The selective use of arteriography is an advance in the management of this vascular condition and is testament to improvements in noninvasive imaging (e.g., duplex, CTA, and MRA) and a better understanding of which patients benefit from renal intervention.

When performed, renal arteriography should include an abdominal aortogram, selective renal artery injections in different planes, and a celiac artery injection with a lateral view if the splenic or hepatic arteries are being considered as the inflow vessels for splenorenal or hepatorenal bypass. The amount of contrast should be minimized in patients with suspected renovascular disease and imaging adjuncts such as CO_2 aortography and intravascular ultrasound (IVUS) aid in this objective.

III. **INDICATIONS FOR INVASIVE INTERVENTION.** The effectiveness of new medical approaches to ARVD, a better understanding of its pathophysiology, and the lack of clinical evidence showing lasting benefit from renal artery stenting have reduced the indications for invasive treatment. For the majority of older patients with ARVD, restoring renal artery patency is not effective in curing hypertension or preserving renal function. The multifactorial nature of hypertension and renal insufficiency make it such that opening the artery is not a long-term solution for most patients.

A. **Renovascular hypertension that is refractory to medical treatment** is the most common indication for intervention. In our practices, we stress the fact that patients with renovascular hypertension also need intensive blood pressure control lifestyle modification (i.e., exercise and weight loss) and cardiovascular risk management (Chapter 6) before and after any intervention. **Such management requires close attention and follow-up after intervention to assess for clinical and technical adequacy (i.e., whether the blood pressure improved and the revascularization is patent).** In most cases, the patient is best served by a multidisciplinary team, which may include vascular and hypertensive specialists and nephrologists.

Success of renal artery revascularization for hypertension depends on the etiology of the disease and the age of the patient. The best results, open or endovascular, have been reported in younger patients (<50 years old) with FMD or focal atherosclerotic lesions and preserved renal function. Additionally, renovascular hypertension caused by bilateral disease often responds more dramatically with a better long-term result than patients with unilateral disease. Long-term cure of hypertension occurs in only about 10% of patients while around 70% of patients will have at least transient improvement in blood pressure as defined by the need for fewer antihypertensive medications. **In contrast, older patients with chronic hypertension and diabetes, both of which damage the renal parenchyma over**

time (e.g., hypertensive nephropathy and diabetic nephropathy), have less convincing and sustained improvement.

In most cases, the initial treatment modality is endovascular
angioplasty with or without stent placement. The most favorable renal
disease treated with endovascular means is FMD of the renal artery. In
this setting, percutaneous transluminal balloon angioplasty is technically
successful in more than 95% of cases and provides a durable treatment. In
cases of FMD, angioplasty without stent placement is preferred and may
even provide satisfactory treatment in patients where the FMD extends
into the first-order renal artery branches. The endovascular approach to
renovascular hypertension caused by atherosclerotic occlusive disease
includes placement of balloon-expandable stents in nearly all cases.
Because much of this disease is felt to originate in the lumen of the aorta,
care is taken to overlap the stent into the aorta slightly to account for and
adequately treat this disease.

B. **Preservation of renal function** through renal artery surgery or angioplasty
has received much attention, and clinical studies examining the effectiveness and limitations of both methods have been reported. **The challenge
is to identify patients most likely to benefit from invasive therapy and then to
perform the therapy with a low rate of technical complication without causing
further decrement in renal function.** Today, most clinical evidence *does not*
support open operation or endovascular stenting to preserve renal function in the majority of patients with ARVD. However, there are categories
of renal artery disease that deserve special consideration such as patients
with bilateral, high-grade renal stenoses, or severe stenosis of an artery to
a solitary functioning kidney (e.g., prior nephrectomy or nonfunctioning
contralateral kidney).

**Studies have identified the utility of measuring and following kidney size
over time with duplex as one indicator of renal deterioration.** The normal size
of the adult kidney, measured as the length from the superior to the inferior pole, is 10 to 14 cm. Kidney lengths are usually an average of three
or four measurements to account for slightly oblique and therefore less
accurate views. Renal size of less than 10 cm suggests atrophy and should
be investigated with additional studies (e.g., serum creatinine, creatinine
clearance, MRI/MRA). A decrement in size of more than 1 to 2 cm over a
2-year period indicates significant loss of renal parenchyma and should
also be further evaluated.

**Renal resistive index (RRI) measured by duplex has been advocated by
many as an indicator of intrinsic or parenchymal renal function, independent of
large vessel renal disease.** As such, RRI has been shown to identify patients
who may respond favorably to large vessel revascularization, open or
endovascular. The formula for RRI is RRI = peak systolic velocity – end
diastolic velocity/peak systolic velocity. The normal RRI is 0.6 to 0.7, and
an index of greater than 0.8 is highly resistive, which suggests significant
intrinsic renal disease often from chronic hypertension or diabetes. High
resistive indices (i.e., RRI > 0.8) indicate chronic, and possibly irreversible,
parenchymal damage that is less likely to respond to large-vessel reconstruction (i.e., unlikely to improve with open or endovascular treatment of
the arterial stenosis). Conversely, those with a lower renal-resistive index
have preserved intrinsic renal function that is more responsive to treatment of main renal artery occlusive disease. Although appealing as a noninvasive indicator of those who may respond to renal angioplasty or open
revascularization, RRI has not borne out to be useful in all clinical studies.

In most studies of patients with large-vessel ARVD examining the
effectiveness of renal artery angioplasty, stenting has not conveyed a lasting benefit to blood pressure control. Some studies have shown a transient
benefit in the reduction of number of blood pressure medications, and a

number of uncontrolled studies have shown benefit in stenting to slow the rate of decline in renal dysfunction. However, the effectiveness at preventing progression of renal dysfunction has not borne out in more recent randomized, multicenter clinical trials on the topic. As has been previously noted in this chapter, the challenge is to identify the subset of patients with renal artery occlusive disease who may benefit from intervention. In addition to a RRI of less than 0.8, 3 to 4 other clinical factors have been consistently shown to be associated with success of renal artery intervention:

1. Nondiabetic patients
2. Treating bilateral severe stenoses
3. Preserved renal size of greater than 9.5 cm
4. A serum creatinine of less than 2.5 mg/dL

C. **Surgical correction** of aneurysm or occlusive disease of the aorta may necessitate preservation of a main or accessory renal artery. Accessory renal arteries less than 3 mm in size can usually be ligated without significant loss of renal function, while larger accessory arteries should be preserved. Maintaining patency of accessory renal arteries may require reimplantation or bypass during open aortic surgery or modification of endovascular techniques to avoid covering the arteries of interest.

D. **Other renal artery problems** requiring renal artery reconstruction include renal artery aneurysms or renal artery trauma, which can result in dissection, aneurysm, or arteriovenous fistula. Renal artery aneurysms greater than 2 cm in diameter should be repaired as they are thought to cause hypertension, distal embolization, and/or thrombosis. CTA is the study of choice to characterize renal artery aneurysms and injuries. Rupture of a renal artery aneurysm is thought to be more likely during pregnancy, so women of childbearing age with aneurysms should be considered with a lower threshold for elective repair. Embolism of the renal artery presents with acute flank pain and often hematuria. Renal arteriovenous fistulas are difficult surgical problems, especially when they are in the renal parenchyma and should be treated with endovascular techniques (e.g., coil embolization or small covered stent) depending upon location. Intrarenal arteriovenous fistulas may also be treated with endovascular coil embolization.

IV. **SURGICAL OPTIONS.** Improvement of blood pressure and preservation of renal function are the primary goals of any operation on the renal arteries. Nephrectomy is done only when no other method of saving a good kidney appears possible and that kidney appears to be responsible for significant hypertension (i.e., also referred to as a **"pressor kidney"**). **Open renal artery reconstruction falls into two categories, bypass and endarterectomy.** A variety of autogenous and synthetic graft materials are available for renal artery bypass procedures, while endarterectomy has the advantage of not requiring a bypass conduit. Figures 15.1 and 15.2 illustrate preferred methods of renal artery revascularization. Autogenous grafts, such as those of saphenous vein, are preferable to synthetic materials. Factors that increase the risk of operative morbidity and mortality are elevated baseline creatinine levels (>3 mg/dL), increased age, and associated cardiac dysfunction. Operative mortality from open renal artery revascularization is between 3% and 5%.

A large series of open renal artery reconstructions from Wake Forest University showed that a majority of patients underwent bilateral renal artery repair, and nearly half (41%) had renal reconstruction as part of an open aortic repair for either aneurysm or occlusive disease. The indication for treatment in this series was renovascular hypertension, and 85% of patients had hypertension cured or improved with an overall improvement in renal function in this select group. In a second study from Massachusetts General Hospital, which examined open renal artery reconstruction for preservation of renal function, the operative approach was as

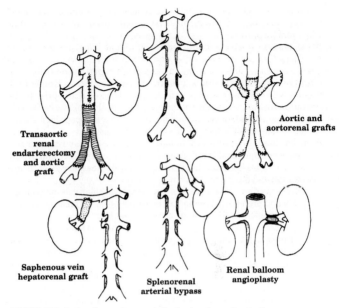

FIGURE 15.1 Options for renal revascularization for atherosclerotic disease.

follows: aortorenal bypass (38%), extra-anatomic bypass (e.g., hepatorenal or splenorenal bypass) (38%), and endarterectomy (24%). Similar to the Wake Forest report, 32% underwent combined aortic and renal reconstruction. Long-term preservation of renal function was noted in 70% of patients with improved results in patients with lower baseline creatinine levels (<3.2 mg/dL) and those undergoing bilateral repair.

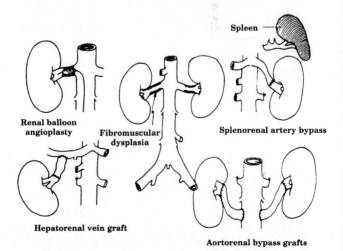

FIGURE 15.2 Options for renal revascularization for fibromuscular disease.

V. **PREOPERATIVE PREPARATION.** Before renal artery revascularization, blood pressure and renal function must be stabilized as much as possible (Chapters 7 and 8).

A. **Blood pressure.** Most patients have significant hypertension, which increases the risk of myocardial and cerebrovascular events. As was stressed earlier, solid treatment and control of hypertension before and after the revascularization is a central tenant of success. One consideration is to reduce or stop diuretic therapy 24 to 48 hours prior to the operation so that chronically contracted intravascular volume can be corrected slowly. Beta-blockers should not be abruptly stopped since discontinuation may result in tachycardia and myocardial ischemia.

B. **Renal function.** About one-third of patients undergoing renovascular surgery have chronic renal insufficiency (creatinine >2 mg/dL), and several factors can cause deterioration in their creatinine clearance prior to hospitalization and during preoperative evaluation.

   1. Vigorous diuretic therapy can cause intravascular volume contraction and prerenal azotemia (i.e., elevation of serum creatinine).

   2. **ACE inhibitors or ARB therapy disturbs renal blood flow autoregulation by decreasing efferent arteriolar resistance, which is needed to provide a perfusion gradient to the glomerulus.** In theory, use of these medications in those who also have inflow stenosis to the kidney (e.g., renal artery stenosis) can worsen serum creatinine. It turns out that only a small percentage of patients with renovascular disease do not tolerate ACE inhibitors or ARBs. Starting an ACE inhibitor or an ARB should be done cautiously and should include checks of blood pressure and serum creatinine. A minority of patients will not tolerate the therapy. **A solid level of clinical evidence supporting the benefit of ACE inhibitors in reducing overall cardiovascular morbidity and mortality outweighs the limited risk of renal dysfunction.** In those who manifest renal dysfunction with initiation of therapy, the ACE inhibitor should be stopped, and the creatinine will return to baseline in 7 days.

   3. Another frequent cause for an acute rise in serum creatinine is **contrast nephropathy related to arteriography or CT angiography.** The vascular provider must be mindful when ordering and performing imaging studies. Fortunately, with hydration and observation, most episodes of contrast nephropathy will resolve over several weeks. Renal revascularization should be delayed until creatinine levels return to baseline following such an event.

VI. **OPEN OPERATIVE PRINCIPLES**

A. **Incisions.** Proper operative exposure is one of the most important aspects of renal artery surgery. A midline xiphoid-to-pubic bone incision provides good access to both renal arteries. An upper transverse or subcostal incision may be used but does not provide good exposure of the distal aorta or iliac system. A left splenorenal arterial anastomosis can be constructed through a low, left thoracoabdominal incision (bed of the tenth rib) or a left subcostal incision.

B. **Proximal renal lesions.** For central lesions, the midline retroperitoneum is opened over the aorta. On the left side, the renal vein can be mobilized by ligation and division of the **adrenal, gonadal, and left renolumbar branches of the left renal vein.** On the right side, the vena cava must be mobilized and retracted to expose the proximal right renal artery.

C. **Middle or distal lesions.** For mid or distal lesions on the right, the duodenum must be reflected by a Kocher maneuver to expose the distal right renal artery. On the left side, the splenic flexure of the colon can be mobilized in a similar fashion.

D. **Renal protection.** Several steps can be taken to reduce the effect of transient ischemia and reperfusion on the kidney(s).

1. Intravenous hydration with a balanced salt solution (e.g., Ringer's lactated solution, 100 to 125 mL/h) is started several hours before surgery.
2. Heparin (5,000 units) is given intravenously before clamping the renal artery.
3. Mannitol (12.5 to 25.0 g) is administered early in the procedure. If a good diuresis is not achieved with mannitol then intravenous furosemide may be used.
4. The kidney may be cooled with 200 to 300 mL of a perfusate if anticipated ischemic time is greater than 45 minutes. A combination of 1 L of Ringer's lactated solution, 18 g mannitol, 20 mg heparin, and 500 mg methylprednisolone chilled to 3°C in saline slush is an example of one such solution.
5. Low-dose (2 to 3 μg/kg/min) dopamine causes renal vasodilatation, which may help minimize vasomotor nephropathy. Starting intravenous dopamine in the operating room before renal artery clamping and continuing it for 12 to 24 hours following the reconstruction is a commonly used approach.

E. **Type of anastomosis.** The proximal anastomosis is constructed first. Then, the distal anastomosis is made end-to-end by the spatulation technique. The suture material is usually 6-0 or 7-0 polypropylene. For a particularly difficult anastomosis, the suture line may be interrupted. Low-power magnifying loops and a high-intensity headlight are essential in most renal artery reconstructions.

F. **Intraoperative assessment of graft patency.** The simplest method to ascertain blood flow is examination of the graft or renal artery with a sterile continuous-wave Doppler. Biphasic signals should be present. Intraoperative duplex has proven to be a quick and reliable method for detecting technical problems after renal artery grafting or endarterectomy. Problems are detected in about 10% of reconstructed arteries, and most of these are correctable and result in outcomes that are similar to those of patients with normal intraoperative ultrasound studies.

VII. **POSTOPERATIVE CARE.** In the immediate postoperative period, intravascular volume must be maintained to ensure adequate urine output. This often requires monitoring central venous and possibly even pulmonary artery pressure use of for a brief period of time to ensure adequate filling pressures and volume repletion. Low-dose dopamine is continued for renal vasodilation, and dobutamine is administered to patients with marginal cardiac output (<3 L/m²). Generally, we strive to maintain a urine output of 1 mL/kg/h. Some patients have a massive or hyperdiuresis (>200 mL/h) and require urinary replacement (0.5 mL of crystalloid per milliliter of urine) for 12 to 24 hours to avoid volume depletion. Diuretics are usually not necessary and should be avoided in the first 24 hours. When a question arises about the early patency of the reconstruction, we obtain a renal duplex ultrasound, which can also be obtained prior to discharging the patient from the hospital. Any subsequent recurrence of hypertension or deterioration of renal function requires a repeat ultrasound and/or angiographic study. Percutaneous transluminal angioplasty may be performed on an anastomotic stenosis in an attempt to salvage a failing graft. Open reoperation of a stenotic or thrombosed renal graft can achieve a successful result in only about 50% of patients.

VIII. **RENAL BALLOON ANGIOPLASTY AND STENTING IS THE INITIAL CHOICE FOR RENAL INTERVENTION EXCEPT IN CASES IN WHICH OPEN AORTIC SURGERY IS NECESSARY.** Because of it less-invasive nature and low morbidity and mortality, the endovascular approach to renal artery disease now mostly preferred when an intervention is indicated. Physicians who treat hypertension and renal insufficiency must be informed about this technique and understand which patients are candidates. **As a vascular specialist, one should understand the premise that just because renal artery stenting can be performed doesn't mean it *should* be performed.**

Typically, endovascular renal artery intervention is accomplished through a transfemoral approach using only a 5 or 6 French sheath (Chapters 9 and 10). Selection of the renal artery is facilitated by pre-shaped guide catheters, such as the renal double curve (RDC) or the Cobra I or II (CI or CII). Once the renal artery has been identified, selection of the orifice can be accomplished using a 0.035-inch hydrophilic wire and 4 or 5 Fr catheter, or in some cases simply a 0.014-inch wire with a distal embolic protection device (Chapters 9 and 10). Renal interventions over a wire with distal embolic protection have been shown in some series to reduce the damaging effects of distal embolization from the atherosclerotic lesion into the kidney parenchyma. Intervention with a distal embolic protection device represents a technologic development that, as is the case with smaller profile devices and newer generation stents, has advanced this therapy. Most atherosclerotic renal artery lesions are treated with a premounted, balloon-expandable stent on a 0.014-inch over-the-wire delivery system. IVUS is also used as an adjunct to evaluate renal stenosis and renal artery diameter in some cases. In certain situations, IVUS may minimize use of contrast material by evaluating the poststent position and expansion, eliminating the need for completion arteriography.

IX. **RECENT PROSPECTIVE CLINICAL STUDIES ON THE EFFECTIVENESS OF RENAL ARTERY INTERVENTION:** Several prospective, multicenter trials comparing renal artery revascularization to optimal medical therapy for the treatment of ARVD have been completed in the past decade. In addition to providing results on the initial success and limitations of different treatment modalities, the studies provide insight into the long-term, natural history of this condition. A full review of these, and other single-center studies, is beyond the scope of this chapter. However, in general terms, the findings of these studies show that for most patients, renal artery revascularization is no better than best medical management in preventing the longer-term end points of renal insufficiency and refractory hypertension.

It is important to point out that each of the studies has limitations in their methodology, and several did identify certain subsets of patients who experienced apparent or at least transient benefit from renal artery revascularization. As such, the provider who is consulting on patients with ARVD should become familiar with the specifics of these trials and tailor their results to the individual patient being evaluated.

ASTRAL Study: In 2009, the Angioplasty and Stenting for Renal Artery Lesions (ASTRAL) investigators published a study entitled *Revascularization Versus Medical Therapy for Renal-Artery Stenosis* in the New England Journal of Medicine. The ASTRAL study was led by investigators and centers in the United Kingdom, and it randomized 806 patients with renal artery stenosis to either endovascular revascularization (i.e., stenting) with medical therapy or medical therapy alone. The median follow-up of the study was almost 3 years, but the primary outcome was a surrogate for renal function projected to 5 years. The study showed that both groups of patients experienced a reduction in blood pressure but failed to demonstrate a positive effect of renal artery stenting. ASTRAL identified a 9% procedure-related complication rate in the stenting group, half of which was characterized as serious.

The limitations of ASTRAL include its having incorporated patients with lesser degrees of renal artery stenosis (i.e., those who may not have stood to be benefited from stenting), and it excluded some patients with disease with a "high likelihood" of requiring revascularization (i.e., patients with stenosis deemed too severe to undergo randomization). The 9% procedure-related complication rate was also viewed as having been unrealistically high by many.

CORAL Study: The Cardiovascular Outcomes in Renal Atherosclerotic Lesions (CORAL) study was published by the CORAL investigators in the New England Journal of Medicine 2014 under the title *Stenting and Medical Therapy for Atherosclerotic Renal-Artery Stenosis.* This U.S. study randomized 967 patients with either hypertension or chronic kidney disease secondary to renal artery stenosis to medical management with or without percutaneous renal artery stenting. Compared with the ASTRAL study, CORAL attempted to include only patients with significant (>80%) renal artery stenosis.

With an average follow-up of more than 3.5 years, CORAL found no difference between groups in the occurrence of renal or cardiovascular events (i.e., progressive renal insufficiency, permanent need for dialysis, stroke, myocardial infarction, or heart failure). Blood pressure did not differ significantly between those receiving medical management and those receiving medical management with stenting, although there was a trend toward a benefit to stenting in patients with higher degrees of renal artery stenosis. CORAL was also the first large clinical study to demonstrate the potential of biomarkers (i.e., urine albumin, creatinine, etc.) as a way to determine which patients are to most likely to benefit from renal artery stenting. The procedure-related complications in CORAL were 0.2% to 2.2%.

The criticisms of CORAL were that both groups of patients had a similar improvement in blood pressure once the trial began, suggesting that neither was initially optimized, which may have introduced bias in favor of medical treatment. The trial design also meant that roughly 4% of patients screened were withdrawn by the physician, many of whom had renal artery stenoses deemed severe enough to require stenting (i.e., considered too severe to randomize in the study).

STAR Study: Another prospective, multicenter study worth noting is the *Stent Placement in Patients with Atherosclerotic Renal Artery Stenosis and Impaired Renal Function* or STAR study published in the Annals of Internal Medicine (2009). STAR randomized 140 patients with creatinine clearance of less than 80 mL/min per 1.73 m^2 and a renal artery stenosis of greater than 50% from 10 European medical centers. Patients were randomized to receive optimal medical management (antihypertensive treatment and a daily statin and 80 mg aspirin) or medical management with stent placement. The end points of the STAR study were a 20% or greater decrement in creatinine clearance and cardiovascular morbidity and mortality. There was no difference between groups in progression to the primary (or secondary) end points, and there was a 3% serious complication rate among those receiving stenting. Although the STAR study had limitations, including a number of false positives in the screening process (i.e., patients falsely identified as having renal artery stenosis greater than 50% by duplex), it concluded that stenting had no effect on progression of impaired renal function and recommended optimizing medical treatment and avoidance of renal artery stenting.

Summary: Renal artery disease is a common condition encountered by the vascular provider and, in its severe forms, can lead to renovascular hypertension and decrement in renal function. ARVD is a marker for more widespread arterial occlusive disease and cardiovascular death, and it is associated with the social risk factors such as tobacco use, obesity, and sedentary lifestyle. Symptomatic ARVD frequently occurs in conjunction with significant other medical comorbidities such as chronic essential hypertension and diabetes mellitus.

The majority of patients initially referred for assessment of renal artery disease do not need extensive imaging or intervention but can be assessed with duplex ultrasound of the renal arteries and kidney and basic chemistry studies such as serum creatinine and creatinine clearance. More extensive or chronic forms of renal artery disease, or those occurring in young patients in whom there is concern for congenital disease or FMD, may require contrast imaging (CTA or MRA). Lifestyle risk factor modification and optimizing antihypertensive medications are successful in managing hypertension, and even renal insufficiency, in most cases. Patients with refractory or severe blood pressure problems (or decline in renal size or function) should be considered in a multidisciplinary forum for an intervention.

The bulk of rigorous clinical evidence—in the form of prospective, randomized, multicenter studies—fails to support the role of routine intervention (open or endovascular) to achieve lasting improvements in blood pressure or renal function in patients with ARVD. The provider who is evaluating these patients should become familiar with the ASTRAL, CORAL, and STAR trials as well as other studies that have evaluated the role of intervention in the management of this condition. Because subsets of patients with renal artery disease do benefit from large vessel revascularization (open or endovascular), the provider should apply the findings of these clinical studies to the individual patient (ideally as part of a multidisciplinary evaluation) in order to achieve optimal outcomes (i.e., patient-centered management strategy).

Selected Readings

Glodny B, Glodny DE. John Loesch, discoverer of renovascular hypertension, Harry Goldblatt: two great pioneers in circulation research. *Ann Int Med.* 2006;144:286-295.

Bax L, Woittiez AJ, Kouwenberg HJ, et al. Stent placement in patients with atherosclerotic renal artery stenosis and impaired renal function (STAR): a randomized trial. *Ann Intern Med.* 2009;150(12):840-848.

Wheatley K, Ives N, Gray R, et al.; on behalf of the ASTRAL (Angioplasty and Stenting for Renal Artery Lesions) Investigators. Revascularization versus medical therapy for renal-artery stenosis. *N Engl J Med.* 2009;361:1953-1962.

Cooper CJ, Murphy TP, Cutlip DE, et al. Stenting and medical therapy for atherosclerotic renal artery stenosis (CORAL). *N Engl J Med.* 2014;370:13-22.

Textor SC, Lerman LO. Paradigm shifts in atherosclerotic renovascular disease: where are we now? *J Am Soc Nephrol.* 2015;26(7):2074-2080.

Davis RP, Pearce JD, Craven TE, et al. Atherosclerotic renovascular disease among hypertensive adults. *J Vasc Surg.* 2009;50:564-571.

Mousa AY, AbuRahma AF, Bozzay J, Broce M, Bates M. Update on intervention versus medical therapy for atherosclerotic renal artery stenosis. *J Vasc Surg.* 2015;61(6):1613-1623.

Coleman DM, Eliason JL, Stanley JC. Arterial reconstructions for pediatric splanchnic artery occlusive disease. *J Vasc Surg.* 2018;pii:S0741-521(18):30269-6. doi: 10.1016/j.jvs.2017.12.070

Lobeck IN, Alhajjat AM, Dupree P, et al. The management of pediatric renovascular hypertension: a single center experience and review of the literature. *J Pediatric Surg.* 2017;pii: S0022-3468(17):30833-3. doi: 10.1016/j.jpedsurg2017.12.008.

Expert Panels on Urologic Imaging and Vascular Imaging. American College of Radiology (ACR) appropriateness criteria renovascular hypertension. *J Am Coll Radiol.* 2017;14(11S):S540-S549.

Campese V, Adenuga G. Renovascular disease: is there still a role for revascularization? *Clin Nephrol.* 2018;89(4):229-240.

Mousa AY, Campbell JE, Stone PA, Broce M, Bates MC, AbuRahma AF. Short- and long-term outcomes of percutaneous transluminal angioplasty stenting of renal FMD over a ten-year period. *J Vasc Surg.* 2012;55:421-427.

16 Mesenteric Ischemic Syndromes

Intestinal ischemia comprises a small portion of all peripheral vascular problems. Although aortic atherosclerosis may involve the origins of the mesenteric arteries, intestinal collateral blood flow usually is adequate enough to prevent symptomatic, chronic intestinal ischemia. Likewise, arterial emboli can obstruct mesenteric arteries, but more commonly they flow by the visceral vessels and lodge in the leg arteries. Consequently, these anatomic and hemodynamic features make intestinal ischemia less common than chronic claudication or acute ischemia of the lower extremities.

For several reasons, acute or chronic intestinal ischemia remains one of the most challenging problems of peripheral vascular surgery. The diagnosis should be entertained based upon clinical suspicion or a lack of other clear etiology for the patient's problems. It is not unusual for someone who has complained of nonspecific abdominal pain to have had a detailed evaluation of their gastrointestinal tract and yet be referred for consideration of arterial insufficiency very late in their course. Failure to recognize that a patient has some form of intestinal ischemia is one of the main reasons for the modest results obtained with intervention. Patients often are operated on too late to salvage the ischemic intestine or, many times, to save the patient's life. Even when intestinal ischemia is recognized and treated expeditiously, many patients still succumb because of serious underlying medical problems. The best results have been achieved in patients with chronic mesenteric ischemia (CMI) who undergo intestinal revascularization before severe weight loss or acute thrombosis occurs. Catheter-based techniques have lower morbidity than open surgical revascularization and are often the preferred first-line therapy, with surgery reserved for younger patients with fewer comorbidities or when catheter-based interventions have failed.

In this chapter, we emphasize early recognition of intestinal ischemia. **Delay in diagnosis represents one of the primary failings in the care of these patients.** Also, we highlight features of treatment and some of the decision-making needed in the proper care of these patients.

MESENTERIC ARTERY ANATOMY

Certain anatomic features of the mesenteric circulation determine symptoms and influence management of intestinal ischemia. The celiac axis supplies the foregut, the superior mesenteric artery (SMA) the midgut, and the inferior mesenteric artery (IMA) the hindgut. Anatomically, the foregut includes the distal esophagus through the second part of the duodenum, the midgut extends from the second part of the duodenum and includes the entire small intestine and proximal 2/3 of the colon, and the hindgut is the descending colon and rectum. Although the three major mesenteric arteries supply specific territories, they normally intercommunicate by excellent collateral channels. These collaterals enlarge when a proximal mesenteric artery is stenotic or occluded. **The primary collateral pathways between**

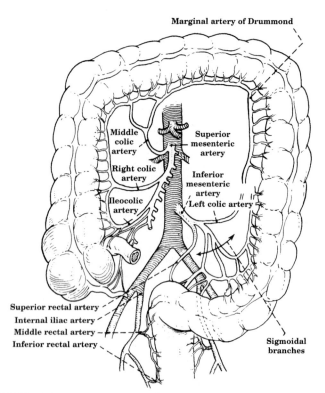

FIGURE 16.1 Anatomy of the colonic arterial supply. Collateral channels play an important role for blood flow to the small and large intestine. The pancreaticoduodenal arteries supply collaterals between the celiac and SMA and are important when one is severely diseased (not shown). When the IMA is diseased or occluded by atherosclerosis, viability of the left colon may depend on collateral flow from the SMA via the marginal artery of Drummond.

the celiac and superior mesenteric arteries are via the gastroduodenal artery to the pancreaticoduodenal arcade that connects with the SMA. The IMA has several main sources of collateral flow when it is obstructed. The middle colic branch of the SMA connects around the transverse colon to the marginal artery of Drummond, a continuation of the left colic branch of the IMA (Fig. 16.1). The IMA also receives collateral flow via the middle hemorrhoidal artery, a branch of the internal iliac artery (Fig. 16.2). In some instances, a more direct connection in the left mesocolon develops more centrally from the marginal artery. This is known as the arc of Riolan or meandering mesenteric artery (Fig. 16.3). These abundant collateral channels for mesenteric circulation explain the clinical observation that intestinal angina usually does not occur until at least two of the three main mesenteric arteries have severe occlusive disease. **Mesenteric ischemia generally refers to the limitation of blood flow to the midgut; therefore, the SMA is invariably affected.** Mesenteric ischemia is differentiated from ischemic colitis, which can occur from IMA disease and insufficient collaterals, but more often results from nonocclusive ischemia and small vessel disease.

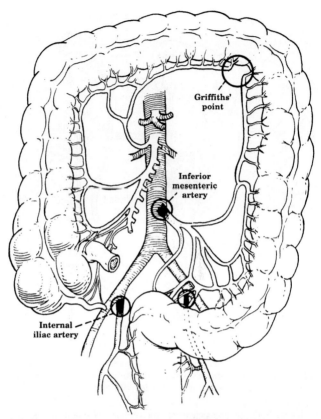

FIGURE 16.2 Critical arterial inflow points for the left colon. If occlusive disease or operative reconstruction obliterates flow through both internal iliac arteries and the IMA, the colon may become severely ischemic. Colonic ischemia is more than likely in this situation if the superior mesenteric-inferior mesenteric collateral connections are not developed or injured at Griffiths' point.

CLINICAL PRESENTATION

Intestinal ischemia is classified as either chronic or acute. However, the presentations may overlap, since chronic mesenteric stenosis can progress to acute thrombosis and intestinal infarction.

I. **CHRONIC MESENTERIC ISCHEMIA (CMI)** often eludes early diagnosis because the chronic abdominal pain is attributed to some other GI disorder. Frequently, the patient has undergone a multitude of diagnostic investigations of the gallbladder, liver, and alimentary tract with ultrasounds and CT imaging, contrast swallows, and upper and lower endoscopies. Because of progressive weight loss, some patients are mistakenly thought to have cancer. Certain clinical features, however, should raise suspicion of chronic intestinal ischemia. Characteristic symptoms are abdominal pain and significant weight loss.

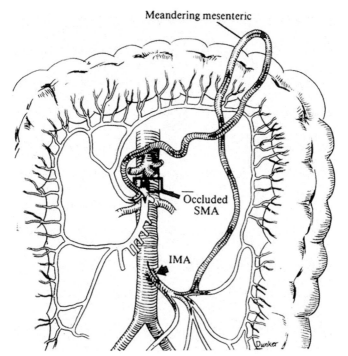

FIGURE 16.3 Direct connection in the mesocolon between SMA and IMA can develop for purposes of collateral flow. This is known as the Arc of Riolan or the meandering mesenteric artery. SMA, superior mesenteric artery; IMA, inferior mesenteric artery.

A. Classically, the **chronic abdominal pain** is intermittent and postprandial. It usually is localized to the epigastrium and has a dull ache, crampy, or colicky quality that begins 30 to 60 minutes after eating and may persist for a few hours. Patients may have associated abdominal bloating or diarrhea.

B. **Involuntary weight loss** eventually occurs because the patient associates eating with pain. Consequently, a "food fear" develops. While actually avoiding food altogether is rare, oral intake often is modified until liquids become the primary nutrient.

C. Physical findings of chronic intestinal ischemia are limited primarily to **weight loss** and an **abdominal bruit**, which is present in over half of individuals. Since the weight loss usually is insidious over several months and many patients with atherosclerosis have abdominal bruits, the significance of these nonspecific findings often is overlooked when the patient initially presents.

D. CMI should be suspected in any adult who has chronic abdominal pain, progressive weight loss, other signs of generalized cardiovascular disease, and a negative workup for more common GI disorders. Some 70% of patients with CMI have been diagnosed with peripheral vascular disease in other territories. They are usually younger than standard aneurysmal or occlusive disease patients (mid-sixties) and are smokers, and over half are women. These features collectively should lead to the following simple questions of patients suspected of having CMI: (a) Do you have abdominal pain after meals? (b) Have you experienced significant weight loss in the past 1 or 2 months?

II. **ACUTE MESENTERIC ISCHEMIA (AMI)** has three main etiologies: thrombosis of an arterial stenosis, embolism, and nonocclusive small vessel insufficiency. Very rarely, venous mesenteric thrombosis may occur. Although the initial symptom for all these etiologies is abdominal pain, the clinical setting often suggests the most likely underlying cause. The frequency of each etiology may vary among medical centers, but generally acute intestinal ischemia is caused by thrombosis in 40% of cases, embolism in another 40%, and intestinal hypoperfusion in 20% of cases.

A. **Severe generalized abdominal pain that is disproportionate to the physical findings** remains the classic presentation of AMI. Nausea, vomiting, or diarrhea may follow shortly after the onset of symptoms and are very common. Although the abdomen may have diffuse tenderness, bowel sounds may be heard, and peritoneal signs usually are absent. The only early laboratory abnormality may be a mildly elevated white blood cell count. With these findings, the clinician must entertain the possibility of AMI and undertake steps to alleviate it. Aggressive radiologic and surgical intervention at this point can salvage the ischemic intestine in about 50% of such patients.

Significant leukocytosis and acidosis with elevated serum lactic acid are late findings and herald a more protracted ischemic course. If intestinal ischemia remains unrecognized, physical findings will change as intestinal necrosis develops—which can happen within 6 to 8 hours of the onset of abdominal pain. Bloody diarrhea may occur, although often it is not present. Hypovolemia becomes evident as fluids are sequestered in the ischemic intestinal wall and surrounding tissues. Fever, peritoneal signs, and shock occur as sepsis becomes established. When intestinal ischemia has advanced to this point, the likelihood of salvaging the ischemic intestine of the critically ill patient is less than 15% to 20%.

B. The **clinical setting** and the patient's past medical history usually suggest the etiology of AMI. If chronic intestinal angina preceded acute symptoms, thrombosis of a mesenteric artery stenosis is the most likely etiology. Emboli should be suspected when atrial fibrillation is present or if the patient has had previous cerebral or lower extremity thromboembolism. Nonocclusive mesenteric ischemia (NOMI) occurs in the setting of low cardiac output. The most common predisposing conditions for NOMI are myocardial infarction, congestive heart failure, renal or hepatic disease, hemodialysis, certain drugs, classically digitalis and diuretics, or any major operation that leads to hypovolemia or hypotension in a patient with atherosclerosis.

DIAGNOSTIC TESTS

When AMI is suspected, thin slice (1 mm) CT angiography is advised as a rapid screening examination. CTA has the advantage of being able to visualize not only the arteries but also the intestine or other intra-abdominal pathology. The intestine may appear normal early on but can show pneumatosis intestinalis and ascites with advanced ischemia. Thin slices are important to capture degree of occlusion and small thromboemboli in these medium-sized visceral vessels.

The evaluation of possible CMI usually includes other diagnostic tests to investigate the patient's symptoms—commonly endoscopy or barium studies of the upper and lower GI tract. Abdominal ultrasound and CT scanning may also reveal hepatobiliary disease or occult tumors such as cancer of the pancreas or lymphoma of the retroperitoneum. Thin slice CT angiography is a good screening tool for significant visceral segment atherosclerosis and will demonstrate important collateral patterns. However, a CT with thicker slices may only provide limited images of the visceral vessels as the heavy calcification present in chronically diseased vessels can make the presence of stenosis or even occlusion difficult to judge. Contrast-enhanced MRA is also a helpful diagnostic tool that avoids the radiation of CT; however, this technology may overcall the degree of narrowing.

Duplex scanning is a very accurate and noninvasive method of interrogating mesenteric blood flow patterns. Similar to other arteries, velocity and waveform parameters are used to discriminate between normal subjects and those with visceral artery stenosis. It is normally performed in the fasting state, as the postprandial state increases flow to the gut and therefore the velocity in the SMA, that could lead to false positives. General findings on fasting examination suggesting ≥70% stenosis include **celiac PSV greater than 200 cm/s, EDV greater than 55 cm/s, reversed hepatic/splenic arterial flow; SMA PSV greater than 275 cm/s, EDV greater than 45 cm/s.** Studies may be indeterminate when performed by less experienced sonographers or in patients with obscuring bowel gas or larger body habitus. A good quality Duplex with normal velocities is 99% predictive for the absence of mesenteric disease and should not require further study. The extent of diagnostic workup for patients presenting with chronic abdominal pain obviously must be individualized, yet advances in CTA, MRA, and duplex scanning has provided a relatively quick, easy, and effective way to discriminate those who should have arteriography.

Arteriography is typically reserved for cases in which CTA is unavailable, unclear, or in order to pursue catheter-based treatment. An arteriogram with lateral views of the aorta to show the mesenteric artery origins is the definitive method. Arteriography can facilitate treatment with percutaneous angioplasty and stenting. If needed, vasodilating drugs and thrombolytic agents can be delivered selectively into the mesenteric circulation.

MANAGEMENT

Treatment for mesenteric ischemia also can be organized into the two broad categories of chronic and acute ischemia.

I. **CHRONIC MESENTERIC ISCHEMIA** can be relieved only by correction of the occlusive lesions. There is no effective medical therapy. However, asymptomatic mesenteric disease does not warrant intervention. Surgical correction is very effective at reestablishing flow, but in recent years, balloon angioplasty and stenting has become the most common method of revascularization.

A. One aspect of perioperative care, **nutritional status**, deserves special emphasis. Since CMI leads to progressive weight loss, some patients are chronically malnourished and have no nutritional reserves for a major abdominal operation. In general, one should not delay revascularization for prolonged nutritional repletion but proceed expeditiously to intestinal revascularization before the patient with progressive chronic ischemia suffers an acute catastrophic bowel infarction. It is not uncommon for these patients to have atrophied bowel mucosa due to the chronic ischemia. Even after revascularization, adaptation may take several days to weeks. Nausea, vomiting, and colicky pain may be precipitated by full early feeding. Parenteral nutrition with early, slow enteral feedings may be essential.

B. **There are two basic surgical options** for mesenteric revascularization: bypass grafting or endarterectomy. Over the years, different authors have preferred one technique over the other. Either supraceliac (antegrade) or infrarenal (retrograde) aortomesenteric bypass grafting is the procedure of choice for most patients (Fig. 16.4). The direct retrograde configuration has been hindered with the problem of graft kinking and, therefore, a "lazy C-loop" graft of reinforced prosthetic should be used. The optimum method of mesenteric revascularization, however, highly depends on the number of vessels occluded and the condition of the abdominal aorta in each patient. Indeed, the optimal number of vessels to be revascularized is controversial. Some centers espouse single vessel (SMA) and others multiple vessel (usually SMA and celiac) reconstruction. Transaortic endarterectomy has also been successful for multiple, focal visceral occlusive lesions at the origins of the mesenteric arteries. Combined infrarenal aortic replacement with retrograde prosthetic bypasses to mesenteric arteries may be performed when either severe aortic occlusive or aneurysmal disease coexists with CMI. However, combining mesenteric revascularization and aortic replacement carries a high mortality rate (10% to 20%) in these cachectic patients. Alternatively, catheter-based techniques may be combined with open surgery to limit morbidity (e.g., SMA stenting prior to open AAA repair).

Regardless of which method of revascularization is selected, early relief of intestinal angina is achieved in over 90% of patients. Graft patencies reveal primary rates of 60% to 80% with primary-assisted 5-year patencies of over 90%. Late survival in these patients who are burdened with atherosclerosis is 60% to 75% at 5 years. In general, we believe the best long-term results have been obtained by revascularization of at least two occluded or stenotic vessels. Yet others believe this to come at a cost of extra morbidity and mortality owing to the more significant dissection, fluid loss, and operative time. Since revascularization of a single mesenteric occlusion often offers relief to most patients, complete revascularization must be weighed against the patient's overall condition, prognosis, and other technical factors.

Endovascular therapies are less-invasive alternatives for the treatment of CMI. The early morbidity and mortality of catheter-based techniques for mesenteric disease is lower than that of surgery. However, the compromise may be durability. Five-year primary patency and primary-assisted patency rates of mesenteric angioplasty and stenting are reported to be approximately 50% and up to 80%, respectively. Many physicians perform mesenteric angioplasty and stenting as first-line therapy for CMI, reserving open surgical bypass for endovascular failures (Fig. 16.5).

II. Successful management of **acute mesenteric ischemia (AMI)** usually begins with rapid imaging to define the mesenteric anatomy. CTA has become so refined that the absolute need for arteriography has been lessened (Fig. 16.6). Optimal therapy for AMI cannot be determined unless the clinician knows whether the problem is thrombotic, embolic, or hypoperfusion-related. This may sometimes be confusing, and the answer may not be apparent until during therapy or afterward.

A. **Thrombosis** usually is apparent on imaging by obstruction of the SMA at its origin from the aorta. The SMA is the most clinically relevant artery involved by thrombosis. Specifically, CTA can show chronic disease and calcification with superimposed darker-appearing thrombus. Aortography may show a flush occlusion of the vessel, with minimal distal filling of branches. Systemic heparin is indicated to prevent clot propagation. Broad-spectrum antibiotics covering intestinal flora are administered. It is common for these patients to have a history of symptoms consistent with CMI suggesting mesenteric stenoses.

Emergency intervention should be undertaken to assess bowel viability and to revascularize the obstructed artery. Resection of nonviable intestine without revascularization of the remaining small bowel is

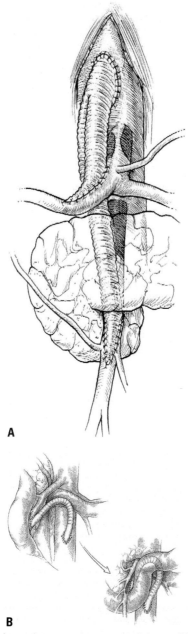

A

B

FIGURE 16.4 (A) Antegrade two-vessel aortomesenteric bypass. **(B)** Retrograde "lazy" c-loop reinforced ePTFE single-vessel aortomesenteric bypass demonstrates no kinking after bowel repositioning.

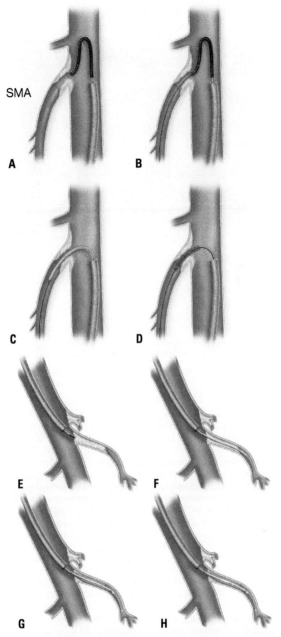

FIGURE 16.5 The SMA can be approached percutaneously from either a femoral (**A–D**) or brachial approach (**E–H**). A long sheath is positioned near the origin of the vessel. A multipurpose or Sos type catheter is used to engage the vessel, and a wire is advanced into the distal SMA. The stenosis is predilated with a small balloon. A balloon-expandable stent is deployed over the stenosis, ideally protruding a couple of millimeters into the aorta to cover "spillover" plaque. (From **A–D** Darling RC, Ozaki CK. *Master Techniques in Surgery: Vascular Surgery: Arterial Procedures.* Philadelphia: Wolters Kluwer Health; 2016, with permission.)

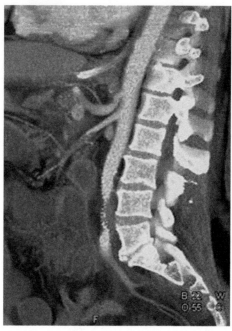

FIGURE 16.6 Computed tomography arteriography image revealing SMA embolus beyond the first several branches. This is seen as contrast attenuation compared to the aorta and more proximal SMA.

associated with a high incidence of further intestinal infarction and death. **Generally the bowel should be revascularized before intestinal resection.** This allows for interrogation of the bowel with known perfusion in order to assess viability. An exception to this rule is resection before revascularization when a segment of intestine is grossly gangrenous or perforated and the abdomen is considered contaminated. Revascularization may be performed with either catheter-based techniques or open surgical approach. In the operating room, thrombosis of the SMA should be suspected with significant palpable atherosclerotic burden at its origin and no palpable pulse nor continuous-wave Doppler signal. A single aortomesenteric bypass is sufficient in these seriously ill patients. The simplest procedure is usually a retrograde infrarenal aortomesenteric or an ileo-mesenteric bypass to the SMA. When bowel contamination is present, a vein graft is preferable to a synthetic material. Despite technical successes, the overall mortality for emergency treatment of AMI is 40% to 60%.

Intestinal viability can be difficult to judge based on appearance alone. Fluorescein can be injected in a peripheral vein followed by immediate examination of the bowel under an ultraviolet Wood's light in a darkened operating room. A viable bowel has a smooth or uniform fluorescence, whereas nonviable bowel has decreased, patchy, or no fluorescence. A continuous-wave Doppler can be used to interrogate the mesentery and antimesenteric border of the bowel. Peristalsis also suggests viability. When it appears that the bowel may survive, it may be left alone and a second-look operation performed within 24 hours to reassess the intestinal viability. Not infrequently, the patient's physiologic status is best served by revascularization, bowel resection, discontinuity with open abdomen, ICU resuscitation, and a second-look operation and restoration of intestinal continuity. **Second-look operations should be routine if *any* bowel had questionable viability at the initial operation.**

B. **Emboli** usually lodge a few centimeters beyond the origin of the SMA at the level of the first jejunal branches *sparing the proximal jejunum* (Fig. 16.7A). Emboli are usually cardiogenic in nature. The SMA is the mesenteric

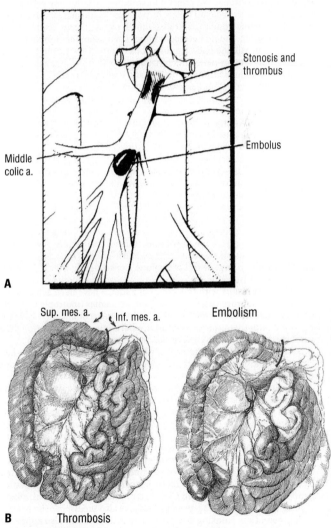

FIGURE 16.7 (A) Commonly occurring locations of thrombosis and embolism in the SMA. **(B)** Note the spared proximal jejunum in-gut ischemia due to acute embolization, as opposed to that with involved proximal jejunum due to acute thrombosis of SMA stenosis.

artery in which emboli are most likely to lodge, due to its acute takeoff from the aorta. Novel catheter-based techniques may effectively remove the clot with aspiration thrombectomy, thrombolysis, and/or angioplasty and stenting. Operative differentiation suggesting embolism over thrombosis can be suggested by new onset of cardiac arrhythmia, ischemic sparing of the proximal jejunum, and a soft SMA origin and surrounding aorta (Fig. 16.7B). Surgical embolectomy is performed by a mesenteric artery arteriotomy and Fogarty catheter. Some prefer a transverse arteriotomy. The weight of the edematous bowel, however, may lead to tearing of the arteriotomy. We prefer a longitudinal arteriotomy with patch angioplasty closure. Should inflow be poor and inadequately established with embolectomy due to arterial stenosis, bypass is now readily done. Again, vein grafts should be used if there is significant contamination of the abdomen. Milking back the thrombus of the SMA branches, branch embolectomy and on-table direct thrombolytic therapy, and heparin are all options to reduce thrombus burden and improve flow after SMA main trunk embolectomy. Emphasis should be made on temporizing damage control surgery with abdominal vacuum packing, resuscitation, and second-look operation.

Still, by adhering to the above-mentioned principles, between 10% and 15% of those with AMI will have midgut infarction at exploration and only comfort measures will have to be instituted. Of those in whom operative measures and salvage are pursued, approximately, half will require bowel resection at initial operation and the other half subsequent bowel resection at the second look. Some may require more review operations until bowel viability is finalized.

C. **Nonocclusive mesenteric ischemia (NOMI)** generally is seen in critically ill patients who have low cardiac output. They often are poor risks for any surgery and many times are so labile that transport to the angiographic suite or operating room is a major undertaking. Their arteriograms show peripheral mesenteric vasoconstrictions and a "chain of sausages" appearance, but with no large-vessel occlusions. Consequently, the entire intestine is diffusely ischemic.

The best results with this group of patients have been achieved by measures to improve cardiovascular hemodynamics (inotropic support) and to vasodilate the mesenteric vasculature. The recommended splanchnic vasodilator therapy is papaverine. Catheter-directed papaverine at 30 to 60 mg/h can be accomplished percutaneously, in an attempt to incite this vasodilation. The catheter is placed in the SMA. In general, when peritonitis develops, abdominal exploration is necessary, but very poor outcomes are expected.

Ischemic colitis is a localized process that typically affects the descending colon and is often seen in elderly patients with other comorbid diseases. The most common etiology is small vessel disease and a remarkable sensitivity of the colonic vasculature to the renin-angiotensin axis. In contrast to mesenteric ischemia, ischemic colitis is usually managed with fluids and antibiotics, with colectomy performed for refractory cases with transmural ischemia. Revascularization surgery is rarely required.

D. **Mesenteric venous thrombosis** is an extremely rare entity. It may be incited by hypercoagulable states, low mesenteric flow states such as congestive heart failure, cirrhosis, or Budd-Chiari syndrome. Intra-abdominal inflammatory conditions such as diverticulitis may also predispose the patient to this condition. Smoking and prior venous thromboses also appear to place patients at a higher risk. **Seventy percent of these thromboses involve the superior mesenteric vein proper with one-third in the splenic vein and one-third with thrombus burden in the portal vein.** CT venography and duplex are used for diagnostic purposes. Full anticoagulation is considered the standard of care with open surgical exploration reserved for cases with concern for ischemic bowel as a result of massive venous congestion and **venous gangrene.** The location of the SMV makes it less accessible to standard angiographic techniques. There are poorly defined roles for endovascular or surgical thromboembolectomy and thrombolysis.

E. **Median arcuate ligament syndrome** is controversial as an etiology for actual intestinal ischemia, as the pathophysiology results from isolated compression of the celiac axis. This creates a functional stenosis of the celiac axis, but as mentioned, should not create significant ischemia because of the rich collateral network via the pancreaticoduodenal vessels. Some extrinsic compression of the celiac axis by the median arcuate ligament is common, particularly in women, but most experts question its functional importance. Symptoms may be attributable to irritation of the nerve ganglion that overlies the celiac artery. Division of the median arcuate ligament and nerve plexus, with or without patch angioplasty of the celiac stenosis or an interposition graft, may alleviate symptoms. Patients with this compressive syndrome should not be stented, as the ligament is likely to compress or crush the stent.

Selected Readings

Atkins MD, Kwolek CJ, LaMuraglia GM, et al. Surgical revascularization versus endovascular therapy for chronic mesenteric ischemia: a comparative experience. *J Vasc Surg.* 2007;45:1162-1171.
Single-center comparison of 80 patients treated with either open or endovascular intervention.

Bjork M, Koelemay M, Acosta S, et al. Management of the diseases of mesenteric arteries and veins: clinical practice guidelines of the European Society of Vascular Surgery (ESVS). *Eur J Vasc Endovasc Surg.* 2017;53:460-510.
Comprehensive guidelines on contemporary management of mesenteric arterial and venous pathology.

Blauw JT, Bulut T, Oderich GS, et al.; on behalf of the Dutch Mesenteric Ischemia Study Group. Mesenteric vascular treatment 2016: from open surgical repair to endovascular revascularization. *Best Pract Res Clin Gastroenterol.* 2017;31:75-84.
Modern management of acute and chronic mesenteric ischemia is effectively summarized.

Hebert GS, Steele SR. Acute and chronic mesenteric ischemia. *Surg Clin N Am.* 2007;87:1115-1134.
Overview of diagnosis, imaging, and treatment for mesenteric ischemia.

Kolkman JJ, Geelkerken RH. Diagnosis and treatment of chronic mesenteric ischemia: an update. *Best Pract Res Clin Gastroenterol.* 2017;31:49-57.
Synopsis of the physiology and diagnosis of mesenteric ischemia.

Mitchell EL, Moneta GL. Mesenteric duplex scanning. *Persp Vasc Endovasc Ther.* 2006;18(2):175-183.
Duplex criteria for mesenteric stenoses reviewed.

Park WP, Cherry KJ, Chua HK, et al. Current results of open revascularization for chronic mesenteric ischemia: a standard for comparison. *J Vasc Surg.* 2002;35:853-859.
Series from the Mayo Clinic of 98 patients over a decade treated with surgical revascularization.

Pillai AK, Kalva SP, Hsu SL, et al.; Society of interventional radiology standards of practice committee. Quality improvement guidelines for mesenteric angioplasty and stent placement for the treatment of chronic mesenteric ischemia. *J Vasc Interv Radiol.* 2018;29(5):642-647.
Current indications and endovascular treatment for CMI from the Society of Interventional Radiology.

17

Upper Extremity Vascular Disorders

In the spectrum of vascular diseases, upper extremity arterial problems, including vasospastic disorders, are relatively uncommon. When pain, numbness, coolness, or ulcers involve the fingers or hand, patients generally seek early medical attention. Such symptoms restrict many normal activities and quickly raise the patient's fear of permanent loss of hand function.

The underlying causes of arm ischemia and vasospastic disorders are diverse. For simplicity, they may be organized into the broad groups of emboli, atherosclerotic or aneurysmal occlusions, trauma, and small vessel arterial occlusive disease. In the initial evaluation, the clinician must determine which group the patient fits into and then diagnostic tests can be selected to define the specific underlying etiology. This chapter emphasizes principles of management after a clinical diagnosis has been established.

COMMON CLINICAL PRESENTATIONS

Although there are multiple etiologies for upper extremity arterial ischemia, including vasospastic disorders, the clinical presentations are relatively few.

I. **RAYNAUD'S PHENOMENON** is a description of a clinical presentation or syndrome that suggests vasospasm. The underlying causes are numerous (Table 17.1). Certain clinical features help differentiate Raynaud's phenomenon from other vasospastic disorders, such as acrocyanosis and livedo reticularis (Table 17.2).

A. **Raynaud's phenomenon defines an episodic vasoconstriction of the small arteries and arterioles of the extremities.** The episodes generally are initiated by cold exposure or emotional stimuli. The symptoms of acrocyanosis and livedo reticularis are constant, although they may increase with exposure to cold.

B. **The phenomenon usually follows a predictable sequence of color changes in the digits and/or hand: pallor (i.e., white), followed by cyanosis (i.e., blue), and then rubor (i.e., red).** The pallor occurs when skin perfusion is minimal due to intense vasoconstriction of small arterioles in the hand and digits. As cutaneous flow resumes, it is sluggish, beginning with poorly saturated blood leading to the bluish color of cyanosis. Finally, when cutaneous flow resumes, a hyperemic or reperfusion phase occurs causing the skin to be warm and ruborous. Attacks usually are accompanied by numb discomfort of the fingers although pain generally is not severe unless ulcerations are present. In contrast, acrocyanosis occurs mainly in women and is characterized by continuous bluish discoloration of the hands and occasionally of the lower extremities. Livedo reticularis also is a continuous vasospastic condition consisting of a mottled or reticulated reddish-blue discoloration of the lower extremities and occasionally of the hands.

C. **Raynaud's phenomenon is localized** to the fingers, toes, and occasionally nose and ears. Attacks are limited most commonly to the upper extremities and rarely involve only the toes.

TABLE 17.1   Etiologies of Raynaud's Phenomenon

Systemic diseases or conditions
Collagen vascular diseases (e.g., scleroderma)
Cold agglutinin disease and cryoglobulinemia
Myxedema
Ergotism
Macroglobulinemia
Nerve compressions
Carpal tunnel syndrome
Thoracic outlet syndrome
Occupational trauma
Pneumatic hammer operation
Chain saw operation
Piano playing
Typing
Arterial occlusive disease

D. The chance of ulceration or gangrene of the tips of the digits depends on the underlying etiology.
   1. **Primary Raynaud's** is the term applied to Raynaud's phenomenon that has no clear association with any systemic disease. It rarely results in tissue necrosis and usually occurs in young females (70% of cases). It

TABLE 17.2   Differentiation of Vasospastic Disorders

Characteristics	Raynaud's Phenomenon	Acrocyanosis	Livedo Reticularis
Sex	Primarily women (70%–80%)	Primarily women (90%)	Men or women
Age	Young adults (15–35 y)	Young adults (15–35 y)	Any age
Color change	Pallor, cyanosis, rubor	Diffuse cyanosis	Mottled cyanosis or rubor
Location	Fingers, toes, sometimes face	Usually hands, sometimes feet	Usually legs, sometimes arms
Duration	Intermittent	Continuous	Continuous
Effect of cold exposure	Increased symptoms	Increased symptoms	Increased symptoms
Skin ulceration	Occurs when collagen vascular disease (e.g., scleroderma) is present	None	Rare

has been suggested that, before the diagnosis of primary Raynaud's is made, the following criteria should be met:

1. Bilateral, symmetric Raynaud's phenomenon is present.
2. There is no evidence of large vessel arterial occlusive disease.
3. There is an absence of gangrene or significant trophic changes.
4. Symptoms should be present for a long period, usually 2 years, without evidence of any other systemic disease.

2. **Secondary Raynaud's** is the term applied when a local or systemic disease appears to be the precipitating factor for this complex of symptoms. In rare cases, Raynaud's phenomenon can also occur in relation to large vessel arterial occlusive lesions in the upper extremity. Gangrene or ulceration of digits is more common in these patients, especially when they have scleroderma, which is the most common collagen vascular disease associated with Raynaud's phenomenon. Raynaud's phenomenon is the initial symptom in 30% of cases and eventually affects 80% of patients with scleroderma. The common rheumatic diseases associated with Raynaud's phenomenon include mixed collagen vascular disease (80%), systemic lupus erythematosus (30%), dermatomyositis/polymyositis (20%), and rheumatoid arthritis (10%). It must be remembered that Raynaud's phenomenon may exist for years before some underlying systemic collagen vascular, immunologic disease, or large vessel occlusive disease is diagnosed.

3. Acrocyanosis is not associated with skin ulceration. **Livedo reticularis** may occur with ulcerations, generally when some systemic disease (e.g., periarteritis nodosa) is present or atherosclerotic microembolism is evident.

II. **TISSUE NECROSIS** includes gangrene and poorly healing ulcerations of the digits. It is not uncommon for patients to dismiss small ulcers caused by microemboli as inconsequential bruises or sores of the finger, not recognizing their more serious etiology. If Raynaud's phenomenon precedes the onset of tissue necrosis, other symptoms and signs of underlying systemic disease should be sought. In the absence of Raynaud's phenomenon, evidence of large vessel occlusive disease, emboli, or small vessel arterial occlusive disease associated with occupational trauma must be sought.

A. **Large vessel occlusive disease** of the arm usually is localized to the subclavian or axillary arteries and is commonly caused by atherosclerosis, often at the origin of the left subclavian. These plaques may manifest in small distal emboli, digital ulcers, or nail bed splinter hemorrhages. Some patients with subclavian stenosis experience arm tiredness and fatigue with mild exertion, particularly when the dominant arm is affected. Severe occlusive disease in the proximal subclavian artery may also result in **subclavian steal**, a condition in which posterior circulation symptoms develop due to retrograde "steal" of vertebral blood flow to supply the upper extremity (Fig. 3.1).

Chronic subclavian artery trauma related to thoracic outlet syndrome also may eventually lead to vessel damage with stenosis, subclavian aneurysm formation, embolization, or distal occlusion. Thoracic outlet compression may also cause extensive acute deep venous thrombosis of the arm (i.e., axillo-subclavian or effort thrombosis) with pain, discoloration and edema, and rarely venous gangrene that may be initially mistaken for arterial ischemia. A less common etiology of proximal upper extremity arterial occlusion is thrombosis of an axillary artery aneurysm caused by years of crutch use. Finally, postmastectomy irradiation of the axillary area can result in axillary-subclavian arterial stenosis years after radiation treatment.

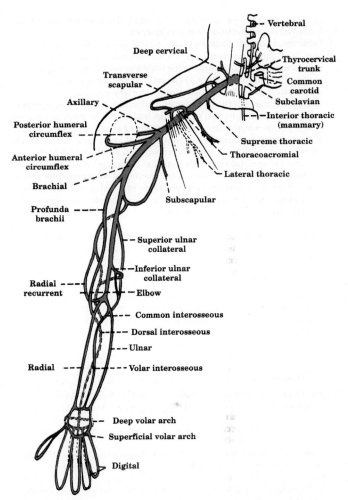

FIGURE 17.1 Arterial anatomy of the upper extremity. The collateral circulation of the arm is well developed, and, consequently, proximal large vessel occlusion seldom results in distal extremity necrosis and amputation.

B. **Emboli** to the upper extremity or digits may originate from the heart, aortic arch, innominate artery, or the subclavian, axillary, or brachial arteries. In cases of significant arm ischemia caused by arterial emboli, the heart is the origin in the majority of cases (e.g., atrial fibrillation, cardiomyopathy, valvular disease). The use of anticoagulation in patients with atrial fibrillation reduces the risk of thromboemboli. Nonetheless, breakthrough emboli can occur despite anticoagulation or when patients are taken off of their anticoagulation. The lower extremity is the most frequent location for cardiac emboli to lodge. Abnormalities in the proximal arterial network (thoracic aortic thrombus, subclavian or axillary stenoses, or aneurysms) are less often responsible for upper extremity emboli. Finally, radial or ulnar artery trauma usually from indwelling arterial lines can lead to embolization into the digital arteries.

C. **Small vessel arterial disease** associated with occupational hand trauma may cause significant hand and/or digit ischemia. Occupations involving repetitive vibration or trauma to the fingers or palmar surface of the hand predispose some individuals to spasm, thrombosis, or aneurysms of the ulnar, radial, or digital arteries. The ulnar artery is especially susceptible to local trauma over the hypothenar eminence, where it is fairly superficial and easily compressed against the underlying pisiform and hamate bones. **The term hypothenar hammer syndrome has been applied to this form of posttraumatic digital ischemia.** Activities that may lead to hand ischemia are operation of the pneumatic hammer, lathe, or chain saw. In industry, the term **vibration-induced white finger** has been applied to posttraumatic digital ischemia. Unlike the lower extremities, **atherosclerotic disease** of the distal upper extremity arteries (i.e., brachial, radial, and ulnar) is uncommon but may occasionally be seen in patients with uncontrolled diabetes and end-stage renal disease.

III. **ARM CLAUDICATION** is an unusual presentation of arm ischemia. In general, exertional arm fatigue is more commonly caused by neurologic compression at the cervical spine or thoracic outlet. Because of excellent collateral blood flow around the shoulder, subclavian occlusive disease often is asymptomatic or only mildly symptomatic (Fig. 17.1). However, active adults, especially manual laborers, may experience arm claudication from subclavian or brachial artery stenosis. Patients with a diagnosis of **giant cell arteritis** may develop long-segment stenoses of the subclavian and axillary arteries, with subsequent upper extremity claudication that can usually be managed medically.

DIAGNOSTIC TESTS

Patient history and physical examination provide most of the information necessary to diagnose the general type of upper extremity arterial disease. The following tests may be performed to confirm the clinical impression, to identify underlying etiologies, and to monitor therapy.

I. **DOPPLER VELOCITY FLOW DETECTION.** The continuous wave (handheld) Doppler is a simple means for assessing arm perfusion when pulses are not palpable. The axillary, brachial, radial, ulnar, palmar, and digital arteries can easily be checked for the presence and quality of Doppler signal. Biphasic or triphasic arterial signals are normal, while monophasic or dampened signals suggest significant arterial obstruction. Upper arm and forearm blood pressures can be measured with a routine blood pressure cuff and the Doppler unit and should normally be equivalent within 10 mm Hg. In cases of suspected claudication, arm pressures should be obtained at rest and after 2 to 5 minutes of exercise.

II. **DIGITAL PLETHYSMOGRAPHY OR LASER DOPPLER** flow patterns may provide more detail in the evaluation of digital ischemia and vasospastic disorders. Flat or diminished (<5 mm) pulse volume recordings (PVRs) confirm severe digital flow reduction and are predictive of poor healing in the presence of ulceration. PVRs using digital cuffs and/or laser Doppler flow measurements can be repeated to assess for changes in digital blood flow after initiation of treatment, either operative or nonoperative.

III. **DUPLEX ULTRASONOGRAPHY** provides excellent visualization of most upper extremity arterial segments. The main limitations are the proximal subclavian arteries, especially on the left, which is covered by the bulky clavicle. As with other arterial segments, duplex provides both a B-mode image of the vessel in question and an assessment of blood flow (i.e., velocity) through the segment.

IV. **ARTERIOGRAPHY.** CT angiography or invasive arteriography is helpful in defining the severity and extent of large vessel occlusive disease. Specifically, arteriography defines the location of the occlusive disease and provides information regarding the runoff to the forearm and hand. Arteriography is not necessary to diagnose vasospastic disorders but may be useful to rule out large vessel occlusive disease when Raynaud's phenomenon is complicated by finger ulcers. When performed, arteriography must show the entire upper extremity vasculature from its origin (i.e., innominate on the right and subclavian on the left) to the digital arteries. Failure to obtain complete upper extremity arteriography is a common reason for a missed diagnosis such as digital occlusions due to an ulcerated atheroma in the proximal subclavian artery.

V. **DIGITAL TEMPERATURE RECOVERY TIME** following immersion of the hands in a cold ice-water bath (i.e., cold immersion test) can help establish the diagnosis of Raynaud's phenomenon.

VI. **SYSTEMIC DISEASE WORKUP.** Since systemic diseases so often underlie vasospastic disorders and upper extremity ischemia, a number of screening laboratory tests should be considered. A platelet count should be done, since thrombocytosis can mimic Raynaud's phenomenon. An elevated sedimentation rate should raise suspicion of a systemic illness. Since serum protein abnormalities may be associated with vasospasm, a serum protein electrophoresis should be performed and cryoglobulins, macroglobulins, and cold agglutinins should be checked. Basic immunologic tests should include antinuclear antibody, rheumatoid factor, and lupus erythematosus tests. If scleroderma is suspected, a skin biopsy in an affected area may confirm the diagnosis or a barium esophagogram may reveal characteristic esophageal dysfunction.

MANAGEMENT

In our experience, these guidelines have provided the best assurance of relieving upper extremity ischemia, including vasospastic disorders. Where there are areas of controversy, we offer several different points of view.

I. **VASOSPASTIC DISORDERS**

A. **Primary Raynaud's** usually can be satisfactorily managed by nonoperative methods. Tissue necrosis rarely is a problem; consequently, the patient needs assurance that loss of fingers or their function is not likely to occur if the following guidelines are observed.

    1. **Avoidance of any tobacco use and protection from cold exposure** are the fundamentals of initial treatment. Tobacco leads to vasoconstriction, a fact that can be documented by comparing baseline digital PVRs to tracings taken immediately after the patient smokes several cigarettes. The basics of protection from cold exposure include warm gloves and footwear during cold weather and gloves when working with refrigeration. Maintaining core body temperature by wearing warm clothing over the trunk also helps. For many patients, these simple measures are enough to prevent symptoms from occurring.

2. When vasospasm is not satisfactorily relieved by these simple measures, **medical options** are available and usually provide some benefit. The best results are obtained with calcium channel blockers such as nifedipine or the alpha-receptor blocker prazosin. For some patients, the longer-acting form of nifedipine causes fewer side effects, which can include headache, dizziness, palpitations, flushing, and edema. Evidence suggests that the medication sildenafil (Viagra®, Pfizer Inc., NY) improves microcirculation and symptoms of Raynaud's that are otherwise refractory to vasodilator therapy.

3. **Thermal biofeedback** has demonstrated good results in many patients in whom anxiety and stress play a role in the initiation of vasospastic attacks. After biofeedback training, 80% to 90% of patients can avert an attack of Raynaud's phenomenon, and some can actually increase skin temperature as much as 4°C.

4. The role of **surgical or thoracoscopic sympathectomy** for primary Raynaud's is limited. Few patients should need sympathectomy, since conservative management controls symptoms in at least 80% of patients.

B. **Secondary Raynaud's** due to some underlying systemic disease or large vessel occlusive lesions often is a more difficult problem to manage than primary Raynaud's. Tissue necrosis with exceptionally painful digital ulcers can be a chronic problem in such patients. The fundamentals of therapy remain avoidance of tobacco, protection from cold, and treatment with vasodilators. Patients with secondary Raynaud's and painful digital ulcers may consider thoracoscopic sympathectomy treatment for pain control. Digital sympathectomies have been performed as well with some success.

In instances where secondary Raynaud's is clinically significant and associated with large vessel occlusive disease (e.g., subclavian, axillary, or brachial arteries), such lesions should be treated to maximize perfusion to the arm and hand. This is especially true in cases where noninvasive testing confirms significant ischemia in the forearm and hand or there has been tissue loss in the digits.

C. **Acrocyanosis** does not lead to tissue loss, so treatment is directed at relieving cold-induced symptoms. The conservative management described for primary Raynaud's usually is sufficient.

D. **Livedo reticularis is** also manageable in most cases by conservative treatment. Digital ulceration may occur when livedo reticularis is associated with periarteritis nodosa, lupus erythematosus, or cholesterol embolization. In such cases, sympathectomy may be considered, although results have been variable.

E. **Cold hypersensitivity** may be seen after recovery from frostbite. The affected area may become bluish and have an associated burning pain with even mild cold exposure. Initially, the medical treatment described for primary Raynaud's should be undertaken. For severe cases, regional sympathectomy may provide lasting relief, especially if it is done before pain becomes chronic.

II. **THREATENED LIMB LOSS.** Although vasospastic disorders may cause ulcerations of the tips of the digits, the hand and arm seldom become ischemic. Severe hand ischemia usually is associated with large artery occlusions, emboli, or trauma.

A. **Acute ischemia** generally requires emergency surgical intervention. The history and physical exam usually will identify the cause. If there is a delay for medical stabilization or arteriography, we administer heparin systemically to the patient to prevent thrombus propagation. Patients who develop brachial artery occlusion after catheterization should undergo immediate brachial thrombectomy and repair of the access site often under local anesthesia. Although the patient's hand may initially be relatively asymptomatic, a chronic brachial artery occlusion in these situations can cause bothersome arm claudication in active individuals. Thus, urgent brachial artery repair is preferable to delayed surgery as it can be accomplished with minimal risk and achieve return of distal pulses in nearly all patients.

B. **An arterial embolus to the upper extremity arterial circulation is the most common cause of acute arm ischemia.** The most common source of such emboli is the heart, and most often the embolus lodges in the brachial artery at the takeoff of the profunda brachii artery. Emboli tend to lodge at a branch point and may also settle at the brachial bifurcation to the radial and ulnar arteries, just below the antecubital crease in the upper forearm. These emboli can nearly always be successfully extracted with local exploration and limited Fogarty catheter embolectomy. In cases where the emboli or subsequent thrombus (i.e., clot) has extended into the distal digital arteries, adjuvant thrombolytic agents may be helpful in restoring distal outflow or runoff. Thromboemboli lodged in more proximal arterial segments such as the subclavian or axillary can also be approached through the proximal brachial or distal axillary artery with passage of the Fogarty catheter proximally. In cases of proximal subclavian or axillary artery emboli, transfemoral arteriography with placement of a catheter in the subclavian artery may provide useful diagnostic information and even therapeutic options. Importantly, if the source of the embolus is not the heart but instead an atherosclerotic lesion in the proximal subclavian or axillary artery, these will require adjuvant operative or endovascular treatment to remove the source of the emboli.

C. **Large artery occlusions in the upper extremity circulation** require treatment, either open or endovascular, as they cause significant symptoms. Proximal subclavian stenoses are preferably treated with angioplasty and stenting using a balloon-expandable stent. If the proximal subclavian artery is occluded and/or not amenable to endovascular treatment, a carotid-to-subclavian bypass or transposition of the subclavian artery into the common carotid artery are very effective options with low associated morbidity and mortality. Subclavian artery aneurysm or thrombosis secondary to thoracic outlet syndrome will require resection of the first rib and any cervical rib in conjunction with arterial reconstruction. In contrast, **axillo-subclavian vein thrombosis** secondary to thoracic outlet compression (i.e., effort thrombosis) is treated by catheter-directed thrombolytic infusion and anticoagulation followed by first rib resection. The timing of the first rib resection is somewhat controversial. Some recommend early resection after thrombolysis, while others prefer to anticoagulate the patient for 6 to 8 weeks prior to resection, to allow the surface of the inflamed vein to heal. Thrombosed axillary artery aneurysms are best treated with open operative reconstruction using an interposition graft of saphenous vein or prosthetic material. Saphenous vein is the best conduit for brachial, radial, and ulnar revascularizations.

III. **ARM CLAUDICATION.** As discussed earlier, incapacitating arm claudication is fairly uncommon because of the rich collateral blood flow to the arm. For the few patients who need revascularization, the options, open and endovascular, described above for threatened limb loss are also applicable to relieve claudication.

LONG-TERM PROGNOSIS

The long-term prognosis for most arterial problems of the upper extremity is good. Nonoperative treatment is successful in many patients. Therefore, unless the viability of the extremity is acutely threatened, a period of conservative treatment and observation should generally be followed. The patients with the worst prognosis generally are those with Raynaud's phenomenon secondary to progressive collagen vascular disease or those with extensive distal small vessel occlusion secondary to recurrent emboli or thrombosis.

Selected Readings

Campbell RA, Janko MR, Hacker RI. Hand-arm vibration syndrome: a rarely seen diagnosis. *J Vasc Surg.* 2017;3:60-62.
Case report with excellent description of occupational hand ischemia.
Kurklinsky AK, Miller VM, Rooke TW. Acrocyanosis: the Flying Dutchman. *Vasc Med.* 2011;16:288-301.
Detailed review of the pathophysiology and differential diagnosis of this esoteric diagnosis.
Landry GJ. Current medical and surgical management of Raynaud's syndrome. *J Vasc Surg.* 2013;57:1710-1716.
Comprehensive review of treatment strategies for primary and secondary Raynaud's syndrome.
Potter BJ, Pinto DS. Subclavian steal syndrome. *Circ.* 2014;129:2320-2323.
Clear explanation of the fascinating "subclavian steal" syndrome.
Sanders RJ, Hammond SL, Rao NM. Diagnosis of thoracic outlet syndrome. *J Vasc Surg.* 2007;46:601-604.
Introduction to the three types of thoracic outlet syndrome (i.e., neurogenic, venous, and arterial).
Taylor LM. Hypothenar hammer syndrome. *J Vasc Surg.* 2003;37:697.
Nice illustrations of the hypothenar hammer syndrome.
Thune TH, Ladegaard L, Licht PB. Thoracoscopic sympathectomy for Raynaud's phenomenon—a long term follow-up study. *Eur J Vasc Endovasc Surg.* 2006;32:198-202.
Single-center study about efficacy of sympathectomy for Raynaud's and discussion of potential complications.
Wigley FM. Clinical practice. Raynaud's phenomenon. *N Engl J Med.* 2002;347:1001-1008.
Expert review on differentiating primary and secondary Raynaud's phenomenon and medical management.

A spectrum of venous disorders, from simple varicose veins to venous stasis ulcers, afflicts at least 20% to 25% of the population. The basic pathophysiology and natural history of venous disorders are summarized in Chapter 2. A description of the initial lower extremity venous examination is found in Chapter 4. This chapter focuses on the principles of medical, catheter-based, and surgical therapy.

Varicose veins are one of the most common vascular problems seen in office practice. Most varicose veins are the result of a congenital predisposition to a loss of vein wall elasticity. Subsequent dilatation of the vein leads to valve cusps that can no longer coapt, causing retrograde flow ("reflux") and further degeneration of the vein. Prolonged standing, obesity, and pregnancy make all leg varicosities more symptomatic and exacerbate venous hypertension in the limb.

Most patients who have had deep vein thrombosis will develop some degree of **postthrombotic syndrome**, often years after the initial event. A surprising observation is that 5 to 10 years after lower extremity deep venous thrombosis (DVT), over 80% of patients will develop some symptoms of chronic venous insufficiency (edema, pain, ulceration). The classic physical findings of postthrombotic syndrome are a chronically indurated ankle, dark stasis pigmentation around the ankle, and skin ulceration in some patients.

Thrombosis damages deep venous valves and often leaves them incompetent. A thrombosed vein also does not completely recanalize in many cases, producing obstruction of venous outflow and exacerbation of venous pressure in the lower limb. Consequently, the patient has chronic venous hypertension in the leg when he or she stands with high venous pressures transmitted through perforating veins from the deep to superficial venous system. The calf muscle pump can no longer overcome ambulatory venous pressures. In 20% to 50% of patients with advanced signs of chronic venous insufficiency, no history of DVT is obtainable. In such cases, the etiology of venous stasis changes is either primary reflux or nonthrombotic obstruction.

Chronic venous insufficiency refers to the lower extremity skin changes that result from venous hypertension. The mechanism by which skin changes occur in the presence of venous hypertension is complex and has been the subject of extensive research. Local capillaries leak fibrinous protein that is not adequately removed by fibrinolysis, forming "perivascular cuffs" that contribute to local diffusion of oxygen and nutrients. Leukocytes become trapped and play a role in the local inflammatory process. Red blood cells escape into the tissue and break down causing brown hyperpigmentation (hemosiderin).

Severe manifestations of chronic venous insufficiency can be especially disabling for active ambulatory workers, since leg dependency increases pain and swelling and impedes ulcer healing. Leg symptoms are also worse in patients with chronic venous obstruction than in those with reflux only. In patients with chronic iliofemoral venous obstruction, venous capacitance is increased at rest and cannot compensate during exercise.

The result is severe thigh pain and a sensation of tightness with vigorous exercise, dubbed **venous claudication.** Venous ulceration is a source of significant stress, time away from work, and debilitation in 2% to 4% of the population. Fortunately, proper elastic leg support, skin care, and, in some situations, invasive therapy can alleviate many of the symptoms of chronic venous insufficiency.

I. **THE CEAP CLASSIFICATION** scheme (see Table 2.1) has been adopted worldwide in order to standardize and facilitate communication about chronic venous disorders. Venous disease is defined by clinical class (C), etiology (E), its anatomic (A) distribution in the veins, and the pathologic mechanism (P) of development (reflux or obstruction or both).

A. Clinical presentation of venous disorders relies upon physical examination. C1 disease is evidenced by telangiectasias and/or reticular veins, commonly referred to as **spider veins.** Varicose veins are distinguished by diameter greater than 3 mm and their characteristic protuberance and are seen in C2 disease. Progression to edema and skin changes from venous hypertension is seen with C3 and C4 disease, respectively. Skin changes may be mild such as eczema or dermatitis. **Lipodermatosclerosis** is a localized chronic inflammation and fibrosis of the skin and subcutaneous tissues of the lower leg, occasionally associated with scarring of the Achilles tendon. **Atrophie blanche, or white atrophy, refers to the smooth, stellate scarring that can occur with venous stasis.** The most severe clinical manifestation is venous ulceration. A healed ulcer is seen in C5 disease. An active ulcer with a full-thickness skin defect, most frequently in the ankle region, defines C6 disease.

B. The **etiology** of the venous disease is also used for classification. Venous disease may be **congenital,** as in **Klippel-Trenaunay syndrome,** which appears to be a fetal developmental abnormality. The classic clinical triad includes (a) port-wine stains, (b) hypertrophy of soft tissue and bone with overgrowth of the extremity, and (c) varicose veins. Because of the benign course of this disease, most of these patients do not have surgery and do well with conservative therapy. Occasionally, a more aggressive operative approach may be necessary in patients with large, symptomatic varicosities, especially if hemorrhage or ulceration has occurred. It is important to rule out deep venous hypoplasia, which can be present in these patients, prior to any treatment of superficial varicosities.

Venous disease may also be **primary** from the degeneration of valves and veins, or **secondary** as a result of damage from prior thrombosis (postthrombotic).

C. Anatomically, venous disease can roughly be classified as superficial, deep, and/or perforating veins. The affected veins cannot be accurately defined by physical exam alone. Duplex ultrasound is necessary if precise identification of the involved veins is desired (Chapter 5).

D. The **pathophysiology** of venous disease is from reflux, obstruction, or a combination of the two. Reflux can develop primarily or as a result of postthrombotic degeneration of valves. Obstruction is most commonly a postthrombotic event, and may occur when the affected vein is only partially recanalized. The residual webs and synechiae prevent normal venous flow. Nonthrombotic causes of venous obstruction also exist. For example, **May-Thurner syndrome** is a congenital obstruction of the left iliac vein by the anatomic crossover of the right iliac artery. In some patients, this impingement may result in pain (venous claudication), edema, and a predisposition toward developing left iliofemoral venous thrombosis. It is interesting that over 20% of the population demonstrates this compression in cadaver studies, but only a minority becomes symptomatic (Fig. 18.1).

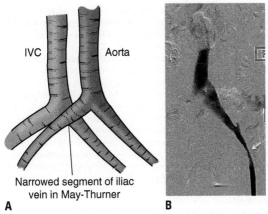

IVC   Aorta

Narrowed segment of iliac
vein in May-Thurner

A   **B**

FIGURE 18.1 May-Thurner syndrome. **(A, B)** Compression of the left iliac vein by the right iliac artery is a normal anatomic variant in 20% of the population in cadaveric study. In some individuals, this compression leads to unilateral leg edema and can predispose to acute iliofemoral DVT in a smaller percentage of patients. Venography in combination with IVUS can be used to detect this problem. (**A** is reprinted from Casserly IP. *Practical Peripheral Vascular Intervention*. Philadelphia: Wolters Kluwer; 2015, with permission; **B** is reprinted from Humphries M. Intravascular imaging. In: Zierler RE, Dawson DL, eds. *Stradness's Duplex Scanning in Vascular Disorders*. 5th ed. Philadelphia: Wolters Kluwer; 2016:438, with permission.)

II. DIAGNOSIS

A. **Clinical presentation.** Varicose veins present with unsightly bulges on the lower extremity and often with associated achiness or heaviness in the legs with prolonged standing. Symptoms may not correlate well with the degree of anatomic defect. Occasionally, a patient will abrade a varicosity, which may cause a rather impressive hemorrhage. A more common complication of varicose veins is superficial thrombophlebitis, which may cause considerable pain and disability but rarely leads to pulmonary embolism. Long-standing varicose veins may also result in chronic ankle induration, stasis dermatitis, and, occasionally, leg ulcerations. Patients with advanced venous insufficiency have skin changes, edema, and ulceration of the lower extremity. Unilateral leg edema in the absence of typical skin changes and with a normal venous duplex should undergo further investigation. This presentation raises the possibility of pelvic tumors, lymphedema, or iliac venous obstruction.

B. **Noninvasive venous testing** is very helpful in the diagnosis of venous disease as described in Chapter 5. Duplex ultrasound is the mainstay of diagnosis. Reflux in the superficial and deep veins can be determined by prolonged valve closure times (>0.5 seconds). Perforator incompetence is determined by reversed or outward flow (deep to superficial) in the perforating veins of the leg. **Duplex has greater than 95% accuracy in the detection of acute venous thrombosis and can also recognize the signs of chronic thrombosis, such as recanalization, collaterals, and more echogenic clot.** Plethysmography can provide a global assessment of the limb's venous function and is generally applied as an adjunct to duplex in more severe cases of chronic venous insufficiency. CT and MR venography are particularly useful in evaluation of the central veins (e.g., iliac veins, subclavian veins), which are less accessible by ultrasound. Occasionally, such imaging will reveal a compressive tumor as the etiology for unilateral limb edema.

Obstructed veins and collaterals can also be seen on high-quality studies. However, both CT and MR can only determine anatomic abnormalities and provide no physiologic evaluation. MR is the test of choice for characterization of venous malformations.

Invasive venography has reemerged as a useful tool to identify and treat patients with chronic thrombotic or nonthrombotic venous obstruction. Venography is also used in conjunction with catheter-directed thrombolysis for acute DVT (Chapter 19). Ascending venography provides a roadmap of the limb and central drainage, such that obstructive lesions can be identified. Descending venography can localize incompetent valves and assess the severity of the reflux. However, even when performed in several projections, venography has low sensitivity for identifying the degree of venous stenosis, intrinsic webs, or compression. Diagnostic venography is frequently combined with intravascular ultrasound (IVUS), an invasive method for gauging venous stenosis in three dimensions.

III. TREATMENT.

A. Noninvasive treatment is appropriate first-line therapy for the majority of chronic venous disorders. The symptoms may range from mild (varicose veins) to severe (ulcers). Patients should be reassured that the presence of chronic venous disease is neither life nor limb threatening. In our experience, these are frequently the unspoken concerns of our patients. Even severe venous ulceration is usually in the dermal layers and does not threaten the limb in the absence of superimposed infection or arterial insufficiency. Chronic venous insufficiency is incurable; thus, it is important that the patient understands that the goal of treatment is to minimize symptoms and prevent ulcer recurrences.

The following measures will promote venous health for patients with chronic venous diseases:

1. Regular use of compression therapy with graduated stockings
2. Elevating the feet and legs for 10 to 15 minutes whenever possible
3. Walking to improve the musculovenous pump of the calf
4. Avoiding trauma to varicose veins
5. Weight reduction for obese patients
6. Avoiding prolonged standing or sitting
7. Consultation with vascular and wound care specialist at the first signs of ulceration or cellulitis
8. Maintaining skin integrity, avoiding cracking and eczema, with proper emollients

    a. Compression therapy is the mainstay of medical treatment for all chronic venous disorders. Graded elastic stockings are available in a variety of strengths, lengths, and styles. Strengths of 20 to 30 mm Hg are most commonly prescribed for varicose veins and milder venous disorders. The stockings alleviate many of the symptoms of leg achiness, heaviness, and swelling. Although below-the-knee stockings are suitable for most patients, some women with varicose veins prefer a prescription thigh-high or panty hose variety. Several companies offer specialized venous stockings and hosiery (e.g., Sigvaris [Winterthur, Switzerland], Jobst [BSN Medical, Charlotte, NC, USA], and Medi [Medi USA Inc., Whitsett, NC, USA]).

    Patients with postthrombotic syndrome and deep venous insufficiency are often affected by **ambulatory venous hypertension**. In such patients venous pressures decrease only 20% to 30% during exercise compared with a 70% decrease in the setting of normal venous function. Venous pressures are highest in the most dependent portion of the leg at the ankle, where most postthrombotic skin changes occur. Although chronic venous hypertension cannot be corrected by elastic leg support, elastic leg support can prevent some of the leg edema. For these patients, strengths of 30 to 40 mm Hg are desirable. Below-the-knee stockings are generally sufficient in most patients for several reasons. First, postthrombotic problems nearly always occur below the knee, where venous pressures are highest. Thigh swelling seldom is a problem after acute DVT has resolved. Second, support hose that come above the knee often bind or constrict the popliteal space, especially if the hose slip down the leg. Third, patients generally do not like a heavy support hose that covers the entire leg. Many patients who are given full-length or panty hose–type heavy support hose will wear them only when visiting their physician for a checkup. However, some patients with vena cava occlusion and severe leg swelling to the waist will need full-leg heavy support hose and will wear them without complaint.

Compliance with compression therapy is particularly important for patients with active or healed venous ulceration. **Active venous ulcers heal at an average of 5 months in 97% of compliant patients compared to 55% of patients who are noncompliant.** Continued compression therapy also significantly reduces the incidence of ulcer recurrence. Several suggestions should be offered to the patient to ensure the proper and comfortable use of graduated support hose. First, the hose should be put on in the morning, prior to ambulation. Otherwise, early leg swelling may begin before the elastic support can control it. This routine usually requires that the patient bathe or shower before going to bed at night. Second, hose may be difficult to slide on the leg, especially for patients who have difficulty applying the stockings due to hand arthritis or poor conditioning. Special stocking-donning devices are commercially available. The stocking can be loaded onto the donning device, which stretches it sufficiently for easier application. A silky liner or light nylon hose worn beneath the heavy stocking can also make application easier. Third, elastic support hose must be properly fitted and made of comfortable, high-quality material, or the patient will not wear them. We encourage patients to contact the fitting shop for adjustments if their new hose do not fit satisfactorily. In general, most support hose will need to be replaced every 6 to 12 months. We will substitute Tubigrip® elastic stockinette (Mölnlycke Health Care, Norcross, GA) in sizes ranging from D through G, or sequential velcro devices (e.g., Circ-Aid), for patients unable to tolerate stockings or with large or unequal leg size. Finally, multi-chamber intermittent pneumatic pumps (e.g., NormaTec, Newton, MA) can be very helpful in the management of patients with refractory venous edema, lymphedema, or venous ulceration.

b. **Leg elevation** remains a simple and effective method of alleviating ankle edema. Patients with chronic venous insufficiency should elevate their legs above the level of the heart for 10 to 15 minutes every 2 to 4 hours during the day. This recommendation may seem impractical for the working individual, but most workers are allowed breaks during their normal work hours at which time elevation can be done. Periodic leg elevation allows most patients to remain comfortable during work. An explanatory note from the physician to the patient's employer often avoids any problem that the patient may encounter by periodically sitting down on the job.

c. **Skin care** is important if dermatitis, local infection, and ulceration are to be prevented. Scaly pruritic skin of the foot or ankle may indicate fungal infection, which is managed by a topical fungicide such as Baza® antifungal cream (2% miconazole nitrate, Coloplast Corp., Minneapolis, MN) or Lotrimin® (1% clotrimazole, Bayer Corp., Whippany, NJ). Flares of stasis dermatitis may be alleviated by short-term use of a topical steroid creams, such as triamcinolone 0.1%, but long-term use can lead to skin atrophy and should be avoided. Routine leg washing should be done with warm water and a mild soap. We discourage soaking the leg, since this may macerate friable skin and increase swelling due to dependency of the extremity. Nonperfumed emollients such as Aquaphor® or Eucerin® (Beiersdorf, Wilton, CT) should be used to treat dry, cracked skin to prevent further breakdown, ulceration, and cellulitis.

d. **Venous ulcers classically occur in the lower third of the leg above the ankle, referred to as the "gaiter distribution."** Most frequently, ulcers occur at the medial malleolus adjacent a medial ankle perforator. Less commonly, they occur on the lateral or posterior calf at the site of the lateral ankle perforator or the mid-posterior calf perforator (Fig. 18.2). The treatment of venous ulcers utilizes all of the principles listed previously; however, supplementary measures may be needed to treat refractory ulcers. A compressive bandage should be applied over the ulcer dressing (Fig. 18.3). A semirigid bandage can provide a greater amount of continuous compression than a stocking, and is a good adjuvant technique for nonhealing ulcers. **The Unna boot is the most well known of these semirigid, multilayer bandages.** The three-layered boot is applied by a medical professional. The innermost layer is a medicated paste gauze that contains calamine, zinc oxide, glycerin, sorbitol, and magnesium aluminum silicate. The second layer is gauze, followed by an outer elastic compression wrap. The boot hardens and can be left on for a week, although more frequent checks (e.g., every 2 to 3 days) of the leg should be performed in diabetic patients or those with resolving cellulitis. The advantage of a boot is that continuous compression is applied and patient compliance is enforced. An absorbent dressing can be applied to the ulcer before applying the boot. The Profore system (Smith and Nephew, London, UK) is a four-layer, commercially available bandage that works by the same principles and is also effective for venous stasis. Meticulous wound care under the supervision of dedicated health care professionals is central to the successful treatment of venous ulcers. Various ointments, salves, and dressings are available for comprehensive wound care. Clean, granulating wounds should be treated with a hydrogel or hydrocolloid dressing to maintain a moist healing environment, whereas wounds with large amount of necrotic tissue should undergo manual sharp debridement. Treatment with an enzymatic debriding ointment such as collagenase may also be beneficial, but some patients experience discomfort or burning with application. Wounds with large amounts of serous drainage should be treated with application of absorbent dressing or powder, such as calcium alginate. All of these dressings can be applied underneath a compression stocking or boot, although we would caution not to use the Unna boot or Profore systems in the setting of active infection or cellulitis. If the ulcer appears

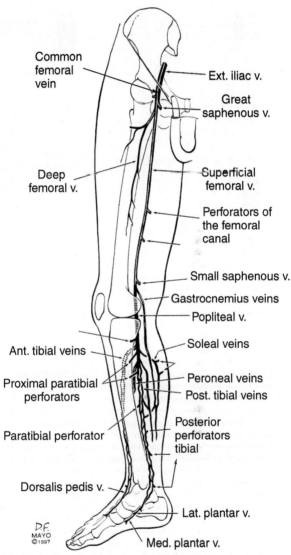

FIGURE 18.2 Location of the major lower leg perforators. The perforating vein sites on the medial leg, especially the upper, middle, and lower posterior tibial perforators (formerly called Cockett's perforators), are common locations for postthrombotic venous ulcers. Ulcers seldom occur at the posterior and lateral venous perforators.

infected, evidenced by foul odor, surrounding cellulitis, fever, or increased drainage, a quantitative culture can be taken or a short course (5 to 7 days) of empiric antibiotics prescribed. Routine use of wound swabs is discouraged, as a multitude of flora will grow from every open wound.

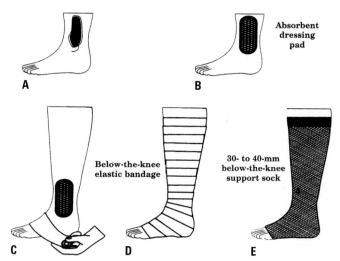

A

B Absorbent dressing pad

C Below-the-knee elastic bandage

D

E 30- to 40-mm below-the-knee support sock

FIGURE 18.3 Application of a compressive bandage for a venous ulcer. **(A)** The ulcer should be washed with warm water and mild soap. In general, topical antibiotics should be avoided since they may cause topical allergic reactions. For grossly infected ulcers, the infection should be controlled before the bandage is applied. **(B)** A soft absorbent pad should be placed over the ulcer. **(C–E)** The leg from the foot to the knee is wrapped with a compressive dressing: an Unna's paste boot bandage, and Ace wrap, or a 30- to 40-mm below-the-knee support stocking.

B. **Invasive therapies** can be used to treat chronic venous insufficiency that is refractory to compression therapy or in patients who are unable or unwilling to comply with compression. Indications for treatment include (a) cosmetic concerns, (b) symptoms of achiness, heaviness, pain, or edema, (c) bleeding from friable varicose veins, (d) recurrent superficial thrombophlebitis, and (e) venous ulceration. The type of treatment is guided by the severity and location of venous reflux and/or occlusion, as defined by the preintervention duplex. Additional tests such as venous plethysmography, venography, and IVUS are obtained in more complex cases, such as those with suspected iliac vein obstruction or who may require deep venous interventions. Duplex is unnecessary in patients with only spider veins. All patients should obtain well-fitted compression hose, which are worn for at least several weeks after venous intervention and indefinitely for patients with history of venous ulceration. Preoperative prophylaxis against DVT with 5,000 units of subcutaneous heparin should be considered in patients at higher risk for periprocedural DVT. Risk factors include older age, obesity, hormone replacement or oral contraceptives, smoking, and history of previous DVT.

1. **Sclerotherapy** is the injection of a sclerosing agent into the varicose vein to damage its endothelium to cause an aseptic thrombosis, which organizes and closes the vein. We use sclerotherapy as primary treatment for C1 disease, that is, spider veins (0.1 to 2 mm) and reticular veins (2 to 4 mm). Foam sclerotherapy can also be used to obliterate small residual varicosities that persist after treatment of great saphenous reflux. **Sclerotherapy will have limited long-term success in patients with untreated saphenous or deep system reflux; therefore,**

patients with more significant C2 and greater disease should first be evaluated by duplex ultrasound. Complications of sclerotherapy include hyperpigmentation, skin necrosis, thrombophlebitis, and allergic reactions.

The essentials of safe and effective sclerotherapy are as follows:

   a. Relative contraindications to sclerotherapy include use of anti-coagulants, ABI < 0.7, veins on the foot, and history of strong allergic conditions.

   b. No more than 0.5 mL of the sclerosant should be used in any one injection site. We prefer 0.5% polidocanol (Asclera®, Merz Pharma GMbH and Co. KGaA, Germany) loaded into 1-cc syringes with a tuberculin needle (30 g). When mixed with air, this agent can be used as a foam to treat larger varicosities as well as C1 disease.

   c. The injections are done while the patient is reclining, not standing. The sclerosant is retained in the vein segment by compressing it above and below the injection site for about 1 minute. The injection is stopped if the patient complains of severe local pain, since this suggests extravasation of the sclerosant outside the vein. **It is particularly important to have the leg elevated when using foam sclerotherapy to avoid migration of air into the deep venous system or centrally.**

   d. A compressive elastic bandage is applied, and the patient is actively ambulated immediately. This ambulation helps the musculovenous pump of the calf to wash out any sclerosant that may have leaked into the deep venous system. Patients are asked to wear compression stockings for at least 1 week following an average injection in small veins.

2. **Surgical and endovascular treatment of varicose veins.** The treatment of saphenous vein reflux is indicated for symptomatic varicose veins (aching, hemorrhage, superficial thrombophlebitis). The best surgical candidates are active, healthy patients who are not overweight. Some patients simply desire removal of the varicose veins for cosmetic reasons. Occasionally, primary varicose veins lead to leg ulcers. In addition, there is evidence that correction of the superficial reflux in patients with combined superficial and deep reflux improves venous hemodynamics. **In a large randomized controlled trial (ESCHAR), eliminating superficial reflux in combination with compression therapy reduced venous ulcer recurrence, although healing rates were not improved compared to compression alone.**

   a. **Saphenous vein stripping** is the surgical ligation and removal of the great saphenous vein for reflux. Before the operation, the correct limb is marked with an indelible felt-tipped pen and the varicosities are marked while the patient stands. A small incision is made at the groin, and the saphenofemoral junction is exposed and ligated along with each of its five or six tributaries. Starting from the groin, a disposable stripper is passed through the vein. The distal vein is tied to the stripper and then removed by pulling the vein through its subcutaneous tunnel. Whether to strip to the knee or to the ankle level is somewhat controversial given the proximity of the saphenous nerve to the vein at and below the knee. Stripping the vein to the ankle has a higher rate of saphenous nerve injury, and the decision depends on the degree of disease in the below-knee great saphenous vein. At the ankle, the great saphenous vein should be exposed medially and slightly anterior to the medial malleolus. Careful exposure at the ankle includes identifying and separating the saphenous nerve from the vein to lessen the incidence of nerve injury resulting in numbness in the foot. Traditional vein stripping has been largely replaced by less invasive endovenous ablation techniques, which demonstrate comparable improvement in venous insufficiency with decreased recovery time. We prefer vein stripping over ablation for select patients with large great saphenous veins (>10 to 12 mm) that have higher chance of postprocedure DVT or late recanalization.

b. **Endovenous ablation** is a percutaneous technique for treating superficial saphenous vein reflux, and has emerged as the preferred choice over vein stripping. Patients with a very large or tortuous saphenous vein, segmental occlusions due to prior thrombophlebitis, or severe coagulopathy may not be good candidates for endovenous ablation. The entire procedure is performed under ultrasound guidance. The great saphenous vein is accessed percutaneously, a sheath placed over the wire into the vein, and the laser or radiofrequency fiber positioned in the vein distal to the saphenofemoral junction. We begin the ablation 1.5 to 2 cm distal to the junction, as beginning closer can lead to transmission of energy into the deep venous system and increase the risk of DVT. A good rule is to position the fiber just distal to the superficial epigastric vein, as this allows the stump of the saphenous vein to drain rather than acting as a potential "blind stump" for thrombosis. Dilute tumescent anesthesia is injected around the saphenous sheath for analgesia and to insulate the skin and adjacent nerves against injury. The procedure can be performed in an office setting with minimal sedation. Endovenous ablation is highly successful at occluding the saphenous vein and improving symptoms of chronic venous insufficiency. When appropriate, the short saphenous vein and anterior accessory saphenous vein can also be treated with endovenous ablation.

c. **Stab phlebectomy** may be used in combination with stripping or endovascular ablation in order to treat tributary varicosities (Fig. 18.4). In many cases, these are the only varicosities that the patient sees, as the saphenous vein itself may not bulge. Since these procedures are in part cosmetic, the skin incisions should be very small "stabs" over the premarked varicosities. A crochet hook or specially designed vein hook is then used to elevate the varicosity, which is then grasped with a hemostat and plucked out. Some surgeons remove only these obvious varicosities and preserve the great saphenous trunk. This approach is reasonable if the great saphenous vein is competent by duplex. However, most patients with large, symptomatic lower-limb varicose veins have a diffusely incompetent great saphenous vein and will be at high risk for recurrent varicosities if this underlying problem is untreated.

d. **Postprocedural care.** After vein stripping or extensive phlebectomy, the leg is wrapped in a compressive gauze bandage with an elastic wrap from the toes to the groin. As most vein surgery is performed in the outpatient setting, the patient is instructed to keep the operated leg elevated for a night. The next morning, the dressings are removed and a new below-the-knee elastic bandage or stocking is applied. The patient should be counseled to ambulate every 2 hours for 5 to 10 minutes.

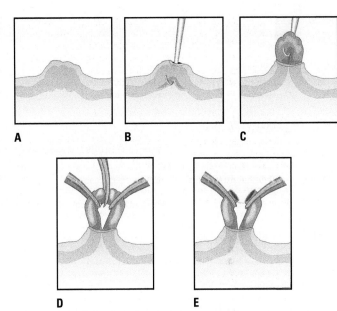

A   **B**   **C**

D   **E**

FIGURE 18.4 The technique of stab phlebectomy to excise varicose tributaries. **(A, B)** The varicosity is visualized and a small stab incision is made directly over it. The dermis is undermined with a small Jacobson hemostat. **(C)** A crochet hook or specially designed vein hook is used to elevate the vein. **(D)** Once above the skin, the vein is grasped with hemostats and divided with scissors. **(E)** Each end is removed by taut traction on the hemostat.

After endovascular ablation, patients are encouraged to ambulate immediately. The patient should return in 2 to 3 days for a duplex, to ensure no interval development of DVT and to reconfirm successful ablation of the vein. The patient is rechecked in the office after 2 to 4 weeks. Elastic support stockings are continued for a minimum of 2 weeks. For some patients, this support is continued for several more weeks to alleviate mild leg swelling and dependent heaviness that may follow lower-extremity venous procedures.

8. **Complications.** Wound cellulitis, hematomas, and bruising can occur after vein stripping or endovenous ablation. Bruising and pain are more common after laser than radiofrequency ablation. Below-the-knee stripping or inadequate tumescence with ablation procedures can increase the risk of saphenous nerve injury resulting in temporary paresthesias or numbness in the foot. Recurrent reflux can present through the saphenous vein or through accessory veins years after ablation and neovascularization after saphenous stripping can result in new pathways of reflux and varicosities. Endovenous heat-induced thrombosis (EHIT) is a particular issue that can occur in up to 6% of patients after ablation. EHIT is classified by the degree of extension of thrombus into the saphenofemoral junction (Table 18.1). For this reason, most patients undergo surveillance duplex several

Class	Definition	Treatment
Class I	Extension of thrombus up to SFJ	Follow-up DUS monthly until clot regresses into GSV
Class II	Thrombus protrudes into the CFV;	<50% cross-sectional area
		Anticoagulation for 7–10 days and follow-up serial DUS until conversion to EHIT I
Class III	Thrombus extends into the CFV;	>50% cross-sectional area
		Standard DVT treatment full anticoagulation 3–6 months
Class IV	Occlusive DVT of the CFV	Standard DVT treatment full anticoagulation 3–6 months

SFJ, saphenofemoral junction; DUS, duplex ultrasound; GSV, great saphenous vein; CFV, common femoral vein; DVT, deep venous thrombosis.

days and again 1 month after the procedure. Careful positioning of the tip of the fiber caudal to the saphenofemoral junction, adequate tumescent insulation around the saphenous vein, and early ambulation may reduce the risk of DVT.

3. **Surgical and endovascular treatment of advanced venous disease.** Patients with severe swelling, pain, and ulcers merit comprehensive investigation when conservative measures are insufficient. Chronic venous disease can be palliated but not cured. Patients are regularly educated about use of compression garments, walking program and strength training for calf muscle pump, skin and ulcer care, and weight loss. Goals of care should be explained and realistic, such as conversion from C6 disease to C5, and maintaining a healed leg. Management of advanced venous disease starts with a thorough history to elucidate duration of symptoms, postthrombotic or primary disease, and methods of treatment to date. A venous duplex is performed to elucidate deep, superficial, and/or perforator vein reflux and presence of chronic venous changes (postthrombotic veins). Typically, superficial venous reflux, if present, is the "low hanging fruit" that can be addressed with ablation or stripping techniques. However, many patients suffer with recalcitrant disease and warrant more complex treatment.

   a. **Intervention for perforator vein incompetence** can be considered in patients with advanced venous (C5 or C6) disease. Perforators often occur at the sites of ulceration, and interruption of venous hypertension at this level may be necessary to achieve healing. Clinical trials have examined the role of perforator treatment, but treatment of superficial venous reflux is often concomitant, which makes the true efficacy of perforator treatment unclear. A pathologic perforator vein is generally considered to have a diameter greater than 3.5 mm, outward reflux greater than 500 ms, and location adjacent an open or healed ulcer. **Subfascial endoscopic perforating vein surgery (SEPS)** can be performed in patients with incompetent perforating veins and venous ulceration.

This open surgical technique involves insufflation of the lower leg with division of these branches under direct vision. Less invasive alternatives for perforator treatment include ablation and sclerotherapy. Patients who undergo perforator vein treatment must continue to wear below-the-knee elastic support hose, as the procedure does not correct the deep venous hypertension due to valvular incompetence.

b. **Endovascular treatment** of iliac vein obstruction has been lauded in recent years as a minimally invasive and highly successful modality for treatment of advanced venous insufficiency. **Venous outflow obstruction may be nonthrombotic or postthrombotic in nature.** Perhaps the most common cause of nonthrombotic venous obstruction is May-Thurner syndrome. This condition is the result of excessive compression of the left iliac vein by the crossover of the right iliac artery and usually occurs in young women. Nonthrombotic lesions may include wall fibrosis, webs, and extrinsic compression. Venography is insensitive for the detection of nonthrombotic lesions, and IVUS has emerged as the gold standard for confirming iliac venous obstruction. In the presence of deep venous reflux and iliac obstruction, the management is geared towards treatment of the obstruction. **In a report of 982 iliofemoral stents placed for primary venous obstruction, 6-year patency rates are 79% with assisted primary patency achieving 100%.** Patients with postthrombotic iliofemoral venous obstruction treated by stenting also have commendable long-term results, although not quite as good as those for primary obstruction. Relief of pain, swelling and ulcer healing with endovascular stenting of iliac venous obstruction were achieved in 58% to 89% of patients in summation of clinical studies.

The technique of iliofemoral venous stenting can be used for nonthrombotic or postthrombotic disease. Several tenets of care are mentioned:

1. Venous access should be obtained below the presumed obstruction. The femoral vein can be accessed in the upper thigh with the leg flexed slightly at the knee and abducted outward. This technique allows for imaging through the level of the common femoral vein (CFV) and a stent can be extended distally into the CFV if necessary. Alternatively, popliteal venous access can be obtained with the patient prone. CFV access may be suitable for a high iliac stenosis such as May-Thurner compression or vena cava lesion.

2. Venography is performed in AP and oblique views. IVUS frequently detects lesions not seen on venography, and a greater than 50% reduction in cross-sectional area of the stenotic vein in comparison to adjacent normal vein is considered significant.

3. Venous angioplasty alone is rarely durable due to recoil of veins, and stenting of iliofemoral lesions is preferred.

4. Large self-expanding stents such as Wallstent™ (Boston Scientific, Marlborough, MA) are used in the iliocaval system with typical diameters ranging from 14 to 20 mm.

Postprocedure care after venous stenting is similar to many angiographic procedures. However, the puncture site locations are unique and often deeper in the leg, necessitating meticulous attention to postprocedure hemostasis. Stenting of nonthrombotic disease can usually be managed with antiplatelet therapies, whereas recanalization of chronic thrombotic veins usually is managed with postprocedure anticoagulation. Often, iliac venous stents can be visualized by Duplex ultrasound for surveillance. Symptoms of increased leg edema or pain are difficult to discern from baseline chronic venous disease but can be an indication of stent restenosis or thrombosis. These concerns should be investigated, and follow-up venography and IVUS may be necessary when Duplex is nondiagnostic.

c. **Open surgery for chronic deep venous insufficiency** is performed at specialized centers and only for severe cases failing other therapies. Direct repair of venous valves (valvuloplasty) is most effective for primary venous reflux. Valve transfer (e.g., axillary to femoropopliteal) may be superior to valvuloplasty for incompetent, severely damaged valves as a result of postthrombotic syndrome. The presence of venous obstruction is associated with more debilitating symptoms (swelling, venous claudication) than is that of reflux alone, and most often occurs as a result of incomplete recanalization after DVT. Unilateral iliofemoral obstruction can be treated with a crossover femoral-femoral bypass using the saphenous vein (Palma method). This procedure is now considered second-line therapy after failed endovascular reconstruction. Open venous reconstructions are technically demanding operations with modest long-term success, thus limiting their applicability to well-selected and motivated patients.

Selected Readings

Glovicczki P, Comerota AJ, Dalsing MC, et al. The care of patients with varicose veins and associated chronic venous diseases: clinical practice guidelines of the Society for Vascular Surgery and the American Venous Forum. *J Vasc Surg.* 2011;53:2S-48S.

Glovicczki P, Hollier LH, Telander RL, et al. Surgical implications of Klippel-Trenaunay syndrome. *Ann Surg.* 1983;197(3):353-362.
An original description of the management of KTS in children from the experts at the Mayo Clinic; includes historical pictures.

Barwell JR, Davies CE, Deacon J, et al. Comparison of surgery and compression with compression alone in chronic venous ulceration (ESCHAR study): randomised controlled trial. *Lancet.* 2004;363:1854-1859.
Elegant, landmark study demonstrated a high prevalence of superficial venous reflux in patients with venous stasis ulcers and decreased 12-month ulcer recurrence after treatment of superficial reflux.

O'Donnell TF Jr, Passman MA, Marston WA, et al. Management of venous leg ulcers: clinical practice guidelines of the Society for Vascular Surgery® and the American Venous Forum. *J Vasc Surg.* 2014;60:3S-59S.
Up-to-date guidelines for venous ulcers—detailed document that covers the evaluation and medical and interventional treatment from international experts.

Meissner MH, Gloviczki P, Bergan J, et al. Primary chronic venous disorders. *J Vasc Surg.* 2007;46(suppl):54S-67S.
Review of pathophysiology and treatment of venous insufficiency with emphasis on the superficial system.

Meissner MH, Eklof B, Smith PC, et al. Secondary chronic venous disorders. *J Vasc Surg.* 2007;46(suppl):68S-83S.
Review of pathophysiology and treatment of venous insufficiency with emphasis on the deep system.

Neglén P, Hollis KC, Olivier J, Raju S. Stenting of the venous outflow in chronic venous disease: long-term stent-related outcome, clinical, and hemodynamic result. *J Vasc Surg.* 2007;46:979-990.

9-year experience with venous stenting of 982 limbs authored by pioneers of venous stenting.

Raju S, Neglen P. Chronic venous insufficiency and varicose veins. *NEJM*. 2009;360: 2319-2327.

Straightforward synopsis including excellent tips and tricks for management of CVI.

Raju S. Best management options for chronic iliac vein stenosis and occlusion. *J Vasc Surg*. 2013;57:1163-1169.

Summary of clinical studies about iliac vein stenting for both nonthrombotic and post-thrombotic lesions; data are nicely displayed in tabular format.

Lohr JM, Bush RL. Venous disease in women: epidemiology, manifestations, and treatment. *J Vasc Surg*. 2013;57:37S-45S.

Discussion of superficial venous disease with additional information specific to female patients.

Ozvath KJ, Moor CJ. Venous occlusive disease in women. *J Vasc Surg*. 2013;57;46S-48S.

Concise analysis of venous obstruction and thromboembolism in women.

19 Venous Thromboembolism and Hypercoagulable Conditions

The current clinical approach to acute venous thromboembolism (VTE) focuses on prevention, rapid diagnosis, and treatment. A better understanding of the pathophysiology of deep venous thrombosis (DVT) and pulmonary embolism (PE) has resulted in more aggressive preventive measures. The limitations of the physical examination in accurate diagnosis of VTE have culminated in the development of efficient, noninvasive methods for detection. Newer anticoagulant medications and regimens offer alternatives for prevention and treatment. Clinical trials will define the role of catheter-directed thrombolysis in the treatment of DVT. Inferior vena cava filters have a niche role in the prevention of PE.

A. **Risk factors** for VTE may be organized conveniently around **Virchow's etiologic triad: stasis, hypercoagulability, and endothelial injury.**

   1. **Stasis.** Prolonged immobilization of the lower extremities is perhaps the single most important event that precedes DVT. At bed rest, blood tends to pool in large, valveless venous sinuses of the calf muscles. The soleus venous plexus normally drains anteriorly into the tibial veins. Consequently, if the body is supine, blood pools in the calf muscles unless these muscles contract to empty the calf veins. Historically, ^{125}I-labeled fibrinogen studies show that calf vein thrombosis often begins while the patient is supine on the operating table.

   Venous stasis in the calf may be prevented by elevation and intermittent or continuous mechanical compression of the leg. Simply elevating the leg 15 to 20 degrees improves emptying of major leg veins but may not completely empty the soleus venous sinuses. Likewise, graduated compression stockings may hasten flow in the tibial veins but not completely empty the soleus plexus where clots often begin. **Several studies have confirmed that intermittent pneumatic leg compression reduces postoperative DVT, especially when combined with pharmacologic prophylaxis.** However, patients may not be consistently compliant with wearing these devices, finding them uncomfortable, unwieldy, or unimportant. Early mobilization and ambulation should be encouraged in all patients able to bear weight. Finally, one of the simplest, yet most effective, methods of preventing calf vein stasis is to have the patient exercise the legs (plantar flexion) against a footboard for 5 minutes every hour. This exercise not only promotes venous flow but actually may enhance fibrinolytic activity, which clears small clots. We have found that patients will exercise regularly when the importance of these exercises is explained to them and encouragement is given after the operation. Patients at higher risk for thromboembolism generally receive pneumatic compression devices on the lower extremities and/or some type of anticoagulant therapy, such as low-dose heparin or low molecular weight heparin (LMWH) (Table 19.1).

TABLE 19.1 Anticoagulants Used for Prophylaxis and Treatment of Venous Thromboembolism

Trade Name	Generic	DVT Prophylaxis	Treatment for Acute DVT/PE
Unfractionated heparin			
	Heparin sulfate	5,000 unit sc 1–2 h preoperatively; then 5,000 unit sc q8–12h	80 unit/kg IV bolus and 18 unit/kg/h IV infusion (adjust for aPTT ratio 1.5–2.5×)
LMWH			
Fragmin (Pfizer, New York, NY)	Dalteparin	2,500 unit sc 1–2 h preoperatively; 5,000 unit sc daily	100 unit/kg sc q12h or 200 unit/kg sc daily
Lovenox (Sanofi-Aventis, Bridgewater, NJ)	Enoxaparin	40 mg sc q24h or 30 mg sc q12h	1.5 mg/kg sc q24h or 1 mg/kg sc q12h
Direct thrombin inhibitors			
Pradaxa (Boehringer Ingelheim, Ingelheim am Rhein, Germany)	Dabigatran	150 mg PO BID[a]	150 mg PO BID (after 5–10 d of parenteral anticoagulant)
Argatroban (GlaxoSmithKline, London, UK)[b]			2 mcg/kg/min IV (adjust to aPTT ratio 1.5–3×)[c]
Anti-Xa inhibitors			
Arixtra (GlaxoSmithKline, London, UK)	Fondaparinux	2.5 mg sc q24h[d]	7.5 mg sc q24h
Eliquis (Bristol-Myers Squibb, New York, NY)	Apixaban	2.5 mg PO BID[e]	10 mg PO BID × 7 d, then 5 mg PO BID
Xarelto (Bayer HealthCare AG, Leverkusen, Germany)	Rivaroxaban	10 mg PO daily (after 6 mo of anticoagulation)[e]	15 mg PO BID × 21 d, then 20 mg PO daily (with food)

sc, subcutaneous; IV, intravenous; PO, by mouth; LMWH, low molecular weight heparin; BID, twice a day.
Adapted by authors for simplicity; guidelines vary for orthopedic, general surgery, and medical patients. The clinician should seek specific guidelines on pdr.net before prescribing.
[a]Prophylaxis for recurrent DVT; different regimens advised post hip or knee replacement.
[b]Parenteral anticoagulation for heparin-induced thrombocytopenia.
[c]When used as bridge to warfarin, argatroban is continued until INR exceeds 4.0.
[d]Initiate 6 to 8 hours after hemostasis achieved for abdominal surgery, hip or knee replacement.
[e]For prevention of recurrent DVT and prophylaxis after hip or knee replacement.

2. **Hypercoagulability.** Inherited or acquired coagulation defects predispose to thrombosis (clotting). Acute lower extremity DVT is the most common presentation for patients with some abnormality of coagulation. Arterial thrombosis in situ may also occur as a result of coagulation disorders but is more often a consequence of underlying atherosclerotic disease.

TABLE 19.2	Inherited Thrombophilia Disorders

Antithrombin deficiency
Protein C deficiency
Protein S deficiency
Activated protein C resistance
Factor V R506Q (Leiden) mutation
Hyperhomocysteinemia
Prothrombin gene variant (20210A)
Hypoplasminogenemia
Dysfibrinogenemia

a. **Inherited hypercoagulability.** Of all patients with a hypercoagulable condition, a genetic or familial cause can be identified nearly 40% of the time. Of these, the most common inherited hypercoagulable state is the factor V Leiden mutation. Screening for these hypercoagulable states is appropriate in certain patients with recurrent, idiopathic DVT (Table 19.2).

Antithrombin (aka antithrombin III) deficiency is an autosomal dominant disease, and its prevalence is 1 in 2,000 to 5,000 people. Antithrombin is synthesized by liver cells (hepatocytes) and inactivates thrombin as well as other coagulation factors. Its activity is greatly enhanced by heparin. Two types of antithrombin deficiency exist, the most common resulting from decreased synthesis of a biologically normal molecule. These patients have functional levels of circulating antithrombin that are only 50% of normal. The second type of antithrombin deficiency is less frequent and results from a functional deficiency associated with specific molecular abnormalities in the molecule involving the heparin or thrombin-binding domains.

Antithrombin deficiency is suspected when patients have recurrent, familial, and/or juvenile deep vein or mesenteric venous thrombosis. Such an event often occurs in conjunction with another predisposing event such as injury, pregnancy, immobilization, or use of oral contraceptives. Deficiency may also be suspected by the inability to anticoagulate a patient with intravenous heparin. Such patients may require large doses of heparin to achieve anticoagulation or may, paradoxically, require treatment with fresh frozen plasma (FFP) that contains antithrombin in order for the heparin to be active. Acquired antithrombin deficiency may also be seen with liver and kidney disease, sepsis, oral contraceptives, and some chemotherapeutic agents.

Deficiencies in protein C and S are inherited as autosomal dominant traits and are most frequently heterozygous. Because both proteins are natural inhibitors of the coagulation cascade, their absence fosters a hypercoagulable state. The prevalence of protein C deficiency is 1 in 200 to 300. Homozygous forms of protein C or S deficiency are associated with extreme, highly lethal forms of thrombosis in infancy, termed **purpura fulminans**. Both protein C and S deficiencies have been associated with a condition referred to as **warfarin-induced skin necrosis.** In this disorder, skin necrosis begins within days of initiation of warfarin therapy (Coumadin). Its pathogenesis is related to a transient, severe hypercoagulable state related to an exaggerated protein C deficiency caused by warfarin. It is treated with intravenous heparin, administration of vitamin K, and/or plasma protein C concentrates.

Acquired protein C and S deficiencies occur with activation of inflammatory response syndromes, such as sepsis. In such conditions, the complement system is up-regulated, and C4b-binding protein (present in the activated complement system) binds and inactivates protein S, creating a relative protein S–deficient state. Acquired deficiencies may also be present in liver disease, pregnancy, postoperative states, and nephrotic syndrome.

Factor V Leiden. In 1994, a point mutation in factor V of the coagulation pathway was identified by Bertina et al. in Leiden (the Netherlands). This genetic mutation at position 506 of the factor V polypeptide is called *factor V Leiden*, resulting in activated protein C resistance (APC resistance) and an associated hypercoagulable condition. Factor V Leiden mutation has been demonstrated in 40% to 60% of patients with familial thrombosis and is considered the most common form of hypercoagulable condition in people of European and Asian descent.

Similar to protein C or protein S deficiencies, patients who are homozygous for factor V Leiden have a much higher risk of thrombosis than patients who are heterozygous for the mutation. The most common manifestation of APC resistance is DVT. In contrast to persons who are homozygous for protein C or protein S deficiency, some persons homozygous for factor V Leiden never experience thrombosis.

As with other inherited hypercoagulable conditions, the development of thrombosis in APC resistance is affected by the coexistence of other genetic or circumstantial risk factors (Virchow's triad). The most common factors affecting APC-resistant individuals are oral contraceptive use, pregnancy, injury, and surgery. Women who are heterozygous for factor V Leiden and use oral contraceptives have a near 30-fold increase in risk for venous thrombosis; women who are homozygous have a several hundred-fold increase in risk for similar events. The factor V Leiden mutation appears to be more commonly associated with venous thrombotic events than with arterial thrombosis.

Hyperhomocysteinemia. Abnormalities in the metabolism of homocysteine result in increased circulating levels of this sulfur-containing amino acid (>14 µmol/L). Additionally, acquired hyperhomocysteinemia may occur as a result of deficiencies of vitamin B_6, vitamin B_{12}, or folate. Hyperhomocysteinemia is present in 5% of the population and is associated with early atherosclerosis and, less commonly, venous thrombosis. Elevated homocysteine levels act primarily by causing endothelial dysfunction and platelet activation. Although homocysteine levels can be corrected with B vitamin and folate supplementation, reduction in number of adverse cardiovascular events has not been demonstrated to correlate with this treatment.

Prothrombin gene 20210 mutation. A mutation on position 20210 of the prothrombin gene was discovered in 1996 and was referred to as the *prothrombin variant*. This mutation results in overproduction of the factor **prothrombin (factor II)**, causing an increased tendency to form clot. Heterozygous prothrombin mutations are found in about 2% of the Caucasian population and 0.5% of the African American population and are present in 20% of patients with familial venous thrombophilia. Having the prothrombin mutation increases one's risk of venous thrombosis and thromboembolism (by two to three times) but may also predispose to arterial thrombosis, although to a lesser degree.

Plasminogen is a proenzyme that is released into the bloodstream and converted to the active form **plasmin** by an enzyme called **tissue plasminogen activator (tPA)** that is secreted by endothelium of the blood vessels. Plasmin plays an important role in maintaining blood fluidity by breaking down fibrin clots in an action referred to as **fibrinolysis**. Individuals with disorders of the plasminogen and fibrinolysis pathways have high rates of venous and arterial thrombosis often at an early age.

b. **Acquired hypercoagulability** (Table 19.3)

Smoking. The nicotine and carbon monoxide in cigarette smoke cause endothelial dysfunction with increased platelet deposition and lipid accumulation. Smoking decreases the production of prostacyclin, a potent vasodilator and inhibitor of platelet aggregation, and increases blood viscosity. These and other effects make smoking the *most common acquired hypercoagulable condition* and contributor to arterial and venous thrombosis.

Oral contraceptives/pregnancy. Exogenous estrogens are associated with an increased risk for venous thrombosis as well as coronary and cerebral arterial thrombotic events. Estrogens are associated with decreased antithrombin and protein S activities and increases in activated factors VII and X. Estrogens are also associated with decreased levels of thrombomodulin and reduction in protein C activity. Pregnancy is associated with an increase in nearly all of the clotting factors, an increased platelet count, and a decrease in protein S activity. In addition, pregnancy is associated with decreased antithrombin. These factors combined with venous stasis from the uterus compressing venous drainage of the legs lead to at least a fivefold increase in venous thrombosis during pregnancy.

Antiphospholipid syndrome (APS) is also referred to as **Hughes syndrome** after the rheumatologist Graham R.V. Hughes, who

TABLE 19.3	Causes of Acquired Hypercoagulable Disorders

Cigarette smoking
Pregnancy
Oral contraceptives
Hormone replacement therapy
Heparin-induced thrombocytopenia
Antiphospholipid syndrome
Malignancy
Antineoplastic medications
Myeloproliferative syndromes
Hyperhomocysteinemia
Inflammatory bowel disease

described the syndrome while working at St. Thomas's Hospital in London. Antiphospholipid syndrome is defined by clotting complications in the setting of positive circulating antibodies to negatively charged proteins that bind to phospholipids in the bloodstream. The two specific classes of antibodies can be diagnosed using the assay for either **anticardiolipin antibody** or **circulating lupus anticoagulant.** The target for the anticardiolipin antibody appears to be a negatively charged protein called B_2 glycoprotein-1, while the target for the lupus anticoagulant is prothrombin (factor II). The assay for anticardiolipin antibody is most sensitive and specific for the diagnosis of APS. Circulating lupus anticoagulant may be independent of an underlying collagen vascular disorder (primary APS) or part of the connective tissue disease such as *systemic lupus erythematous (SLE)*, in which case it is referred to as secondary APS. As many as 50% of those with SLE or lupus-like disorders have either the circulating lupus anticoagulant or antiphospholipid antibodies.

Antiphospholipid antibodies are present in 1% of the population, more so in women and older individuals. The most common arterial event in patients with APS is ischemic stroke, while the most common venous event is DVT. Antiphospholipid antibody syndrome is also known to cause pregnancy-related complications, including late-term miscarriage likely due to a thrombotic event. The pathogenesis of thrombosis in individuals with APS is not well understood but has been suggested to involve autoantibodies that inhibit endothelial cell prostacyclin or that interfere with thrombomodulin-mediated protein C activation.

Malignancy. The association of malignancy and venous thrombosis is well recognized. One of the first recognized patterns of this association was that of superficial thrombosis in patients with adenocarcinoma of the bowel or pancreas or cancers of the lung (**Trousseau's syndrome**). Patients who develop DTV and have no other identifiable risk factors have a 10% chance of having an undiagnosed cancer. The hypercoagulable state associated with malignancy is due to interaction of tumor cells and their products with host cells leading to elimination of normal protective mechanisms that the host employs to prevent thrombosis.

Tumor cells may induce procoagulant properties such as secretion of tissue thromboplastin, which is a constituent composed of protein and phospholipid that is widely distributed in the tissues. Tissue thromboplastin serves as a cofactor with factor VIIa to activate factor X in the extrinsic coagulation pathway, and its secretion in the setting of malignancy may contribute to a relative hypercoagulable condition. Additionally, tumor cells may cause release of proteases, which activate clotting factors. Patients with malignancy may also have increased levels of factors V, VIII, IX, and X. Cancer patients frequently have other risk factors that place them at risk for thrombosis, such as chemotherapeutic treatment, indwelling central venous catheters, and limited mobility.

Antineoplastic drugs. Chemotherapeutic agents have been associated with vascular abnormalities such as thrombotic thrombocytopenic purpura, **Budd-Chiari syndrome**, myocardial infarction, and venous thrombosis. Thrombotic events are related to hypercoagulable states caused by the effect of these drugs or their metabolites on vascular endothelium.

Myeloproliferative syndromes. At least three myeloproliferative disorders have been associated with thrombosis and hypercoagulable conditions likely secondary to increases in blood viscosity. The disorders, **polycythemia vera, essential thrombocythemia,** and **agnogenic myeloid metaplasia,** may also affect platelet function either directly or indirectly. In addition to association with extremity venous thrombosis, the myeloproliferative disorders predispose individuals to mesenteric, hepatic, or portal venous thrombosis. This type of hypercoagulable state rarely manifests as arterial thrombosis unless combined with other previously described thrombotic risk factors.

3. **Vein injury.** During elective operations, meticulous attention must be given to the gentle dissection and handling of veins. Large vein injuries should be repaired by fine lateral suture technique, and ligation should be avoided. The surgeon also must avoid prolonged **compression** of the vena cava or other large veins with retractors or packs. Experimental studies have also documented endothelial tears that occur in extremity veins remote from an elective operative site. These endothelial lesions may become the focus of DVT. Indwelling venous catheters injure endothelium and create a nidus for thrombus formation.

B. **Prevention** of venous thrombosis

Thrombophilia exists in patients with one or more additive risk factors that in combination may or may not reach a thrombotic threshold. In a hospitalized setting, patients can be identified as high risk for developing DVT based on the number of identified risk factors. High-risk patients include those who have experienced (a) previous VTE; (b) lower extremity trauma (e.g., hip fracture) and other orthopedic surgery of the hip, knee, or lower limb; (c) major pelvic operations (e.g., open prostatectomy or gynecologic operations); (d) prolonged bed rest or extremity immobility (e.g., stroke or back surgery); (e) acute myocardial infarction; (f) chronic congestive heart failure; and (g) malignancies (e.g., pancreatic, lung, gastrointestinal cancers), as well as those on (h) oral contraceptives. Early ambulation, pneumatic compression devices, and foot pump exercises are advisable for most patients. In addition, prophylactic, low-dose anticoagulation does offer high-risk patients significant protection against VTE. An easy calculation of the Caprini score identifies a patient as "low," "moderate," or "high" risk for DVT and can help determine who will benefit from the addition of pharmacologic prophylaxis.

Several anticoagulant agents are available: LMWH, low-dose unfractionated heparin (UFH), warfarin, and direct Xa inhibitors (fondaparinux). Of course, the risk of anticoagulant therapy in surgical patients is bleeding, but major bleeding complications are rare if therapy is properly delivered and monitored and certain contraindications are observed. **These contraindications include an active peptic ulcer, intracranial or visceral injury, hemorrhagic diathesis, gastrointestinal bleeding, severe hypertension, and gross hematuria or hemoptysis.**

1. **Adjusted-dose warfarin** can be an effective prophylaxis for venous thrombosis; however, there is not widespread acceptance of this strategy. The dosage may be difficult to regulate, and an excessively prolonged prothrombin time is associated with increased bleeding complications. Recommendations from the American College of Chest Physicians only include warfarin prophylaxis as an option for elective hip or knee surgery patients.

2. **Unfractionated heparin (UFH)** has received widespread attention for its use in the prevention of fatal postoperative PE. Compared to those who receive no prophylaxis, heparin-treated patients experience a 40% reduction in nonfatal and a 64% reduction in fatal PE. The **usual** dosage has been a loading dose of 5,000 units given subcutaneously, 2 hours prior to operation, and then 5,000 units every 8 to 12 hours until the patient is ambulatory. Low-dose heparin binds to and **enhances antithrombin activity with minimal to no change in coagulation tests** although bleeding and wound complications may be slightly higher in patients on prophylactic heparin. Therefore, the use of prophylactic heparin should be reserved for those at increased risk of thromboembolism, including patients with prior VTE, those immobilized for long periods, and those subjected to major surgical procedures.

3. **Low molecular weight heparin (LMWH)** has three potential advantages over UFH: (a) effective prophylaxis with once-daily administration, (b) improved efficacy, and (c) a lower frequency of bleeding. LMWHs have higher bioavailability and extended half-life compared to UFH. Compared to UFH, LMWH has greater anti-Xa activity than anti-IIa activity, which may reduce the risk of bleeding complications without compromising efficacy. Several randomized clinical trials have demonstrated that LMWH is as effective as and as safe as unfractionated heparin in the prophylaxis against VTE.

4. Data showing efficacy of **antiplatelet agents or dextrans** for VTE prophylaxis are equivocal, and their use for this purpose is not supported by current guidelines.

5. **Fondaparinux is a synthetic pentasaccharide that acts exclusively as a factor Xa inhibitor.** With a long half-life, dosing is once a day subcutaneously, although renal excretion limits its use in patients with renal insufficiency. Fondaparinux is currently approved for VTE prophylaxis in orthopedic and general surgery patients. This agent has shown improved efficacy compared to LMWH in patients after hip or knee surgery, although bleeding risk may be slightly higher.

C. **Diagnosis.** Patient history and physical examination frequently are unreliable in establishing an accurate diagnosis of either acute DVT or PE. **In fact, about 75% of patients who are evaluated for suspected venous thrombosis or PE do not have these conditions.** Since either condition requires systemic anticoagulation, with its potential complications, we recommend the following approach to ensure that an accurate diagnosis is established.

1. **Superficial thrombophlebitis** generally is recognized by the physical findings of a tender superficial venous cord in the upper or lower extremity. Usually, there is no deep vein involvement. If the process extends to the groin, extension into the deep femoral system may be present. Duplex is the best method to ascertain thrombotic involvement of the common femoral vein, which may occur in 5% to 40% of patients and sometimes in the contralateral leg. It is noteworthy that a given percentage of these patients may be hypercoagulable due to an inherited or acquired condition, and a careful personal and family history should be obtained with this in mind. Superficial thrombophlebitis not infrequently affects a preexisting varicose vein, and vein removal (**ambulatory phlebectomy**) may be indicated in recurrent cases.

2. **DVT** is suggested by leg pain, swelling, and tenderness. Since these findings are not specific for venous thrombosis, treatment generally should not be started without confirmation by duplex examination. **Phlegmasia alba dolens and phlegmasia cerulea dolens** are dramatic

clinical presentations of DVT manifested by massive leg swelling with white or blue discoloration, respectively. Rarely, these may progress to venous gangrene.

  a. Compression **duplex ultrasonography** is highly sensitive (sensitivity, 90% to 100%) for detecting proximal femoropopliteal vein thrombosis but is less sensitive (60% to 90%) for detecting calf vein thrombosis. Noninvasive studies have limitations especially in the pelvic veins, below the knee, and in the profunda femoris vein. Also, duplex may be difficult to interpret if the patient had a previous DVT that has not recanalized. If the results of noninvasive tests are normal, other etiologies for the leg symptoms are investigated. CT venography, MR venography, or invasive venography is reserved for those rare patients with equivocal duplex results and an elevated clinical suspicion of DVT, such as with isolated iliac vein thrombosis.

  b. Plasma D-**dimer** is a fibrin-specific product, and therefore a marker of fibrinolysis, which may be elevated with venous thrombosis. The D-dimer test has emerged as a useful screening test to rule out DVT. **In outpatients with a low clinical likelihood of DVT and a normal d-dimer level, the negative predictive value exceeds 99% and duplex is probably unnecessary.** A positive D-dimer does not necessarily mean the patient has a DVT, as positive values can be seen in a number of acute or chronic medical conditions such as malignancy, immobility, pregnancy, and recent surgery.

3. **PE is a condition in which thrombus (i.e., clot) has migrated or embolized through the right heart and into one of the pulmonary arteries obstructing flow of unoxygenated blood to that segment of lung.** Depending upon the size of the pulmonary embolus, it may cause significant strain on the right heart and often presents with chest pain, dyspnea, and, occasionally, hemoptysis. The source of the emboli is nearly always the leg or pelvic veins. Similar symptoms may occur with myocardial ischemia, bronchitis, pneumonia, or pleurisy, so PE must be confirmed by other tests. Given that the mortality of untreated PE is great, it is important to maintain a high index of suspicion and to have a low threshold for pursuing diagnostic testing and early treatment with anticoagulation.

  a. Although hypoxia demonstrated on **arterial blood gas testing** is common with PE, a low arterial PO_2 is not diagnostic. Other laboratory tests may be abnormal but often are inconclusive. **Electrocardiographic abnormalities** may include a rhythm disturbance and ST segment depression or T-wave inversion, particularly in leads III, aVF, V1, V4, and V5. These findings are indicative of myocardial ischemia associated with acute PE. **The classic finding of S1, Q3, T3 (S wave in lead I, Q-wave, and T-wave inversion in III) is uncommon unless the PE causes acute right heart strain.** In many patients, the only ECG finding is sinus tachycardia. The ECG is most important to rule out an acute myocardial infarction as the cause of chest pain. The chest radiograph may look normal, although in seriously ill patients it may show infiltrates from pneumonitis or atelectasis. An x-ray is therefore important to examine for other potential pulmonary pathology.

  b. **Helical CT angiogram** (CTA) is a rapid and acute method for the detection of pulmonary emboli for emergency room and hospitalized patients. CTA is able to directly visualize the location of emboli, whether they are in the central, segmental, or subsegmental branches. The appearance of the lung parenchyma and chest structures is noted in addition to the pulmonary vasculature. CTA may demonstrate a differential diagnosis (e.g., effusion, pneumonia) to more fully explain the clinical situation. Helical CTA has sensitivity and specificity of 90% to 100%. The limitations of CTA are mostly in the detection of small subsegmental emboli, although the newest scanners can detect these with great accuracy. By timing contrast injection and performing delayed imaging, CT venography of the legs and pelvis can also be added to the initial PE scan. This adjuvant imaging provides even greater sensitivity to the examination by identifying deep venous thromboses.

c. **Ventilation/perfusion lung scanning (V/Q scan)** has largely been replaced with helical CTA for diagnosis of PE, due to greater speed and specificity with CTA. However, occasionally, a patient is unable to undergo CTA due to severe dye allergy, renal insufficiency, or limited hospital resources. V/Q scan uses a radioisotope to identify areas of disproportionate lung perfusion that may occur as a result of PE. False-positive V/Q tests may occur in patients due to preexisting lung pathology such as asthma, emphysema, chronic bronchitis, pneumonitis, or neoplasm. Consequently, the chest radiograph should be checked before a lung scan to identify any disease process that may affect the scan. In properly performed and interpreted scans, normal results essentially exclude a significant pulmonary embolus. High-probability scans predict the presence of PE in about 90% of patients. However, the majority of V/Q scans fall into the "intermediate probability" category, often necessitating further diagnostic testing.

d. **Pulmonary arteriography** is an invasive method for diagnosis of PE that was for many years considered the "gold standard" but has been supplanted by thin slice CTA. One must remember that most pulmonary emboli resolve over a period of days to several weeks, and, consequently, a pulmonary arteriogram may look normal after a while. Pulmonary angiography is rarely performed for pure diagnostic reasons due to a 3% to 4% risk of complications but has regained popularity in the setting of catheter-directed thrombolysis for treatment of massive and submassive PE.

D. **Treatment.** In Chapter 2, we emphasize that the natural history of DVT and PE may be altered by anticoagulation. In certain situations, catheter-based and/or surgical intervention also may help the patient. **Specifically, catheter-directed thrombolytic therapy has added another important alternative to managing serious DVT and PE.**

1. Treatment of **superficial thrombophlebitis** depends on the extent of the phlebitis and the general health of the patient. Elastic support, local heat, and an anti-inflammatory medication (e.g., aspirin or a nonsteroidal anti-inflammatory agent) may relieve localized superficial **phlebitis.** The inflammation results in erythema that resembles cellulitis; however, infection is rarely present and antibiotics are generally not indicated. Resolution may take 7 to 14 days. A short course of anticoagulation is recommended for superficial thrombophlebitis extending over 5 cm in length or extending to the saphenofemoral junction, given a higher risk of DVT and PE in these patients. The patient with recurrent superficial thrombophlebitis of their varicose veins can benefit from removal of the affected veins. We will typically

wait 4 to 6 weeks to allow the inflammation to subside before performing ambulatory phlebectomy (Chapter 18). Rarely, suppurative thrombophlebitis can result from an intravenous line infection and should be treated with antibiotics, warm compresses, and occasionally resection or open drainage of the vein to prevent septicemia.

2. For **established DVT,** standard therapy is initiated with a form of heparin followed by a longer course of warfarin. Alternatively, a novel oral anticoagulant can be prescribed (Table 19.1). The goal of anticoagulation is to prevent the propagation of thrombus or embolism to the **pulmonary** circulation. Anticoagulation does not dissolve the present clot but allows the patient's inherent fibrinolytic system to eliminate the thrombus over months.

   a. **Continuous heparin infusion** has been associated with fewer bleeding complications than intermittent intravenous therapy. The patient is systemically heparinized with an intravenous bolus of 5,000 to 10,000 units (80 to 100 units/kg), followed by a continuous infusion based on a weight-based protocol (usually 1,000 to 1,500 units/h). Although the ideal method of monitoring heparin therapy is debatable, an activated partial thromboplastin time test (aPTT) is the standard in most hospitals. Anticoagulation is considered adequate when these test values are at least 1.5 to 2.0 times the pretreatment values. It is extremely important to achieve therapeutic levels within 24 hours, as subtherapeutic levels have been associated with recurrent thromboembolism in randomized trials. There is a common misconception that an aPTT greater than twice normal (usually >100 seconds) is associated with more bleeding complications. On the contrary, clinical trials demonstrate a lack of association between a supratherapeutic aPTT (ratio of 2.5 or greater) and the risk of clinically important hemorrhage. Antifactor Xa assays are an alternative and more accurate method of measuring heparin efficacy but are more expensive and not readily available at many hospitals.

   Platelet counts should also be checked at least every other day, since heparin may induce thrombocytopenia. **Heparin-induced thrombocytopenia (HIT)** generally is recognized at least 3 days after onset of therapy and appears more commonly in patients with prior heparin exposure. HIT occurs with an incidence of 1% to 5% with UFH and can result from an immune reaction to the heparin-platelet complex. The development of antibodies to heparin is independent of patient age, gender, amount, or route of heparin exposure. **A smaller percentage of patients with antiplatelet antibodies experience profound platelet aggregation and clumping that can lead to the devastating syndrome of HIT with thrombosis.** This condition can result in paradoxical arterial and venous thrombosis despite heparin therapy. In any patient with a decreased platelet level on heparin, antiplatelet antibodies should be checked. The treatment of HIT is to stop all heparin, including heparin flushes and heparin-coated lines, as this condition is not a dose-dependent phenomenon. **If continued anticoagulation is necessary, the direct thrombin inhibitor argatroban can be used (Table 19.1).**

   b. **LMWH** has been proven in clinical trials to be equally effective as UFH in the treatment of DVT. LMWHs have several advantages over UFH. Their bioavailability is better due to lesser plasma protein binding. The dosage is a convenient once or twice per day, subcutaneously. LMWHs act more specifically on factor Xa, rather than thrombin, which may lessen the risk of bleeding. LMWHs are weight based and do not need monitoring of levels, which avoids the frequent blood draws that are needed for monitoring UFH. **The incidence of heparin-induced thrombocytopenia with LMWH is ten times less than that with unfractionated heparins.** Outpatient treatment is also practical for selected cases of first-time, uncomplicated DVT in conjunction with the initiation of warfarin therapy. Unfractionated heparin can be used for complicated venous thrombosis, suggested by significant symptoms, large thrombus burden, or recurrent thrombosis. In these more complicated cases of DVT, admission to the hospital allows for leg elevation, observation for phlegmasia, and consideration of catheter-directed thrombolysis in appropriate candidates.

c. **Oral anticoagulation with warfarin is started during heparin therapy and is continued for 3 months.** During this period, the deep veins usually recanalize slowly. Since warfarin inhibits coagulation by inhibiting liver synthesis of vitamin K–dependent clotting factors (II, VII, IX, X), which have long half-lives, anticoagulation with oral agents requires several days of therapy before the patient is anticoagulated. Additionally, warfarin inhibits the synthesis of the anticoagulant protein C, which has a fairly short half-life causing a relative prothrombotic state during the first several days after starting warfarin. Heparin therapy during these first few days keeps the patient anticoagulated until eventually all of the vitamin K–dependent factors have been effectively inhibited.

To standardize the prothrombin time (PT) for oral anticoagulation, the **World Health Organization has developed an international reference (INR) thromboplastin from human brain tissue and has recommended that the PT be expressed as this INR.** With the past conventional use of rabbit brain thromboplastin reagents, a PT ratio of 1.3 to 1.5 (16 to 20 seconds) corresponds to an INR of 2.0 to 3.0. Clinical trials support less intense oral anticoagulation therapy (INR of 2.0 to 3.0) for most conditions requiring anticoagulation.

As previously mentioned, when warfarin is started, protein C levels fall more quickly than the other vitamin K–dependent factors resulting in a transient prothrombotic state. Patients with underlying protein C deficiency may be particularly at risk for warfarin-induced skin necrosis, which appears typically on the breasts, buttocks, and thighs. The safest method of instituting warfarin therapy is the nonloading technique, administering an average dose (we suggest 5 to 7.5 mg) orally each day until INR is in the therapeutic range. Dose alterations can be made, keeping in mind that a particular dose of warfarin is not reflected until the peak effect 36 to 72 hours later. A heparin "bridge" should be initiated prior to warfarin in order to counteract warfarin's transient thrombogenicity and in order to begin to treat the clinical thrombosis. **The target INR for warfarin should be 2.0 to 3.0 for at least 24 hours before stopping the heparin.** A more prolonged INR places the patient at increased risk of bleeding complications. Warfarin may be continued longer or indefinitely in patients with ongoing risk factors for VTE. For patients who cannot take warfarin (e.g., pregnant women), full-dose subcutaneous LMWH may be administered for extended periods of time.

d. Practitioners have rapidly adopted **novel oral anticoagulants (NOACs)** as an alternative to warfarin and even the preferred treatment for uncomplicated DVT. These medications have quick-onset, reasonable safety profiles and do not require laboratory monitoring. **Rivaroxaban and apixaban are direct factor Xa inhibitors** that can be used to treat DVT immediately, without a requirement for heparin overlap. **Dabigatran is a direct thrombin inhibitor** that is more often used for stroke prophylaxis due to nonvalvular atrial fibrillation but is also approved for VTE after a period of parenteral anticoagulation. Caution should be used in patients with severe liver or renal dysfunction, as these drugs have not been well vetted for such conditions. Dabigatran is metabolized heavily via the renal system and must be dose-adjusted in renal impairment. One potential downside to NOACs is the lack of a readily available antidote in the event of bleeding, although some clinical trials have noted that the absolute risk of bleeding is lower when compared with warfarin. Warfarin is reversible with administration of vitamin K or FFP that contains vitamin K–dependent coagulation factors. The antidote to heparin is protamine, although in larger doses protamine may exhibit a paradoxical anticoagulant effect. Protamine can also have serious adverse reactions and may induce transient hypotension, pulmonary vasoconstriction, and, less commonly, anaphylaxis.

e. **Leg pain and swelling** can range from mild or absent with calf thrombi to severe with larger and more proximal iliofemoral thrombosis. Leg elevation above the level of the heart is important to minimize swelling. Bed rest is no longer considered standard for DVTs, and patients are permitted to ambulate ad lib. Before discharge, patients should be fitted for 30 to 40 mm Hg compression stockings, which are part of a long-term strategy to minimize the morbidity associated with postthrombotic syndrome. **The consistent use of compression hose for several years after proximal DVT is proven in randomized trials to reduce the risk of developing symptoms of postthrombotic syndrome such as skin changes and ulcers.**

f. The role of **catheter-directed thrombolytic therapy for acute DVT** is still debated despite clinical evidence demonstrating its effectiveness in proximal DVT of less than 72 hours in duration. The initial goal of treating DVT is to prevent clot propagation and PE. Although standard treatment with anticoagulation treats this problem, it does not prevent the long-term sequelae of postthrombotic syndrome. Years afterward, only a minority of patients are completely recanalized, whereas most have residual obstruction and valvular damage. **Patients with iliofemoral DVT are particularly at risk for developing severe postthrombotic syndrome.** Intuitively, early lysis of the thrombus would seem beneficial and support for this lies with studies demonstrating that early recanalization more often results in preserved valvular function and vein patency.

The National Venous Registry has reported a large experience from a number of centers using catheter-based techniques of pharmacologic thrombolysis. Complete lysis was achieved in 65% of patients. Among those who had a first-time DVT and experienced complete lysis, 96% maintained a 1-year vein patency. Favorable results are also seen in quality of life questionnaires at follow-up 1 to 2 years later. In a Norwegian randomized trial, **catheter-directed thrombolytic therapy improved 24-month vein**

patency and correlated with lower risk of postthrombotic syndrome. Thrombolysis is contraindicated in patients with recent internal bleeding (within 2 months), cerebrovascular accidents, or other active intracranial disease. It also may cause serious hemorrhage after recent (within about 10 days) major surgery or obstetric delivery, organ biopsy, and previous puncture of a noncompressible vessel. Although life-threatening complications such as intracranial hemorrhage are rare (<1%), careful patient selection is important to minimize this risk. In addition, thrombolytic therapy must be used only by physicians who are completely familiar with its dosage and contraindications and in a setting in which therapy can be continuously monitored. DVT thrombolysis has not been demonstrated to prolong life or reduce risk of PE, nor does it replace the need for anticoagulation after the procedure. Patients with mild edema or limited life expectancy (i.e., advanced malignancy) are unlikely to benefit substantially from thrombolysis, and anticoagulation and support hose is the standard of care for these patients.

The technique of venous thrombolysis is most often used in patients with extensive iliofemoral thrombosis and/or phlegmasia cerulea dolens. With the patient in a prone position, the popliteal vein can be accessed via ultrasound guidance, and a sheath is placed in the femoral–popliteal vein. A thrombolytic catheter (e.g., "soaker hose catheter") with multiple side holes is then positioned within the clot, and lytic agent can be infused at a continuous rate. Recombinant tPA (alteplase) is the lytic agent most commonly utilized at doses of 0.5 to 1 mg/h. Recombinant tPA is derived from the structure of native tPA produced by vascular endothelial cells. This enzyme is critical to the body's own fibrinolytic system by catalyzing the conversion of plasminogen to plasmin. Recombinant tPA is a powerful drug for treating acute thrombosis in a variety of settings (e.g., VTE, arterial thrombosis, myocardial infarction). Low-dose heparin infusion is usually administered through the sheath concomitantly. Venograms are performed over 12 to 24 hour intervals to monitor the success of lysis. During this period, patients are monitored in the ICU, with periodic checks of the aPTT and fibrinogen levels. Bleeding at the sheath site may be treated by holding the lytic agent temporarily. Once lysis is complete, venography and intravascular ultrasound should be used to evaluate for residual stenosis. These stenoses are best treated by venoplasty and stenting, similar to the technique described in Chapter 18. Many clinicians have combined the use of mechanical thrombolysis using one of several commercially available devices with pharmacologic lysis. The mechanical component allows for debulking of the thrombus, can hasten the process of thrombolysis, and may reduce the amount of thrombolytic needed to achieve an acceptable result. Several mechanical thrombectomy devices are available. The AngioJet™ Zelante (Boston Scientific, Marlborough, MA) functions by creating a Venturi effect to break up and then evacuate the thrombus. The EkoSonic™ endovascular system (BTG Interventional Medicine, London, UK) uses targeted ultrasonic waves in combination with clot-dissolving drugs. The Penumbra Indigo® (Penumbra, Alameda, CA) uses an aspiration catheter and separator system connected to high-level, continuous suction.

g. **Subclavian-axillary venous thrombosis** may be associated with central venous catheters or thoracic outlet syndrome. If a catheter is present in the affected vein, it should be removed and systemic heparin administered just as for lower extremity DVTs in order to minimize the risk of PE. Catheter-directed thrombolytic therapy is encouraged in younger patients with thoracic outlet syndrome and effort thrombosis (i.e., **Paget-Schroetter syndrome**). This may be performed via a thrombolysis system inserted through the antecubital or basilic vein into the subclavian vein. Of course, definitive treatment requires surgical correction of the thoracic outlet compression once the vein has been recanalized with the thrombolytic therapy. This operation involves removal of a portion of the first rib, removal of a cervical rib (if present), division of any fibrous or constricting bands, and release of scalene muscle compression (see Fig. 4.1). The timing of thoracic outlet surgery is controversial. While some advocate delay between thrombolysis and surgical treatment of 2 to 3 months, others prefer to treat the thoracic outlet during the initial hospitalization. Regardless, full anticoagulation with warfarin or a NOAC should be continued for a period of at least 3 months after the acute thrombosis.

h. **Surgical thrombectomy** for acute DVT has had limited results over the years. Nonetheless, patients with phlegmasia cerulea dolens who are not candidates for thrombolysis should be considered for this rare procedure. An arteriovenous fistula is performed at the end of the procedure to help maintain long-term venous patency. Neither surgical nor endovascular thrombectomy is a substitute for anticoagulation, as full heparinization followed by conversion to oral anticoagulation must be continued after the procedure to prevent early rethrombosis.

i. The **management of DVT during pregnancy** begins with the establishment of a solid diagnosis, usually made with duplex, although MRV can be useful for cases of proximal DVT. V/Q scan is the test of choice to rule out PE during pregnancy, as it avoids the radiation exposure associated with CTA. **Warfarin crosses the placenta and is contraindicated during pregnancy. Subcutaneous LMW heparin provides an adequate means of full anticoagulation and has a lower risk of osteoporosis and heparin-induced thrombocytopenia when compared to long-term UFH.** Full anticoagulation is accomplished using LMWH during the pregnancy, and then near the time of delivery, the patient is admitted for a "heparin window." The LMWH is stopped, and intravenous heparin, which has a short half-life, is started. The intravenous heparin is stopped prior to the delivery and then restarted following the delivery. Temporary vena cava filters have been used in pregnant women at high risk for PE and must be placed in a suprarenal position in order to prevent compression by the gravid uterus.

3. **PE** is a potentially life-threatening event from acute DVT. Many patients with **clinically silent DVTs experience** PE as their initial clinical presentation. Untreated, the mortality of PE is extremely high. In some situations, such as unexplained and rapid cardiopulmonary demise, there may be a role for empiric initiation of treatment (heparin) until diagnostic testing can be completed.

a. PE also requires systemic heparinization followed by long-term oral anticoagulation. The dosages, methods of administration, and duration of therapy are the same as those used for acute

DVT. **Anticoagulation is intended to prevent further thromboembolism or clot propagation within the lung and does little to resolve an existing thrombus.** In select patients with massive acute PE, intravenous thrombolytic can be administered. One regimen is 100 mg of tPA intravenously over 2 hours. Emergency catheter-directed pulmonary thrombolysis may also have benefit in patients with massive and submassive PE. Rarely, urgent pulmonary surgical embolectomy is indicated for salvageable patients who have documented massive PE and persistent refractory hypotension despite maximum medical therapy. In select patients with chronic organized pulmonary thromboemboli and pulmonary hypertension, elective pulmonary endarterectomy also may improve chronic hypoxia and respiratory disability.

b. The introduction of the Greenfield **inferior vena cava (IVC) filter** in 1972 was a pivotal moment in medical innovation. With a minimally invasive procedure, physicians were able to successfully treat patients who otherwise would succumb to complications of anticoagulation or pulmonary emboli. **Filters are usually deployed in the inferior vena cava below the renal veins and function by capturing thromboemboli and preventing them from traveling to the pulmonary arteries.** Vena cava filters can be placed percutaneously under fluoroscopic or intravascular ultrasound guidance via a femoral or jugular approach.

Over several decades, there has been a substantial increase in the number of IVC filters implanted (Fig. 19.1). Yet, the prevalence of VTE has remained the same in epidemiologic studies. IVC filters are frequently placed for a variety of relative indications outside of the original indications (Table 19.4). The relative simplicity and ease of IVC filter placement has contributed to frequency of usage. The development of retrievable IVC filters has been a significant technologic advance. A retrievable IVC filter is placed when the patient has a temporary condition that precludes standard anticoagulation treatment. The filter can then be

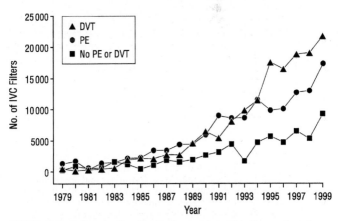

FIGURE 19.1 IVC filter implantation has increased significantly over time, due to availability of retrievable filters and expanding indications. (Credit to Stein PD, Kayali F, Olson RE. Twenty-one year trends in the use of inferior vena cava filters. *Arch Int Med.* 2004;164:1541-1545.)

TABLE 19.4	IVC Filters Are Utilized in Many Clinical Scenarios

Absolute Indications
- Contraindication to anticoagulation with VTE
- PE despite anticoagulation

Relative Indications
- "Free-floating" iliofemoral thrombus
- Poor cardiopulmonary reserve
- Noncompliance with medication
- Severe ataxia or fall risk

Prophylactic indications
- Trauma patients
- Bariatric surgery
- Spinal cord injury
- History of VTE

"Relative" and "prophylactic" reasons for placement should be carefully weighed against potential risk of filters.

removed with a second percutaneous procedure after the period of presumed thrombogenicity is over. The vascular interventionalist grasps a hook at the end of the filter with a snare, collapses the filter, and removes it through a sheath. The window of opportunity for removing these filters is finite and varies among filter type. Most filters must be removed within 1 to 6 months before they become incorporated into the vena cava wall. Alternatively, the retrievable filter can be deliberately left in place as a permanent filter. However, many filters are ultimately not retrieved when patients are lost to follow up or for medical reasons.

The traditional or **absolute** indications for IVC filter placement are **contraindication to anticoagulation or breakthrough PE despite adequate anticoagulation**. Gastrointestinal bleeding, intracerebral hemorrhage, and recent spinal surgery are examples of contraindications to anticoagulation. Contraindications to anticoagulation are not always clear-cut, such as "fall risk" or "history of GI bleed," and careful consideration should be given to the risk of bleeding. Without anticoagulation, edema and pain from DVT can persist and even worsen. **Relative** indications for IVC filter placement may seem intuitive but have not been thoroughly studied. Examples include poor cardiac reserve, free-floating iliofemoral thrombus, and as protection during thrombolysis treatment for DVT. Also unclear is the role for **prophylactic** IVC filters, meaning placement in patients who do not have an acute VTE but are considered "high risk," such as after major trauma or spinal cord injury and around the time of bariatric surgery. Filters placed for prophylactic indications are almost exclusively retrievable IVC filters, but their low retrieval rate and limited follow-up is problematic. Patients receiving prophylactic filters are generally younger and therefore more subject to potential long-term complications from IVC filters. It is clear that the availability of retrievable IVC filters has liberalized the placement criteria.

In the landmark "PREPIC" study, 400 patients with proximal (i.e., not calf) DVTs were randomized such that 50% received an IVC filter and 50% did not. All of the patients were treated with standard anticoagulation for at least 3 months. Although there were fewer pulmonary emboli in the IVC filter group in the short term, importantly at 8 years follow-up, there was no significant difference in fatal pulmonary emboli and no difference in overall survival between groups. Patients who received an IVC filter were more likely to develop recurrent DVT. The PREPIC 2 study investigated the use of **retrievable** IVC filters using similar methodology in "high-risk" patients within the first 3 months of symptomatic PE. When used as an adjunct to anticoagulation, retrievable filters did not further reduce recurrent symptomatic PE. Accordingly, we do not advocate routine use of this "belt and suspenders" approach to VTE.

In general, filter placement is safe and quick and can be performed in an angiogram suite or at the bedside in the intensive care unit. Nonetheless, the decision to place an IVC filter, whether permanent or retrievable, should include a careful consideration of the indications as well as the potential long-term risks of the filter to the patient (Table 19.5). Nearly 1,000 cases of adverse events related to IVC filters have been reported, which prompted the FDA to issue the following warning statement specific to retrievable filters in 2010: "...implanting physicians should consider removing the filter as soon as protection from PE is no longer needed..." In the short term, IVC filters can be misplaced in the iliac vein or in aberrant anatomy, be positioned with excessive tilt, or in improper position relative to the renal veins. Thrombosis of the femoral vein insertion site has been noted but is less frequent with the smaller profile systems. In the long term, recurrent DVT rates of 10% to 30% are higher in patients with an IVC filter, likely due to stagnation of flow. Thrombosis of the vena cava is a devastating complication that can occur in up to 2% of patients with an IVC filter. This event results in massive, disabling lower extremity edema. IVC filter migration is uncommon, but filters have been reported to migrate anywhere along the path of the vena cava up to the cardiac chambers and pulmonary arteries. Filter perforation of the cava is also noted not infrequently as an incidental finding on imaging and can rarely result in bowel perforation or aortic injury. Patients who receive an IVC filter and do not receive anticoagulation for their DVT are at highest risk for developing postthrombotic syndrome, as the leg DVT has been untreated except by the body's own fibrinolytic system.

TABLE 19.5   Potential Adverse Events from IVC Filters

Maldeployment	Rare
Access site bleeding or thrombosis	4%–11%
Penetration	Common[a]
Migration	<1%
Filter fracture	1%–2%
Vena cava thrombosis	<10%
Recurrent DVT	10%–30% higher in patients with IVC filters

[a]Incidental penetration of vena cava on imaging is common, whereas penetration with injury to adjacent structures, that is, aorta and duodenum is rare.

Selected Readings

Caine GJ, Stonelake PS, Lip GY, et al. The hypercoagulable state of malignancy: pathogenesis and current debate. *Neoplasia*. 2002;4(6):465-473.

The epidemiology and pathogenesis of cancer-related thrombosis explained succinctly.

Caprini score for DVT calculator, 2017. Retrieved from: https://www.thecalculator.co/health/Caprini-Score-For-DVT-Calculator-1108.html

Online Caprini score calculator.

Caprini DVT Risk Score, 2017. North Shore University Health System (Version 1.1) [Mobile application software]. Retrieved from http://itunes.apple.com

Mobile application quickly calculates DVT risk.

Decousus H, Leizorovicz A, Parent F, et al. A clinical trial of vena caval filters in the prevention of pulmonary embolism in patients with proximal deep-vein thrombosis. Prevention du Risque d'Embolie Pulmonaire par Interruption Cave Study Group. *N Engl J Med*. 1998;338(7):409-415.

The original "PREPIC" randomized trial studied patients with DVT treated with anti-coagulation, with or without IVC filter placement.

Enden T, Haig Y, Klow NE, et al. Long-term outcome after additional catheter-directed thrombolysis versus standard treatment for acute iliofemoral deep vein thrombosis (the CaVenT study): a randomised controlled trial. *Lancet*. 2012;379(9810):31-38.

Norwegian randomized trial of 209 patients showed efficacy for iliofemoral DVT thrombolysis with end points of vein patency and post-thrombotic symptoms.

Gould MK, Dembitzer AD, Doyle RL, et al. Low-molecular-weight heparins compared with unfractionated heparin for treatment of acute deep venous thrombosis: a meta-analysis of randomized, controlled trials. *Ann Intern Med*. 1999;130:800-809.

Early meta-analysis that compared UFH vs. LMWH for treatment of DVT.

Guyatt GH, Akl EA, Crowther M, et al. American College of Chest Physicians Antithrombotic Therapy and Prevention of Thrombosis Panel. Executive summary: Antithrombotic Therapy and Prevention of Thrombosis, 9th ed: American College of Chest Physicians Evidence-Based Clinical Practice Guidelines. *Chest*. 2012;141(2 suppl):7S-47S.

CHEST 2012 guidelines on VTE with emphasis on prevention. Extensive document with easy to search bullet points.

Johnson CM, Mureebe L, Silver D. Hypercoagulable states: a review. *Vasc Endovasc Surg*. 2005;39:123-133.

Additional information about inherited and acquired thrombophilias for the interested vascular specialist.

Kabrhel C, Mark Courtney D, Camargo CA Jr, et al. Factors associated with positive D-dimer results in patients evaluated for pulmonary embolism. *Acad Emerg Med*. 2010;17(6):589-597.

Although a negative D-dimer is highly predictive for no VTE in outpatients, this article demonstrates the multiple factors that may contribute to a positive D-dimer in a hospitalized setting.

Kearon C, Akl EA, Ornelas J, et al. Antithrombotic therapy for VTE disease: CHEST Guideline and Expert Panel Report. *CHEST*. 2016;149(2):315-352.

Updated expert guideline recommendations for venous thromboembolism diagnosis and management.

LaMuraglia GM, Houbballah R, Laposata M. The identification and management of heparin-induced thrombocytopenia in the vascular patient. *J Vasc Surg*. 2012;55(2):562-570.

Excellent review of the pathogenesis, diagnosis and management of HIT, readily readable for the young clinician.

Meissner MH, Gloviczki P, Comerota AJ, et al.; Society for Vascular Surgery; American Venous Forum. Early thrombus removal strategies for acute deep venous thrombosis: clinical practice guidelines of the Society for Vascular Surgery and the American Venous Forum. *J Vasc Surg*. 2012;55(5):1449-1462.

Hallmark document from joint vascular societies provides specific guidance and evidence for percutaneous venous thrombolysis of acute DVT.

Meissner MH, Wakefield TW, Ascher E, et al. Acute venous disease: venous thrombosis and venous trauma. *J Vasc Surg*. 2007;46:25S-53S.

Excellent discussion of pathophysiology, prevention, and treatment of VTE, including catheter-directed thrombolysis.

Merriman L, Graeves M. Testing for thrombophilia: an evidence-based approach. *Postgrad Med J.* 2006;82(973):699-704.
Concise article on thrombophilias with completion post-test to solidify learning.

Mewissen MW, Seabrook GR, Meissner MH, et al. Catheter-directed thrombolysis of lower extremity deep venous thrombosis: report of a national multicenter registry. *Radiology.* 1999;211:39-49.
Early venous registry data indicating the benefit of catheter-directed lysis (does not include mechanical thrombectomy).

Mismetti P, Laporte S, Pellerin O, et al.; PREPIC2 Study Group. Effect of a retrievable inferior vena cava filter plus anticoagulation vs anticoagulation alone on risk of recurrent pulmonary embolism: a randomized clinical trial. *JAMA.* 2015;313(16):1627-1635.
"Sequel" to the original PREPIC studies, examining specifically the adjuvant usage of retrievable IVC filters.

The PREPIC Study Group. Eight-year follow-up of patients with permanent vena cava filters in the prevention of pulmonary embolism: The PREPIC (Prévention du Risque d'Embolie Pulmonaire par Interruption Cave) randomized study. *Circulation.* 2005;112(3):416-422.
8 year follow-up data from the randomized PREPIC study examined the role for IVC filter placement.

Robertson L, Jones LE. Fixed dose subcutaneous low molecular weight heparins versus adjusted dose unfractionated heparin for the initial treatment of venous thromboembolism. *Cochrane Database Syst Rev.* 2017;(2):CD001100.
2017 Cochrane review attests to lower bleeding risk and recurrent DVT with LMWH.

Spyropoulos AC. Brave new world: the current and future use of novel anticoagulants. *Thrombosis Research.* 2008;123:S29-S35.
Overview of basic pharmacology and clinical trials for the novel oral anticoagulants.

20 Hemodialysis Access

In 1972, an amendment to the Social Security Act provided Medicare coverage for patients with end-stage renal disease (ESRD). The magnitude of the current expenditure is impressive, with over $34.3 billion spent on just over a million patients with various degrees of ESRD in 2011. Nearly 450,000 patients are dialysis dependent in the United States, with diabetes and hypertension identified as the leading causes of ESRD. Patients with ESRD also suffer from a higher incidence of comorbid conditions such as chronic anemia, heart failure, peripheral arterial disease, and metabolic bone disease. The 5-year life expectancy of a patient on dialysis is 25%, with the largest percentage of deaths occurring from cardiac causes. With an aging population of ESRD patients, the magnitude of medical care and economic burden is expected to increase.

Procedures involving dialysis access are the most common vascular procedures in the United States. A well-functioning and durable vascular access circuit is truly a "lifeline" for patients on hemodialysis. Patients with a poorly functioning access or those with percutaneously placed central venous dialysis catheters have increased morbidity and suffer frequent hospitalizations for access-related complications such as thrombosis or infection. Management of vascular access requires the coordinated efforts of health care providers and a well-informed patient. The ideal care paradigm uses a multidisciplinary team of nephrologists, surgeons and interventionalists, dialysis nurses and technicians, diabetes educators, dieticians, and social workers. Patients with ESRD should be referred early to a vascular surgeon, prior to initiating dialysis, in hopes of establishing autogenous access (e.g., native arteriovenous fistula). Unfortunately, one of the most predictable aspects of chronic hemodialysis is the need for additional procedures to achieve, maintain, or restore patency of the high-flow circuit. This chapter focuses on essentials in the patient's initial evaluation and the placement, and revision of hemodialysis access.

I. **INDICATIONS FOR DIALYSIS.** Chronic kidney failure resulting from the decrease in functioning nephrons is measured by the decrement in glomerular filtration rate (GFR) (Table 20.1). A patient's GFR can be estimated from a formula using variables for serum creatinine, age, race, and gender. The degree of kidney failure is categorized using the commonly accepted vernacular for the stages of chronic kidney disease (CKD) 1 through 5. In this system, stage 1 CKD is the least severe (i.e., only mild renal dysfunction) and stage 5 is the most severe (i.e., complete renal failure) (Table 20.1).

The 2015 Kidney Disease Outcomes Quality Initiative (KDOQI) guidelines state that patients who reach CKD stage 4 (GFR of 30 mL/min/1.73 m^2 or less), including those who have imminent need for maintenance dialysis at the time of their first assessment, should receive education about kidney failure and options for its treatment, including kidney transplantation, peritoneal dialysis, hemodialysis, and

TABLE 20.1	Stages of Chronic Kidney Disease and Corresponding Rates of Estimated Glomerular Filtration (eGFR) as well as Common Complications of Reduced eGFR		
Stage	Description	eGFR (mL/min/1.73 m^2)	Complications of Reduced eGFR
1	Kidney damage with normal or increased GFR	≥90	Anemia Hypertension Calcium malabsorption Hyperkalemia Hyperparathyroidism Hyperphosphatemia Left ventricular hypertrophy Metabolic acidosis Volume overload
2	Kidney damage with mild eGFR decrease	60–89	
3	Moderate decrease in eGFR	30–59	
4	Severe decrease in eGFR	15–29	
5	Kidney failure	<15	

conservative treatment. In addition to educating patients with more advanced staged CKD, it is important to inform and prepare their family members and caregivers about options and expectations.

The decision to initiate maintenance hemodialysis should be based on an assessment of signs and/or symptoms associated with uremia, evidence of protein-energy wasting, and the ability to safely manage metabolic abnormalities and/or volume overload with medical therapy rather than on just one specific level of kidney function (i.e., one lab measurement) in the absence of other clinical signs and symptoms.

Although initiating the planning and even the start of hemodialysis is important for patients with stage 4 CKD, nearly all patients with stage 5 CKD (GFR < 15 mL/min) will need dialysis to manage the manifestations of renal failure. The following are some of the most common clinical indicators of renal failure (CKD stages 4 to 5) that challenge the patient and the care team to consider initiating hemodialysis (Table 20.1):

A. **Hyperkalemia (serum potassium > 6 mEq/L),** especially when accompanied by ECG or neuromuscular abnormalities, requires dialysis. Dietary restriction of potassium and potassium-bonding resins may also assist in lowering levels of potassium in the blood.

B. **Fluid overload** is another frequent indication for both acute and chronic dialysis. This includes patients who have not responded satisfactorily to fluid restriction and diuretics. In addition to diffuse, whole body edema, fluid overload often manifests as heart failure and severe shortness of breath.

C. **Worsening acidosis** results from the kidneys' inability to excrete hydrogen and resorb bicarbonate and represents an indication for hemodialysis.

D. **Drug overdose** is a less common indication for hemodialysis, and not one necessarily related to CKD. However, hemodialysis can be used as an emergency or critical care adjunct to acutely manage certain situations of medication overdose.

E. **Uremic signs and symptoms** are the most common indication for chronic dialysis as blood-urea-nitrogen (BUN) and serum creatinine levels rise. Neurologic symptoms related to uremia include lethargy, seizures, myoclonus, and peripheral neuropathy, and it has been shown that mortality and morbidity can be reduced if the BUN level can be chronically maintained below 90 mg/dL.

II. **ACCESS PLANNING.** An initial consideration in dialysis access planning is whether or not the access is intended to be **temporary** or **permanent**. Patients with lesser degrees of CKD (i.e., CKD 1 to 3) who develop acute renal failure will often recover over a period of days, weeks, or even months and may be candidates for temporary access while their condition is assessed and optimized. In contrast, patients who develop acute renal insufficiency in the setting baseline severe CKD (CKD 3 to 5) are likely to require chronic or permanent dialysis.

Patients with CKD stage 4 (GFR of 30 mL/min/1.73 m²) or 5 (GFR of 15 mL/min/1.73 m²) should be referred to a vascular provider, preferably months in advance of needing dialysis. The goal of the initial consultation should be to obtain a history and to perform an exam, with a focus on the potential options for vascular access. This evaluation should allow time for the creation and maturation of an autogenous arteriovenous (AV) fistula when possible (i.e., the "fistula first" approach) (Table 20.2). Even if dialysis access may not be immediately necessary establishing a rapport between the vascular providers, the patient, and his or her family, helps to facilitate realistic expectations regarding the location and durability of any future dialysis access procedures.

A. **A history of prior access procedures and selection of anatomic location for dialysis graft or fistula.** The date, type, and anatomic location for previous access procedures should be recorded during the patient evaluation. Additionally, the dates and methods of failure (e.g., thrombosis, infection, or failure to mature) of previous access maneuvers should be noted.

It is also important to record the location and duration of any previous central venous catheters (tunneled or nontunneled) placed into the subclavian or internal jugular veins as temporary dialysis ports. Patients who have these types of indwelling catheters have a higher probability of having stenoses or occlusions in the subclavian, jugular, and/or innominate veins (i.e., central veins of the upper extremities and chest), which will adversely affect the success and longevity of any subsequent permanent fistulas or grafts placed in the upper extremities.

Whether the patient is right or left hand dominant should also be noted so that consideration can be given for placing the dialysis access mechanism in the nondominant arm. Although it may be more convenient for the patient to have the fistula or graft placed in the nondominant upper extremity, the authors will defer to the upper extremity with the most favorable or suitable venous anatomy, even if this means placing the fistula or graft in the patient's dominant arm.

TABLE 20.2	Selected Guidelines for Vascular Access from the K/DOQI Work Group

1. 50% AVF placement in incident hemodialysis patients (i.e., first-time patients)
2. 40% AVF usage in prevalent hemodialysis patients (i.e., patients who have had dialysis access)
3. <10% prevalent patients with chronic (>3 months) catheter access
4. The order of preference for establishing an AV access circuit
   a. Wrist (radiocephalic) fistula
   b. Elbow (brachiocephalic) fistula
   c. AV graft with PTFE or basilic vein transposition

K/DOQI, National Kidney Foundation Kidney Disease Outcome Initiative; AV, arteriovenous; PTFE, polytetrafluoroethylene; AVF, arteriovenous fistula.

1. **Medical comorbidities** such as poor cardiac function should be determined, as these can limit the long-term success of hemodialysis access. The choice of anesthesia (general, regional, or local) is also be influenced by the presence of these comorbidities. The presence of diabetes should be noted, as this condition is associated with poorer outcomes including a higher risk for hand ischemia due to arterial steal phenomenon following performance of a fistula or graft.

2. The use of **antiplatelet and anticoagulant medications** should be noted, and in some cases, these should be stopped prior to performing a fistula or graft, depending on the type of medication and/or planned operation. These medications are particularly important to note, as patients with more severe forms of CKD are likely to have baseline platelet dysfunction. Generally, aspirin can be continued throughout most, if not all, dialysis access operations, although for those such as a basilic vein transposition that require larger incisions, one may choose to stop the patient's aspirin 3 to 5 days prior to the case. Because clopidogrel (Plavix) is a more potent antiplatelet agent, it should be held 5 to 7 days prior to elective access operations to reduce the risk of bleeding complications such as hematoma. Similarly, because warfarin or medications that are direct thrombin or factor Xa inhibitors provide full anticoagulation, they should be stopped prior to the dialysis access operation.

3. **Smoking negatively influences long-term access patency** and all patients should be encouraged to quit preoperatively and provided access to formal smoking cessation programs if available.

B. **Physical exam** as an important determinant for the hemodialysis access site.

1. **Surgical scars** and location of previous access procedures are noted, including percutaneous or tunneled central venous catheters. **Skin conditions** must be noted for signs of infection or other dermatologic disorders that would impair wound healing following an operation.

2. **The axillary, brachial, radial, and ulnar pulses should be palpated and blood pressure recorded in both arms (Chapter 3).** Diminished pulse strength or a difference in blood pressure of more than 10 mm Hg may indicate proximal arterial occlusive disease (i.e., a proximal arterial stenosis) on the side with the low pressure. The subclavian and axillary arteries in the area of the supra- and infraclavicular fossa should also be auscultated, as the presence of a bruit would suggest an underlying arterial stenosis.

It is critical to diagnose what may be underlying, asymptomatic arterial occlusive disease in the upper extremity (i.e., a proximal or inflow stenosis) *before* performing the access operation as it can lead to **steal phenomenon and hand ischemia** once the arteriovenous circuit is completed and opened. Steal phenomenon results when an otherwise asymptomatic proximal or inflow arterial stenosis that is able to perfuse the extremity at baseline is unable to provide adequate perfusion to both the newly formed fistula and the distal arm and hand once the arteriovenous circuit is opened. Steal is based on the **Bernoulli principle and equation** that defines a decrease in pressure across a fixed stenosis when flow across that stenosis is increased. In the case of a proximal upper extremity stenosis, once the dialysis fistula is created, flow across that stenosis increases dramatically because of the newly created venous circuit. This new and increased flow into the dialysis circuit results in a significant decrease in pressure across the fixed, proximal stenosis and distal to the newly created fistula. This decrease in distal pressure and perfusion renders the distal arm and hand ischemic. Steal following creation of dialysis access circuits can be immediate and dramatic in some cases, or more chronic and subtle in other cases. Depending on its severity, steal phenomenon resulting in symptomatic arm and or hand ischemia requires treatment by either opening or bypassing the original proximal arterial stenosis or by restricting flow in the AV dialysis circuit itself (e.g., banding or ligating the circuit).

3. **Perfusion of the hand should be examined prior to creation of an upper extremity dialysis access site.** Specifically, performance of the **Allen test** provides a good assessment of radial and ulnar artery patency as well as patency of the palmar arch in the hand. This evaluation is especially important when planning for an access configuration that will use the radial artery as the inflow vessel (e.g., radiocephalic fistula). In 85% to 90% of patients, the ulnar is the dominant artery to the hand, and confirmation of this indicates that diversion of flow from the radial artery will not significantly reduce hand perfusion. If the radial artery is found to be the dominant artery, one should consider using a different inflow vessel for the arteriovenous circuit.

   To perform the Allen test, first, the hand should be elevated for a brief period of time. Then, with the patient making a tight fist, the examiner should compress the radial and ulnar arteries simultaneously. Separately, the radial and then the ulnar artery should be released as the examiner observes the opened hand for return of perfusion. If the ulnar artery is dominant, perfusion (i.e., color and capillary refill) will not return to the hand until it is released.

4. **The upper extremities should be examined for swelling or edema,** which would suggest the presence of **central venous outflow obstruction** (e.g., subclavian or innominate veins) (Chapter 4). Just as arterial inflow disease can be exacerbated by creation of a high-flow AV fistula, a central venous outflow obstruction can become quite symptomatic following creation of a high-flow dialysis circuit in the affected arm.

5. The **cephalic and basilic veins** should be inspected for patency and size and palpated for compressibility (normal vein) or firm cords (chronic thrombosis or phlebitis). Application of an upper arm tourniquet to increase distal venous filling is sometimes helpful in delineating veins that may be suitable for use in dialysis access configurations.

6. **When peritoneal dialysis is being considered, the abdomen should be examined for prior surgical scars.** Prior abdominal operations may compromise the placement of a chronic peritoneal dialysis catheter.

C. **Noninvasive vascular laboratory testing** is an important part of the preoperative evaluation for hemodialysis access and has been shown to increase effectiveness and durability of access procedures (Chapter 5).

   1. **Duplex ultrasound** of the upper extremity veins should be performed before dialysis access configuration is considered. Suitable veins for fistula formation can be identified by ultrasound that may be otherwise underappreciated on physical exam. Additionally, direct and indirect evaluation of the central venous system can be achieved by duplex, which is especially important in individuals who have had prior central venous dialysis catheters. **Studies have shown the increased ability of vascular specialists to provide autogenous AV fistulas to patients with the use of duplex ultrasound in the preoperative evaluation phase.** These studies report higher patency rates of fistulas with the use of preoperative duplex, and duplex has also been found to be useful in sorting out patients who have had previous access sites that have failed.

   2. **Measurement of segmental pressures** of the upper extremities can be helpful in select instances if the pulse examination is abnormal or arterial occlusive disease is suspected. Furthermore, duplex assess-

ment of arterial flow can provide anatomic and hemodynamic information in complicated cases. In our experience, when bilateral upper extremity blood pressures are equivalent and the Allen test is normal, significant arterial inflow disease is rarely present.

3. Duplex ultrasound of the **central thoracic veins** can be performed if a proximal stenosis is suspected based on a history of prior venous catheters, arm edema, or prominent venous collaterals. This is relatively sensitive for the detection of subclavian venous stenosis or occlusion, although complete visualization of the axillary, subclavian, and innominate veins can be limited by the structures of the thoracic outlet. Significant stenosis is present in 20% to 50% of patients with a history of dialysis catheters (tunneled or nontunneled) placed in the internal jugular or subclavian veins.

III. **VASCULAR ACCESS OPTIONS.** Hemodialysis works by filtering the patient's blood to remove fluid, electrolytes, and toxins—functions that are normally performed by the kidneys. To achieve this end, the patient must have a high-flow dialysis access circuit established that can withstand repeated trauma from needle cannulation. Establishing a connection between the arterial and venous system is the most effective way to create such a high-flow circuit. A direct connection between an artery and vein (**i.e., AV fistula**) results in enlargement and thickening of the outflow vein. As the vein matures, it undergoes "arterialization," making it strong enough to support hemodialysis. A prosthetic bridge graft can also be used to connect an artery and vein (**i.e., arteriovenous graft**), so that the graft and not a vein is punctured for dialysis. An extremity is the most accessible and common location for either type of dialysis access.

The National Kidney Foundation published evidence-based guidelines for vascular access, referred to as Kidney Disease Outcome Quality Initiative **(K/DOQI)**. This consensus statement has been revised multiple times (most recently in 2015) and should be referred to by providers who care for dialysis patients and perform access procedures. Foremost among these recommendations is an emphasis on maximizing the use of AV fistulas (Table 20.2). Specifically, the initiative recommends that autogenous AV fistulas make up more than 50% of new, permanent hemodialysis operations. Historically, the United States has lagged in the use of native fistulas for hemodialysis, despite statistical analyses controlling for patient characteristics (e.g., obesity, diabetes, age). These findings suggest that practice patterns in the United States may be the major limitation to use of autogenous fistulas as the preferred access configuration. Nonetheless, there is a consensus among clinicians that autogenous fistulas are preferred over prosthetic grafts and percutaneous catheters for hemodialysis, due to greater durability and fewer complications (Table 20.2).

A. **An autogenous AV fistula** is the "gold standard" for hemodialysis access and should be established 1 to 2 months in advance of initiating dialysis. Following creation of the fistula, a 6- to 8-week interval must elapse to allow maturation before it is ready for cannulation. Despite this interval, about 10% to 30% of fistulas fail to mature, a difficult scenario addressed in several of the K/DOQI guidelines. Recommendations are made for optimal vein diameter and time for cannulation as well as direct methods to enhance maturation such as hand exercises, ligation or embolization of fistula side branches, and resting the fistula following needle infiltration. Use of preoperative ultrasound mapping is also important to minimize use of a vein that is too small or inadequate to support flow.

A mature AV fistula provides excellent access for hemodialysis and has the highest patency rates; 60% to 90% 1 year, and 40% to 70% over 3 years. These results are superior to the 40% to 75% 1-year patency and 25% to 50% 3-year patency for prosthetic grafts. Patency also varies according to the location of fistula, vein size, and comorbidities such as diabetes. Secondary interventions such as thrombectomy, angioplasty, and revision may improve longer-term patency by 20% to 30%. **Prosthetic AV grafts require a higher number of interventions than native fistulas to maintain and restore patency, and infectious complications are higher with grafts and percutaneously placed catheters than with autogenous arteriovenous fistulas.** In fact, patients with AV grafts or percutaneously placed catheters have overall higher mortality than those with functioning autogenous fistula, with infectious etiologies accounting for the majority of the difference.

Numerous configurations of AV fistulas are possible in the upper extremity. The hierarchy of fistula placement is typically the nondominant before the dominant arm, and forearm before the upper arm (Table 20.1). However, a more suitable (larger) vein may be selected out of standard sequence in order to increase the longevity of the circuit. Likewise, concern for arterial insufficiency in the arm should prompt further evaluation or selection of an alternative location (e.g., the opposite arm). Common sites for a native AV fistula in the upper extremity are as follows:

1. The original AV fistula was the **Brescia-Cimino fistula**, which remains popular in clinical practice (Fig. 20.1A). The anastomosis is

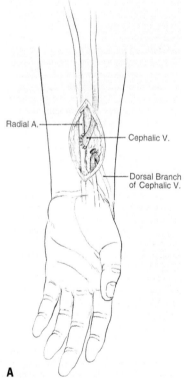

Radial A.

Cephalic V.

Dorsal Branch of Cephalic V.

A

FIGURE 20.1 **(A)** The radiocephalic (Cimino) fistula and brachiocephalic fistula are common forearm and upper arm AVFs, respectively.

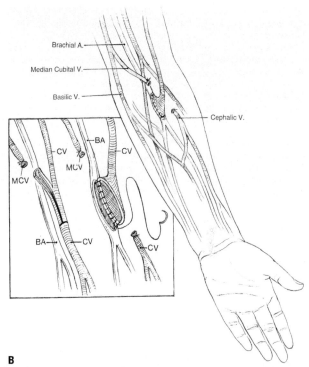

B

FIGURE 20.1 (Continued) **(B)** The anastomosis is constructed from the end of the vein to the side of the artery. After 6 to 8 weeks of maturation, the outflow vein should be dilated and thickened enough to cannulate on dialysis. (BA, brachial artery; CV, cephalic vein; MCV, median cubital vein).

constructed between the cephalic vein and the radial artery at the wrist, most often in an end-to-side fashion and is therefore referred to as a **radiocephalic fistula**. The location of this fistula at the wrist makes it attractive as the initial access procedure, because it does not compromise the more proximal veins or arteries of the arm. Veins that are 2.5 mm or larger by exam or ultrasound can be selected, although smaller veins may used if lower maturation rates can be accepted. The Allen's test should first indicate good ulnar flow to the hand.

2. **Brachiocephalic** fistulas are created in the antecubital region by an end-to-side anastomosis and are often termed a **cephalic vein turndown** (Fig. 20.1B). A few studies have shown superior maturation of brachiocephalic fistulas over those at the wrist. The cephalic vein develops in its superficial location on the lateral aspect of the upper arm, where it can be readily cannulated once the fistula is mature.

3. **A basilic vein transposition** is another option for an upper arm fistula (Fig. 20.2) and can be accomplished via a one- or two-stage operative process. Because the basilic vein lies deep in the medial upper arm, it must be dissected—side branches isolated, ligated, and divided—and "transposed" into a more superficial location in a subcutaneous

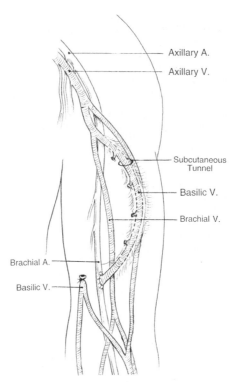

Axillary A.

Axillary V.

Subcutaneous Tunnel

Basilic V.

Brachial V.

Brachial A.

Basilic V.

FIGURE 20.2 The basilic vein transposition is another option for an upper arm AVF in patients with suitable vein. The vein is transposed to a more superficial location in a lateral subcutaneous tunnel.

tunnel on the lateral surface of the upper arm. This process is sometimes referred to as "superficialization of the basilic vein."

In the **single-stage basilic vein transposition procedure**, once all of the side branches have been ligated and divided and the vein is free over its anatomic extent, the distal aspect, at or distal to the antecubital fossa, is ligated and divided. The freed basilic vein is then tunneled superficially on the upper arm such that the distal end of the vein can be sewn, end-to-side, to the brachial artery just proximal to the antecubital fossa.

For the **two-stage basilic vein transposition procedure**, the vein is isolated along its anatomic extent and it is sewn to the brachial artery, leaving the vein in its original, deep and medial, anatomic location for a period of weeks. The second stage of this procedure occurs then weeks later when the arteriovenous fistula is observed to have dilated sufficiently. The second stage of the operation involves rerouting or tunneling the now dilated and functioning arteriovenous fistula to a more accessible, superficial location in the upper arm (i.e., "superficialization of the basilic vein"). Many providers prefer the two-stage procedure as it allows confirmation that the fistula will function effectively before creating the larger soft tissue defect need to tunnel or superficialize the basilica vein. Regardless of whether the one- or two-stage transposition approach is chosen, the basilica vein selected should be 4 mm or larger in order to provide the best chance of fistula maturation.

Because a long incision is required for this operation, regional block or general anesthesia is often used, whereas simpler fistulas such as the radial or brachial cephalic can be performed with local anesthetic and mild sedation. Patients with large arm girth are suboptimal candidates for basilic vein transposition because the length of transposed vein may not be sufficient to route superficially to reach the brachial artery at or just proximal to the antecubital fossa. Additionally, wound complications in patients with obese arms are a concern, which may lead the provider to choose the two-stage transposition approach or select of other access options.

B. **An arteriovenous (AV) dialysis graft** is constructed by sewing a synthetic polytetrafluoroethylene (PTFE) graft between an artery and vein in one of many configurations. One favored configuration is a looped graft placed in the nondominant forearm (i.e., **forearm looped AV graft**) connecting the brachial artery at or near the antecubital fossa to a vein in the same location. In the authors' experience, this loop configuration is preferable to a **straight forearm AV graft** using the radial artery as the inflow and an antecubital vein as outflow, although either method can be attempted with good initial success. Straight forearm grafts have a limited area for puncture and provide challenges associated with sewing a prosthetic graft to what is often a calcified and small-caliber radial artery at the wrist. For this and other related reasons, straight AV forearm grafts seem to have decreased patency compared with forearm loop grafts using the larger brachial artery as the inflow source.

Another choice for an upper extremity graft is an upper arm loop graft between the brachial artery just proximal to the antecubital fossa and the very proximal basilic or axillary vein (i.e., **brachial-axillary AV graft** or "brach-ax" graft). The lower extremity is used only when the upper extremities can no longer accept some type of hemodialysis access. Although grafts can be placed in the groin area (e.g., saphenous vein to proximal femoral artery), infection and soft tissue wound healing is a greater problem than in the upper extremity, and patency rates are limited.

One advantage of prosthetic grafts is that they can be anastomosed to veins that are considered too small for autogenous fistula formation with reasonable patency. Although an autogenous fistula should be created in advance of dialysis in order to allow time for maturation, the same is not true for prosthetic grafts, which can generally be used within 14 days of placement. This advantage notwithstanding, the graft should be examined by the surgeon prior to dialysis, as use prior to graft incorporation can result in subcutaneous hematomas and wound complications. If the patient is not a candidate for an autogenous fistula, the AV graft should be deferred until dialysis is imminent because of the risk of failure in the intervening time period.

C. **A variety of dialysis catheters** are available for acute hemodialysis that provide quick percutaneous access. These catheters may be used for days to weeks depending upon whether or not they are of the long, tunneled configuration or are short and not designed to be tunneled. Infection and central venous thrombosis are complications associated with this form of hemodialysis and limit its long term and repeated usage. **The internal jugular vein is preferable to the subclavian vein** for the site of access, as chronic subclavian vein catheterization is associated with higher rates of thrombosis and/or stenosis and with risk of dysfunctional hemodialysis access in the upper extremity. Prolonged catheterization through the jugular vein can also lead to innominate vein or superior vena cava stenosis, although it is less common than that following subclavian vein cannulation.

1. **The most common dialysis catheters** (e.g., Shiley, VasCath, or Quinton catheters) are short, noncuffed, dual-lumen catheters placed percutaneously using the Seldinger method.

2. **Cuffed dialysis catheters** (e.g., PermCath or VasCath) are longer catheters, which are designed to be tunneled under the skin, and placed when prolonged catheterization (>2 to 3 weeks) is anticipated. Initial vein access is similar to the short, nontunneled, noncuffed catheters, except that these are brought through a subcutaneous tunnel on the chest wall, which offers stability and provides resistance to infection. Tunneled catheters are relatively soft and well tolerated by patients and will often function for weeks or even months. Again, central venous thrombosis and catheter infection are the complications that generally necessitate catheter removal.

D. **Chronic peritoneal dialysis** is another alternative preferred by some patients. This form of dialysis can be performed at home and generally at a lower cost than hemodialysis. The disadvantage of this form of dialysis is the duration of dialysis needed to effectively clear metabolic byproducts, which is generally much longer than high-flow hemodialysis. Another disadvantage of peritoneal dialysis is the possibility of recurrent infection (i.e., bacterial peritonitis). However, peritoneal dialysis is mentioned in the 2015 KDOQI guidelines as an important and viable options for some patients and in certain scenarios, including for patients with difficult upper extremity access for hemodialysis, chronic peritoneal dialysis becomes an important option.

IV. PERIOPERATIVE CARE

A. **The indications for dialysis, the type of dialysis, and potential complications** should be discussed with the patient and family prior to the operation. In particular, infection, thrombosis, and ischemic steal syndrome of the hand should be explained. Additionally, the authors find it useful to establish realistic expectations with the patient and his or her family with regard to patency rates and the need for repeat procedures, including declot procedures, those needed to address steal syndrome and additional attempts for access at alternative sites should the initial attempt to establish an effective AV circuit be unsuccessful.

B. **Prophylactic antibiotics** (e.g., cefazolin 1 g) should be given within 1 hour of the procedure may reduce the risk of infection, especially in cases where a prosthetic graft is being used.

C. Most extremity hemodialysis procedures can be performed under local anesthesia with intravenous sedation. A supplemental axillary block may be necessary, depending upon the location of the access, and general anesthesia may also be preferable in some instances of proximal upper arm cases (e.g., basilic vein transposition or brachial-axillary AV grafts). **It is important for the surgeon to discuss the location of the access and anticipated anesthesia requirements before any such plan is initiated.**

D. Although **anticoagulation** is not mandatory, a small dose of heparin (e.g., 2,000 to 5,000 units) is often used prior to occluding arterial flow and creating the anastomosis. Heparin may reduce the risk of early thrombosis in locations where vasoconstriction may initially cause lower flow rates. Protamine may be used to reverse the heparin effect at the completion of the operation to minimize bleeding, although the authors most often just allow the heparin to dissipate and do not formally reverse anticoagulation using protamine.

E. **Skin incisions** over a prosthetic AV graft should be constructed so there is ample tissue coverage at the end of the procedure. Whenever possible, skin incisions should not be placed directly over the anticipated course of a synthetic graft.

F. When the access has been completed, it is essential to check the **presence of pulses** at the wrist and good perfusion in the hand. Additionally, it is helpful to auscultate flow in the palmar arch with a continuous wave Doppler unit. The loss or diminution of wrist pulses and/or the absence of Doppler flow in the palmar arch are harbingers of postoperative hand ischemia (e.g., steal syndrome).

G. Postoperatively, the extremity should be placed at a **position of comfort.** Generally, it does not need to be elevated. In fact, elevation may exacerbate hand ischemia in patients who have marginal perfusion following placement of the AV circuit. Finally, constrictive bandages or wraps should be avoided, as they may limit flow through the fistula or graft placed in a superficial position.

H. The access configuration—AV graft or autogenous fistula—should be checked for patency within 4 to 6 hours of placement. The two most reliable signs of patency are the presence of a **palpable thrill and audible bruit** heard with a stethoscope over the venous anastomosis and distal vein. A handheld Doppler will not detect flow over a fresh prosthetic graft because porosity in the graft material and air in the tissues impede the Doppler transmission. Once the graft becomes incorporated into the tissues, a Doppler may be effective.

I. Development or maturation of an autogenous fistula may be aided in some patients by performance of daily exercise of the hand (e.g., squeezing a soft, rubber ball).

J. The hand must be checked for symptoms or signs of **ischemic steal syndrome.** The earliest symptom is numbness of the fingers, although in the setting of severe steal, progressive paresis of the intrinsic muscles of the hands will evolve over 24 hours. An absent radial pulse that was previously present is a key physical finding. Additionally, patients with hand ischemia will have monophasic or no Doppler signals over the radial, ulnar, and palmar arteries. **If ischemic steal syndrome is present and progressive, early intervention (i.e., diagnostic and operative reintervention) is indicated.** However, in many cases, steal is more subtle and develops weeks to months after dialysis access placement. In such instances, patients may complain of pain or numbness in the hand only during hemodialysis, when episodes of hypotension exacerbate the symptoms of steal.

Although ischemic steal can usually be diagnosed on clinical grounds alone, additional testing can be helpful. Although less commonly used today, digital photoplethysmography demonstrates dampened arterial waveforms in the fingers in the presence of steal syndrome that improve or return to normal with manual compression of the high-flow, dialysis access circuit. Arteriography should be reserved for severe or progressive forms of steal and is used to rule out an arterial inflow stenoses. **Endovascular techniques such as balloon angioplasty can be used effectively to treat the underlying inflow stenosis responsible for the symptoms of steal.** During diagnostic arteriography, steal is confirmed when compression of the dialysis access circuit results in filling of the forearm and/or digital arteries distal to the access circuit.

Ligation of the hemodialysis access circuit is a straightforward, and terminal, treatment for ischemic steal that eliminates the high-flow fistula or graft and restores perfusion to the hand. This option, however, leaves the patient without dialysis access and should be reserved for very ill patients, or when other options are not feasible. An alternative is to decrease flow through the shunt by "banding," which narrows the flow channel and flow through the circuit by one of several techniques. Small Weck clips can be applied along the side of the proximal access for approximately 1 cm or a PTFE ring of fixed diameter can be placed around access to narrow its lumen. Wrist pulses will usually increase and Doppler signals of the palmar arch will improve if the banding is effective. Banding is imprecise and the ability to achieve a balance between treating steal and occluding the dialysis access circuit is difficult.

A more effective treatment for ischemic steal is referred to as **distal revascularization and interval ligation (DRIL)** (Fig. 20.3). In the upper extremity, DRIL involves bypassing the inflow arterial stenosis using a saphenous vein conduit. This bypass is typically from the very distal axillary or proximal brachial artery (i.e., proximal to the underlying arterial stenosis) to the distal brachial or ulnar artery. The intervening brachial artery segment distal to the fistula anastomosis is ligated to prevent retrograde flow back into the low-pressure AV access circuit. This method of bypass

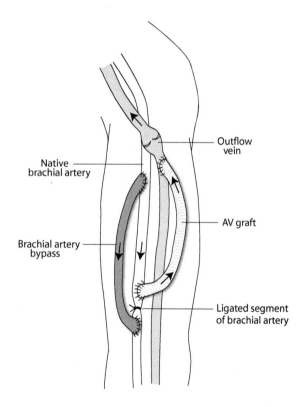

Native brachial artery

Outflow vein

Brachial artery bypass

AV graft

Ligated segment of brachial artery

FIGURE 20.3 The distal revascularization and interval ligation (DRIL) procedure can be used to treat ischemic steal, which occur with an incidence of about 5% with vascular access procedures. In the upper extremity, a brachial-brachial bypass is constructed to restore blood flow to the hand, and the segment of brachial artery between the distal bypass anastomosis and the distal access anastomosis is ligated to prevent steal. Long-term patency of the DRIL is 80% to 90%.

restores flow into the forearm and hand beyond the access site while leaving the dialysis configuration intact.

V. **LATE COMPLICATIONS**. The most important complications that occur with hemodialysis are chronic hand ischemia, infection, arteriovenous circuit dysfunction or failure (i.e., thrombosis), or formation of a pseudoaneurysm from the dialysis graft or fistula.

A. **Infection** is uncommon with an autogenous AV fistula, although synthetic dialysis grafts are more susceptible. Exam findings of erythema, induration, tenderness, and or drainage from or around dialysis graft channel are pathognomonic for infection. Occasionally, a patient will present with a fever of unknown origin and minimal signs of local graft infection. In these instances, a positive blood culture may indicate a more subtle graft infection and duplex ultrasound may identify fluid around the graft. An infected synthetic graft must be removed entirely, although a localized infected segment can occasionally be resected with a new segmental bypass around the infected area.

B. **Pseudoaneurysm** is another relatively common problem of older dialysis access circuits. These occur from repeated puncture over a particular site where the wall of the conduit weakens and fails to seal after one or more of the dialysis sessions. Duplex is the best way to diagnose and characterize a pseudoaneurysm, which can gradually erode through the skin and, in rare instances, lead to bleeding. If large and symptomatic, pseudoaneurysms should be repaired by resection and grafting around the area.

C. **A poorly functioning (or occluded) AV access site** is a common scenario referred to the vascular provider. Essentially, there are two categories of dysfunctional AV access: (a) improper function since placement (e.g., nonmaturation of an autogenous AV fistula) or (b) a failing access site that had previously worked well.

   1. **Diagnosis.** Findings on examination or during dialysis can be useful in sorting out the dysfunctional access site. Reasons for referral often include the following:
      a. Weak or diminished thrill
      b. Significant arm edema
      c. Prolonged bleeding after needle withdrawal
      d. Increased venous pressures
      e. Poor flows during the dialysis run
      f. Inadequate hemodialysis
      g. Difficulty with cannulation

   2. **Etiology.** Failure of an autogenous AV fistula to mature may result from a technical problem; abnormal arterial inflow; or inadequate (small) or damaged vein, or central venous (outflow) stenosis. These causes also account for the majority of early dysfunctional prosthetic AV grafts. In contrast, an AV graft that had been functioning and is now failing or occluded is most commonly affected by a progressive, high-grade stenosis from myointimal hyperplasia, most commonly at the venous outflow anastomosis. Venous outflow problems, whether at the graft anastomosis in the arm, or within a central vein of the thorax, often cause edema and "pulsatility" in the access that can be appreciated on examination. A high-pitched bruit may also indicate venous outflow stenosis.

   3. **Salvage of a dysfunctional AV dialysis access** may be possible under many circumstances (i.e., maintaining assisted patency of the graft or fistula). However, revised access sites have a lower long-term patency compared with nonrevised access sites, even when proper function

is restored. In general, repeated intervention, whether with open or endovascular techniques, to assist with the patency of a poorly functioning access site is the rule, and not the exception.

The standard test for a dysfunctional AV access is duplex ultrasound followed by a **fistulogram (i.e., an angiogram of the AV fistula)** in certain cases. To perform the angiogram, percutaneous access is obtained into the flow channel and a small sheath is placed, generally using ultrasound or fluoroscopic guidance. Contrast dye is injected into the circuit to examine the entire conduit, including the inflow and outflow anastomoses. A venogram of the proximal veins of the arm and chest is also important to look for proximal obstructive lesions, which can also limit fistula outflow and thus its function. Duplex can be performed prior to the fistulogram to identify and localize hemodynamically significant stenoses.

a. **Endovascular techniques** are most commonly used to treat dysfunctional AV dialysis circuits. Myointimal hyperplasia at an anastomosis can be treated effectively in the short- to mid-term with angioplasty using standard, high-pressure, or even cutting balloons. Short segment stenoses in the outflow and central veins are also amenable to PTA with or without placement of a stent. Frequently, additional interventions are needed to maintain patency. The durability of percutaneous treatment for central venous stenosis is limited, reported to be in the wide range of 20% to 70% at 1 year, depending on the length, severity, and chronicity of the offending stenosis.

b. **Open surgical treatment** is also effective for the treatment of dysfunctional AV access circuit and should be tailored to the underlying problem. Open exploration of the stenosis and treatment with patch angioplasty can be used to treat a narrowing at either the arterial or venous anastomosis sites. An interposition graft or an extension bypass (jump graft) to more proximal vein can also be used to address venous outflow stenoses. Open surgical treatment of central venous stenoses is now uncommon as it is associated with higher morbidity and mortality than endovascular techniques.

D. **Thrombosis** is the end stage of a chronically dysfunctional access circuit (graft or native fistula) although occlusion may occur in the absence of previous dysfunction and be due to hypotension, a hypercoagulable condition, or an otherwise ill-defined reason. Once an access site has thrombosed, it cannot be used for dialysis unless a high rate of AV flow can be restored within the access circuit. Although prosthetic AV grafts can often be salvaged by thrombectomy (i.e., removal of thrombus or clot), complete thrombus removal from autogenous AV fistulas is less likely and often leads to rethrombosis.

Thrombectomy can be performed by a variety of techniques. Open surgical thrombectomy using a cutdown onto the graft, a transverse opening of the graft and removal of clot from within the graft with a Fogarty thrombectomy catheter, is often effective. Once the thrombus is removed from and flow restored within the graft, a completion angiogram (i.e., fistulogram) should be performed to evaluate for the underlying problem or defect that led to the thrombosis (i.e., identify the severe venous outflow stenosis). When identified, the causative can be treated at the same operation with an open or endovascular revision. Restoring flow in an occluded dialysis circuit using only endovascular techniques is also common and effective and may include using a mechanical thrombectomy device such as with the AngioJet™ (Boston Scientific, Marlborough, MA, USA) with or without thrombolytic drugs such as a form of tissue plasminogen activator (TPA). In this setting, it is essential to correct any flow-limiting problems (e.g., stenoses) identified in the access configuration following the thrombectomy, in order to prevent immediate rethrombosis of the circuit.

Selected Readings

Casey K, Tonnessen BH, Mannava K, et al. A comparison of basilic versus brachial vein transpositions. *J Vasc Surg.* 2008;47:402-406.

Hu H, Wu Z, Zhao J, et al. Stent graft placement versus angioplasty for hemodialysis access failure: a meta-analysis. *J Surg Res.* 2018;226:82-88. doi: 10.1016/j.jss.2018.01.030.

Koraen-Smith L, Krasun M, Bottai M, Hedin U, Wahlgren CM, Gillgren P. Haemodialysis access thrombosis: outcomes after surgical thrombectomy versus catheter-directed thrombolytic infusion. *J Vasc Access.* 2018:1129729818761277. doi: 10.1177/1129729818761277.

McClafferty RB, Pryor RW III, Johnson CM, Ramsey DE, Hodgson KJ. Outcome of a comprehensive follow-up program to enhance maturation of autogenous arteriovenous hemodialysis access. *J Vasc Surg.* 2007;47:981-985.

Misskey J, Yang C, MacDonald S, Baxter K, Hsiang Y. A comparison of revision using distal inflow and distal revascularization-interval ligation for the management of severe access-related hand ischemia. *J Vasc Surg.* 2016;63(6):1574-1581. doi: 10.1016/j.jvs.2015.10.100.

National Kidney Foundation. KDOQI clinical practice guideline for hemodialysis adequacy: 2015 update. *Am J Kidney Dis.* 2015;66(5):884-930.

Schmidli J, Widmer MK, Basile C, et al. Vascular access: 2018 clinical practice guidelines of the European Society for Vascular Surgery (ESVS). *Eur J Vasc Endovasc Surg.* 2018;55(6):757-818. doi: 10.1016/j.ejvs.2018.02.001.

Tonnessen BH, Money SR. Embracing the fistula first national vascular access improvement initiative. *J Vasc Surg.* 2005;42:585-586.

Yang HT, Yu SY, Su TW, Kao TC, Hsieh HC, Ko PJ. A prospective randomized study of stent graft placement after balloon angioplasty versus balloon angioplasty alone for the treatment of hemodialysis patients with prosthetic graft outflow stenosis. *J Vasc Surg.* 2018;68(2):546-553. doi: 10.1016/j.jvs.2017.12.062.